the
8-week
Healthy
Skin diet

Includes more than 100 recipes for beautiful skin

Karen Fischer

Robert
ROSE

For complete cataloguing information, see page 468.

Disclaimer

This book is a general guide only and should never be a substitute for the skill, knowledge, and experience of a qualified medical professional dealing with the facts, circumstances, and symptoms of a particular case. The nutritional, medical, and health information presented in this book is based on the research, training, and professional experience of the author, and is true and complete to the best of her knowledge. However, this book is intended only as an informative guide for those wishing to know more about health, nutrition, and medicine; it is not intended to replace or countermand the advice given by the reader's personal physician. Because each person and situation is unique, the author and the publisher urge the reader to check with a qualified health-care professional before using any procedure where there is a question as to its appropriateness. A physician should be consulted before beginning any exercise program. The author and the publisher are not responsible for any adverse effects or consequences resulting from the use of the information in this book. It is the responsibility of the reader to consult a physician or other qualified health-care professional regarding his or her personal care.

This book contains references to products that may not be available everywhere. The intent of the information provided is to be helpful; however, there is no guarantee of results associated with the information provided. Use of brand names is for educational purposes only and does not imply endorsement.

The recipes in this book have been carefully tested by our kitchen and our tasters. To the best of our knowledge, they are safe and nutritious for ordinary use and users. For those people with food or other allergies, or who have special food requirements or health issues, please read the suggested contents of each recipe carefully and determine whether or not they may create a problem for you. All recipes are used at the risk of the consumer. We cannot be responsible for any hazards, loss, or damage that may occur as a result of any recipe use. For those with special needs, allergies, requirements, or health problems, in the event of any doubt, please contact your medical adviser prior to the use of any recipe.

Brand Names: Brand names of beauty products are not used in this book because product formulas can change. For up-to-date information of the contents and suitability of brand-name beauty aids, see www.healthbeforebeauty.com

Design and Production: Daniella Zanchetta/PageWave Graphics Inc
Editor: Bob Hilderley, Senior Editor, Health
Copy editor: Sheila Wawanash
Proofreader: Kelly Jones
Indexer: Gillian Watts
Illustration: Kveta (Three in a Box)
Cover image: Lemon/lime stack © iStockphoto.com/Larisa Bozhikova

We acknowledge the financial support of the Government of Canada through the Book Publishing Industry Development Program (BPIDP) for our publishing activities.

Published by Robert Rose Inc.
120 Eglinton Avenue East, Suite 800, Toronto, Ontario, Canada M4P 1E2
Tel: (416) 322-6552 Fax: (416) 322-6936
www.robertrose.ca

Printed and bound in Canada

1 2 3 4 5 6 7 8 9 MI 21 20 19 18 17 16 15 14 13

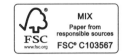

Contents

Part 1: Getting Started

Healthy Skin Diet Basics 5

Quick Guidelines for Developing
    Healthy Skin. 12

Associated Conditions 16

**Part 2: Getting to Know Your
    Skin**

Skin Makeup. 19

Skin Types. 22

Skin Talk 22

**Part 3: Eight Guidelines for
    Healthy Skin**

#1 **Think Green and Friendly:**
    Restoring Your pH Balance. . . . 29

#2 **Moisturize Your Skin from the
    Inside Out:** Eating Great Fats . . .55

#3 **Eat Less:** Controlling Your
    Carbs and Protein 73

#4 **Be a Sleeping Beauty:** Practicing
    Good Sleep Habits 95

#5 **Sweat for 15 Minutes a Day:**
    Exercising for Healthier Skin. . . 101

#6 **Be a Hat Person:** Avoiding
    UV Light Exposure. 109

#7 **Relax:** Making Peace with
    Your Body. 115

#8 **Follow a Good Skin-Care
    Routine:** Selecting Safe and
    Effective Beauty Aids 126

Part 4: Specialized Programs

Acne Care. 147

Cellulite Care 167

Cradle Cap Care 183

Dandruff Care. 186

Eczema Care 200

Psoriasis Care. 232

Rosacea Care 246

Children's Clear Skin Program . . . 263

**Part 5: Being Beautiful and
    Healthy**

Beauty Breathing 281

How to Be Beautiful. 293

**Part 6: The Healthy Skin Diet
    Program**

Planning for the Healthy Skin
    Diet Program 312

3-Day Alkalizing Cleanse. 317

Top 12 Ingredients for the
    Healthy Skin Diet. 323

14-Day Healthy Skin Menu
    & Activity Plan 329

Life after the Healthy Skin Diet . . .340

Part 7: Healthy Skin Recipes

Beverages. 343

Breakfasts 357

Sauces, Dips and Salad
    Dressings 379

Snacks. 387

Chicken Lunches and Dinners . . . 395

Fish and Seafood. 407

Beef and Lamb. 421

Vegetable Main Courses
    and Side Dishes. 429

Desserts and Sweet Treats 451

Appendix: Additives to Avoid . . . 459

Acknowledgments. 460

Resources 460

References 461

About the Nutrient Analyses . . . 468

Index. 469

Part 1
Getting Started

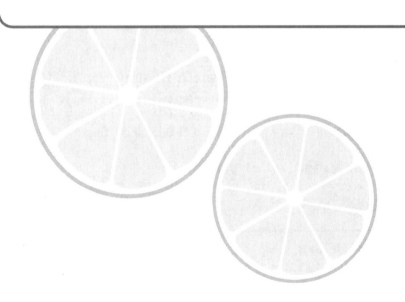

Healthy Skin Diet Basics

What spirit is so empty and blind, that it cannot recognize the fact that the foot is more noble than the shoe, and skin more beautiful than the garment with which it is clothed?

— Michelangelo

You were not born to suffer endlessly from a terrible skin condition, such as acne or psoriasis. You weren't meant to get wrinkles or cellulite prematurely either. You were born for a much better reason than to battle with your skin and feel terrible every time you glance in the mirror. Okay, so this might be an exaggeration, but I want you to not just hope, but know that you can improve your skin quality so you can enjoy having beautiful skin like the genetically blessed.

I know this is true because the skin you have today will be totally renewed within 2 months. Yep. Those wrinkles and that crop of whiteheads will be gone and new skin will be in its place in a matter of weeks, and it can look exactly the same, worse, or better, depending on the building materials and instructions you supply for it.

Whatever your skin condition may be, whether it is quite okay or out of control, you can improve its quality and have fantastic-looking skin within 8 weeks. The Healthy Skin Diet provides eight related guidelines that will take the guesswork out of creating clear skin.

The Healthy Skin Diet is designed to supply your body with the specific building materials it needs to make gorgeous skin. Beautiful skin is created by a body that is functioning properly — by a body that is digesting food thoroughly, eliminating wastes efficiently, and transporting nutrients at lightning speed around the body. Beautiful skin is not something exclusively reserved for the genetically blessed. You do not have to be born with it. You can have it, too.

Perhaps the best way to show you how the Healthy Skin Diet works is to present case histories so you can see and hear real people meeting their own health challenges. I do this throughout the book. But let me start with me. I thought you might like to have a giggle about my "ugly skin" days — and believe me, there were many of them. I also want to show you that you don't have to be blessed with the perfect skin gene —

Did You Know?

Skin Cell Regeneration

The body you have today, all your cells and tissues, will be totally new within a year. Your body turns over six billion cells each day and new ones are made to replace them. The pimple you have right now is not the one you had a month ago, and it is certainly not the same blemish you had last year. You just haven't changed the underlying cause of your skin problems, so they occur over and over again.

and you definitely don't have to settle for ho-hum skin.

This diet is a unique eating and lifestyle plan, designed to fit into your social, working, and home routine so it becomes a healthy way of life rather than a short-term diet scheme that is hard to maintain for a long period of time. The program lasts for 8 weeks but is flexible, so you have no excuses not to complete this short program.

You don't even have to have bad skin to profit from the Healthy Skin Diet plan. This program is fantastic for overall health and well-being. You can be in your 90s or starting school. There is even information for parents with babies suffering from eczema.

CASE STUDY
My Case

I know what it's like to be so uncomfortable in your skin that you wish you were invisible. When I was in high school, I had stick-skinny legs, thin blonde hair, and buck teeth (which braces eventually fixed), so I rarely smiled, and my teenage years saw the beginning of my skin worries with a regular crop of pimples decorating my oily forehead. I was not only shy, awkward, and blemished, I was not well much of the time. I always seemed to have a runny nose or a headache and had dark circles under my eyes.

Maybe I had poor genes, or maybe my health and skin problems occurred because I refused to eat my lunch, declaring in grade 2, "I'm sick of eating sandwiches." From that moment on, I refused to eat homemade lunches. My parents didn't know what to do. I hated healthy food and I was a fussy eater. On occasion a stranger in the street would rudely accuse my mother of not feeding me because I was so skinny and sickly. So, in desperation, my mother gave me lunch money in the hope that I would buy healthy food of my own accord and put on some weight. For the rest of my school years, what did I buy? Meat pies, sausage rolls, french fries, strawberry milk, and cream buns (the ones with extra sugar and jam). I was not quite on the same page as my mom. A vegetable never appeared on my radar screen at school. It was the 1970s and the health food craze was decades away.

At home, I did have some veggies with dinner thanks to Mom's persistence, but I would only eat white bread, as the texture of the brown stuff just didn't feel right in my mouth. Dairy was my addiction. I drank a quart of milk and ate two bowls of ice cream nearly every day.

When I was a teenager, washing the dishes would make my hands peel until they were red, raw, painful, and totally useless, and my face had never-ending red patches.

Inevitably, my childhood eating habits caught up with me as I became increasingly unwell. When I was a teenager, washing the dishes would make my hands peel until they were red, raw, painful, and totally useless, and my face had never-ending red patches. I wasn't much of a help around the house either. Once I used a chemical-based furniture polish to clean the dining room table and I temporarily lost my vision — it was like I was looking through thick gray smoke — and then I vomited. Of course, I suspected I was allergic to manual labor, so I avoided it as much as possible.

In my 20s, I joked that I'd been tired for 10 years, but it was no laughing matter. I went to see various doctors about my constant lethargy and I rattled off a big list of symptoms. Then I would undergo various medical tests that would come back normal. Again and again, I was told there was nothing wrong with me. "But I'm endlessly tired and so damned irritable," I thought, "and haven't you noticed my spotty forehead?" I cut bangs to cover my forehead so I had one less thing to worry about.

One doctor recommended that I should eat healthy food, but he didn't inspire me to investigate further. He had a good point, though: my diet could have been a lot better. This doctor also said I would have more energy if I exercised. Putting on a baggy tracksuit (which practically covered me from head to toe), I went to the gym. But as usual, after one workout I got flu-like symptoms and felt too sick to exercise for the next week. Maybe it was all those toxins being mobilized in my body from years of eating fast food, or maybe it was my lazy side winning the inner battle. Whatever the case, I would predictably lose motivation and go back to my sedentary lifestyle — listening to music in my bedroom as I scoffed strawberry milks.

However, my aversion to exercise sometimes worked in my favor. When I was 25, I had an audition for a TV presenting job, and after I read the scripted dialog, I was asked to talk for a minute about something I hated. Without a moment's hesitation, I chose exercise as my topic. "Exercise is for wacky people! You think about it… To run on the spot on a noisy treadmill for an hour. Ugh! Sounds absurd to me. I say, pass me a tub of ice cream and the remote control!"

> We filmed every Monday, and I was energetic all day, but by Tuesday I was fatigued and the rest of the week I was miserable. I was still getting sick and it affected my work.

To my surprise, I got the job. This ended up being my first (and last) full-time job in television. The show was an afternoon cartoon program, Channel Nine's *What's Up Doc?* (formerly *The Bugs Bunny Show*). We filmed every Monday, and I was energetic all day, but by Tuesday I was fatigued and the rest of the week I was miserable. I was still getting sick and it affected my work. It was no wonder, though: I would eat any junk food that was on set, and the scriptwriter even dedicated a segment to my obsession with chocolate mousse. I think I ate seven tubs of the stuff that day.

During this time, I got a debilitating flu, and a couple of shooting days had to be rescheduled because I could barely speak. I went to see two doctors, and both of them told me that antibiotics wouldn't work because I had a virus, and they said I had to rest and drink plenty of water. I did… and didn't get any better.

Eventually, after 6 weeks of complaining and moping around, I decided to go into the local herbal dispensary to see a naturopath. The shop had always looked a bit too herbal for me, and I had never felt comfortable enough to go inside, but I was really sick of being sick and tired, so I finally took the plunge. The naturopath looked into my eyes with an iridology torch and exclaimed, "You must be so tired!" We discussed my symptoms, my diet and lifestyle, and then she told me about eating healthy food. She said, "You are what you eat." Oh dear, I'm a walking chocolate mousse.

She made me a foul-tasting herbal mixture for my chronic flu, and after 2 days of taking the herbs (and eating slightly more fruits and vegetables) I felt better. I was no longer a zombie extra in a B-grade flick. After my battle with the never-ending flu, which would have been conquered quickly by a half-decent immune system, I decided to learn how to be healthy. I wanted to know what foods could make a difference to my energy levels and I wanted to find out how to look good without makeup. I changed my diet very, very slowly (yes, I'm stubborn). I weaned myself off my dairy addiction, culled the chocolate mousse, and made friends with whole grains.

> After 2 days of taking the herbs (and eating slightly more fruits and vegetables) I felt better. I was no longer a zombie extra in a B-grade flick.

I also took up exercise (once again), but I started slowly and indulged in my body's natural aversion to movement for as long as I could. In my new-found yoga class, I realized I had the flexibility of a brick and the 60-year-olds in the front row had better balance than I did. At least the classes were "beginner-friendly," so I could go at my own pace. Eventually, I got better at exercising and choosing healthy food. It wasn't long before I began to feel better.

I was 27 and pregnant and I had more vitality than when I was a teenager. My complexion also cleared up and I no longer needed to kick-start my brain with a cup of coffee or four. I felt ripped off for all those years — some people get to enjoy health like this all the time!

During this period, I somehow completed a health-science degree and a 3-year nutrition diploma. This introduced me to nutritional biochemistry, which is the study of how nutrients work in the body. This background knowledge has helped me to understand how different diets work and, more importantly, how some diets can be effective (with weight loss in particular) but also be unbelievably harmful to your health and skin.

I didn't become a nutritionist who specialized in skin health because of my own skin dramas. I did it because of my daughter. Two weeks after she was born, she developed a severe case of eczema. Her face and the creases in her elbows and knees were red and painfully itchy. Eczema sufferers can develop asthma if the underlying cause of the inflammation is not treated.

My daughter's eczema persisted until she was 7 months old — until I put her on a "friendly food" diet. This was a difficult diet that only offered temporary relief. Her eczema would come back if the food program wasn't followed strictly. I thought there must be a better way...

> I didn't become a nutritionist who specialized in skin health because of my own skin dramas. I did it because of my daughter.

Scientific Foundation

That would have been the last chapter of my case if, after much research, I had not found an effective long-term solution to my daughter's inflamed skin. For years now she has been eczema-free, and she's able to sleep with her fluffy toys without any irritation from dust mites (she had been diagnosed with dust mite allergy). She can now swim in any type of pool because the chlorine does not sting her skin, and she can eat tomatoes, grapes, and mangos, and all of the other salicylate-rich foods she adores. She can also eat dairy products and go to kids' parties and scoff a few colored lollipops for the first time in her life without getting a flare-up! My daughter and the other eczema sufferers I've treated over the years still have a genetic predisposition to eczema, but they now have a simple health routine to follow that allows them to have a normal and rash-free life.

As fate would have it, my knowledge of skin health would be tested once again when my house was invaded by fleas (thanks to the gorgeous dog from next door). After attempting to get rid of the mites without using harsh chemicals, I eventually flea-bombed the house with a pesticide bought from the supermarket. But after the chemical exposure, I got a small patch of psoriasis on my neck. Within a month the flaky patch had spread down my neck and all over my torso. My skin was scaly,

> After the chemical exposure, I got a small patch of psoriasis on my neck. Within a month the flaky patch had spread down my neck and all over my torso.

dry, and red. It looked so bad, I felt embarrassed when I went for a swim at the local pool. I began to avoid socializing as it continued to spread. I finally devised an anti-psoriasis program. A month later my psoriasis had completely disappeared.

I feel very privileged to be able to pass on my knowledge of skin health to you, especially in a format that allows me to give you all the information you need to create gorgeous skin. Just so you know, this skin health program is evidence-based. I have included references to the medical literature at the end of the book. You can read more about the components of what I now call the Healthy Skin Diet.

Prognosis for Healthy Skin

Just think: with clear, healthy skin you would be able to focus on the rest of your life with confidence rather than worrying about skin-deep first impressions.

Poor genes, enjoying too much of the good life, or having an unhealthy diet as a child can leave you with bad skin. However, we all want to enjoy ourselves and not become Nancy-No-Fun in order to look good. I believe in having fun, and being kind to yourself is an important part of healthy living. There are plenty of scientific studies to back me up. The Healthy Skin Diet is designed so you can have low alcohol and coffee consumption. This enables you to hang out with your friends or have a couple of glasses of red with your partner over dinner if you wish.

As a health-care practitioner, it is my job to make being healthy accessible to you. I do this by not only giving you health information but also by setting activities for you, similar to the ones I've previously given my clients. The activities are your cue to take action and work toward gorgeous skin. I know you can do it!

This takes a bit of effort on your part because, as you may already know, theory alone cannot make your skin beautiful. It's the process of doing that will get you the results you want. Your skin's health is in your hands. And no matter what kind of genes you were lumped with, I hope you now realize that when you follow the Healthy Skin Diet you can have gorgeous skin not unlike the genetically blessed. Of course, you can simply read the book and get some fab skin-care tips. But I'm guessing you want more — gorgeous skin, vitality, and long-lasting results — or else you wouldn't be reading this book right now.

I don't want to just sell you this book so it can gather dust on your bookshelf, either. I want you to follow the complete dietary advice and lifestyle activities involved in the Healthy Skin Diet so you can then enjoy all the benefits of having beautiful skin. Just think: with clear, healthy skin you would be able to focus on the rest of your life with confidence rather

Skin Health Questionnaire

Who can benefit from the Healthy Skin Diet? To see if the Healthy Skin Diet can help you with your skin problems, take this quiz. Circle your answers, add up your numbered responses, and turn to the score card at the end of the quiz to determine if you have a skin problem.

QUESTION	Often	Rarely	Never
Do you suffer from dry skin and skin rashes?	5	3	0
Are you a worrywart and just too busy to look after yourself?	5	3	0
Do you suffer from acne or pimples?	5	3	0
Do you have asthma, arthritis, or arthritic-like pain?	5	3	0
Do you have trouble losing weight?	5	3	0
Do you suffer from allergies and intolerances?	5	3	0
Do you have a dull complexion?	5	3	0
Do you have signs of premature aging?	5	3	0
Do you suffer from premenstrual syndrome (PMS)?	5	3	0
Do you get dandruff, bad breath, or smelly body odor?	4	3	0
Do you have dark circles under your eyes?	4	2	0
Do you have cellulite?	4	2	0
Do you suffer from irritability, mood swings, or depression?	4	2	0
Do you often wake feeling lethargic?	4	2	0
Do you suffer from constipation, gas, bloating, or indigestion?	4	2	0
Have you taken antibiotics in the last 6 months?	3	1	0
Do you crave sugar or bread?	3	1	0
Do you need a coffee pick-me-up or something sweet in the afternoon?	3	1	0
TOTAL SCORE:			

Score Card
Score: 40 +

If your score is more than 40, then you should experience dramatic results from following the Healthy Skin Diet. Still, you should also take a couple of the recommended supplements to speed up the process.

continued...

Score: 29–39

If your score is between 20 and 39, you should benefit greatly from following the Healthy Skin Diet but supplements are optional.

Score: 0–20

If your score is below 20 and you don't have any specific undesirable skin conditions, your skin is probably quite healthy (or you are one of the lucky ones with fabulous genes). Even then, you can use the Healthy Skin Diet as a food and lifestyle guide to help guard against premature aging and preserve those wonderful genes.

than worrying about skin-deep first impressions. I won't tell you not to stress about what other people may think of your skin. I will be honest and say, yes, people can be unkind and leave you wishing you were invisible and, yes, it's really wonderful when acquaintances remember your name or at least compliment you on your gorgeous complexion. You can enjoy this too.

Quick Guidelines for Developing Healthy Skin

The Healthy Skin Diet is an 8-step program you follow for 8 weeks (that's only 2 months) that addresses your lifestyle habits, including diet, exercise, sleep, stress, and general thinking. Take one step at a time rather than trying to handle all the guidelines steps at once so you don't slip back into bad eating, exercise, sleeping, and thinking habits. A healthy attitude is important for the success of this diet.

1. Think Green and Friendly: Restoring Your pH Balance

One of the chief causes of bad skin is acidosis, an imbalance of acid and alkaline elements in your body. Avoiding high acid and eating more alkalizing foods, especially "green" foods, will help restore this fundamental balance.

FAQs
& Short Answers

● ●

These are a few of the questions my patients ask on a regular basis. You likely have other questions to pose. These answers are explained in greater detail elsewhere in the book.

Q. I have rosacea. Is the Healthy Skin Diet suitable for me?

A. Yes. I have developed special programs for severe skin ailments, specifically rosacea (redness of the skin and facial flushing), acne, cellulite, eczema, dermatitis, and psoriasis. Just look up your skin condition in the table of contents or the index. This advice will help you to tailor the Healthy Skin Diet to your own specific needs. For more information, see page 246.

Q. I have a child with skin problems, specifically eczema. Is the program suitable for her?

A. Yes. There are far too many children suffering with eczema, so I have included healthy food and supplement information specifically for these children with eczema and dermatitis, which I call the Children's Clear Skin Program. The Healthy Skin Diet may be suitable for older children who eat the same food as their parents, but for babies who are just starting on solids, there is a list of specific foods for them. I've had wonderful success at eliminating childhood eczema. For more information, see page 263.

Q. Can I follow the Healthy Skin Diet if I'm pregnant?

A. Yes, you can, but be sure to check with your health-care practitioner before taking any supplements. You should avoid vitamin A and liver detoxification supplements, as well as raw fish. You should also take a calcium supplement because this is a dairy-restricted diet.

continued...

Q. I don't like taking supplements — do I need to take any while on the Healthy Skin Diet?

A. No, provided you are following the structured menu plan as part of the Healthy Skin Diet, then you won't need to take any supplements, but be sure to eat nutrient-rich foods.

Q. Can I drink tea and coffee while on the Healthy Skin Diet?

A. During the first 3 days of the diet, it is recommended that you avoid caffeine, but after this time you can enjoy coffee and tea in moderation. If you have a severe skin rash, you should avoid tea and coffee and substitute decaffeinated coffee or dandelion tea until your skin condition clears up. For more information, see page 43.

Q. Will the Healthy Skin Diet help me lose weight?

A. Yes. Even though the Healthy Skin Diet is not specifically designed for weight loss, it will help balance your metabolism, improve fat digestion, and increase elimination of wastes, so you'll lose excess weight if you need to.

Q. Can I still eat at restaurants while on the Healthy Skin Diet?

A. Yes, you can. Restaurant options are listed within the 8-week menu plan. Once you have learned the basic principles of the diet, you'll find it's relatively easy to spot a healthy meal when eating out. Of course, the specially designed recipes in the Healthy Skin Diet are likely to be superior for your skin. I would recommend keeping restaurant trips to a minimum.

Q. Can I find non-diet information in this book that I can use to look after my skin even is my skin looks good and my diet is okay?

A. Yes, there are plenty of skin-care and lifestyle tips that you can follow to improve your skin's appearance even further.

2. Moisturize Your Skin from the Inside Out: Eating Great Fats

Yet another cause of bad skin is an excess of saturated fats and a lack of omega-3 fats, leaving your skin dry. I provide guidelines for separating the bad from the good and the great fats so your skin is moisturized from the inside out.

3. Eat Less: Controlling Your Carbohydrates and Protein

Scientific studies have shown that reducing carbohydrates in your diet will help improve your skin and make way for weight loss, while foods rich in specific proteins have an anti-aging effect on your skin. This guideline identifies carbohydrates low on the glycemic index (sugar content) and protein foods with remarkable anti-aging properties.

4. Be a Sleeping Beauty: Practicing Good Sleep Habits

Tired skin is not healthy skin. The sleep habits I present in this guideline will help make your skin look alive.

5. Sweat for 15 Minutes a Day: Exercising for Healthier Skin

Good muscle tone is a cornerstone of radiant skin tone. This guideline presents an easy-to-follow exercise program that takes no more than 15 minutes a day.

6. Be a Hat Person: Avoiding UV Light Exposure

You know by now that you should avoid extended exposure to ultraviolet light from the sun. In this guideline, I present some tips for self-examining your skin for signs of melanoma and some common-sense strategies for balancing the need for sunlight in generating vitamin D with the dangers of overexposure.

7. Relax: Making Peace with Your Body

Stress and skin don't mix. Tired skin can be enlivened through the positive relaxation strategies presented in this guideline.

New Hope for Good Skin

If you suffer from acne, cellulite, dandruff, eczema/dermatitis, psoriasis, or rosacea, you will be pleased to know that the Healthy Skin Diet has specialized programs tailored for your condition. If you have a child with an undesirable skin condition, you can turn to the Children's Clear Skin Program. If you have another type of skin complaint or no specific skin problem (and you just want to guard against premature aging), there is a section on beauty aids and how to remain beautiful as you age. But first, let's look more closely at our skin.

---

8. Follow a Good Skin-Care Routine: Selecting Safe and Effective Beauty Aids

Among the many beauty aids on the market and the various esthetician programs, some are helpful, some are harmful. In this guideline, I help you to distinguish the good from the not so good.

Associated Conditions

• •

The **Healthy Skin Diet** is an anti-inflammatory eating program that was originally designed for people with eczema. The diet was also found to be effective in eliminating acne, psoriasis, and dandruff, as well as improving mood swings, increasing energy levels, and reducing rosacea. The Healthy Skin Diet promotes production of anti-inflammatory prostaglandins, which makes it ideal also for people with sinusitis, hay fever, asthma, arthritis, and other allergies.

Positive Side Effects

The Healthy Skin Diet has a number of positive side effects beyond skin health for preventing and treating various health conditions.

Heart Health

The Healthy Skin Diet is suitable for people with heart disease and high blood pressure because the diet is low in red meat (two servings or less per week). It is packed full of heart-protective antioxidants. Continue to take your prescribed medications and consult your doctor before taking supplements of any kind, as they may interfere with your drug treatment.

Diabetes and Hypoglycemia

Because the Healthy Skin Diet has many low-carbohydrate and low-fat recipes, it is fantastic for people with blood sugar problems, such as type 2 diabetes and hypoglycemia.

Did You Know?
• • • • • • • • • • • • • • •

Liver Detoxification Phases

The liver has the job of ridding the body of toxins. There are two phases involved in detoxification. Without getting too technical, phase 1 is where waste chemicals and hormones are made water soluble. If retained, these substances can become more toxic. You need phase 2 to finish the job and promote safe removal of these substances. Phase 2 also increases glutathione production, which guards against premature aging.

Conditions That Can Be Helped by the Healthy Skin Diet

Specific Conditions

- Acne
- Cellulite
- Contact dermatitis
- Dandruff
- Dermatitis
- Eczema
- Hives
- Psoriasis
- Rosacea

Associated Conditions

- Aging, premature, with wrinkles
- Abdominal bloating
- Body odor, bad breath
- Yeast and fungal infections
- Complexion dull and sallow
- Eyes, baggy with dark circles
- Fatigue and sluggishness
- Flatulence/gas
- Food intolerances
- Headaches
- Hypoglycemia (food-related)
- Mood swings and irritability
- Poor immunity to colds and flu
- Poor digestion
- Parasites in the bowel
- Premenstrual syndrome (PMS)
- Skin pigmentation
- Weight, inability to lose

Digestion

If you have poor digestion with bloating, embarrassing gas, and constipation, then the Healthy Skin Diet has got you covered. Many of the skin-healthy recipes have ingredients that are natural digestives with the right type of fiber to improve elimination of wastes. When you eat these digestive aids and fiber, you won't get offensive gas, BO, or bad breath! (Wouldn't that be nice?) Parasites and *Candida albicans* can also cause really nasty bowel symptoms and skin problems, but the Healthy Skin Diet is designed to significantly decrease harmful microbes within your bowels. Healthy bowels equal beautiful skin.

Liver Detoxification

The Healthy Skin Diet is designed to improve your liver health because it contains many foods that stimulate phase 1 and phase 2 liver detoxification (especially phase 2). You can feel lethargic and unwell if your phase 1 is high and your phase 2 is compromised. The Healthy Skin Diet works to balance these reactions.

Did You Know?
....

Allergies
Please note that the Healthy Skin Diet is NOT designed to prevent anaphylaxis allergic reactions. Continue to avoid your trigger foods while you are on this diet.

Part 2
Getting to Know Your Skin

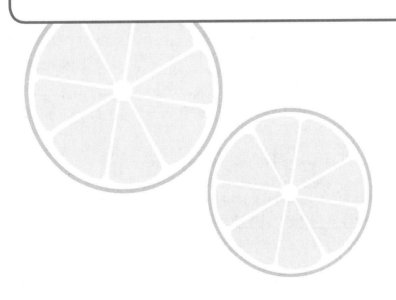

Your skin is the largest organ of your body. Quite frankly, your skin is absolutely essential for your existence. Without it, you would die. Your skin protects you from invading bacteria, it helps to regulate your body temperature, and it keeps your insides from falling out. But you probably don't give a second thought to the role of your skin (why would you?). You are more likely to spend your day thinking about work and worrying about your bills … or checking to see if you have food stuck between your teeth. Thinking or worrying about your skin is not a pressing concern for most people. Your skin only grabs your attention once it lets you down.

Your skin may start to wrinkle. It can become patchy with pigmentation. It might develop rashes and pimples or dimples all the way down your thighs. You wonder what you did to deserve a butt like yours. You sit at the beach, practically covered from head to toe with zinc cream and tie-dyed sarongs, for fear of cellulite mockery and a nasty case of skin cancer. You ask, "Are wrinkles and dimples a normal part of aging?"

STOP! Don't be ridiculous. Your skin is simply telling you that something is amiss on the inside and it is hoping that you pay attention to its early warning signals. Let's start by getting to know some basic skin facts before we look at what your skin might be trying to tell you.

> You sit at the beach, practically covered from head to toe with zinc cream and tie-dyed sarongs, for fear of cellulite mockery and a nasty case of skin cancer.

Skin Makeup

The skin is an ever-changing organ that contains many specialized cells and structures. The skin functions as a protective barrier that interfaces with a sometimes hostile environment. It is also very involved in maintaining the proper temperature for the body to function well. It gathers sensory information from the environment, and plays an active role in the immune system, helping to protect you from disease. The skin is a complicated structure with many functions. If any of the structures in the skin are not working properly, a rash or abnormal sensation is the result. The whole specialty of dermatology is devoted to understanding the skin, what can go wrong, and what to do if something does go wrong.

> If any of the structures in the skin are not working properly, a rash or abnormal sensation is the result.

Anatomy of the Skin

Let's look at the anatomy of the skin and define some key terms for understanding how the skin works — or doesn't work.

Layers of Skin

Your skin is made up of three layers:

1. Epidermis (outside layer)
2. Dermis (middle layer)
3. Subcutaneous layer (inner layer)

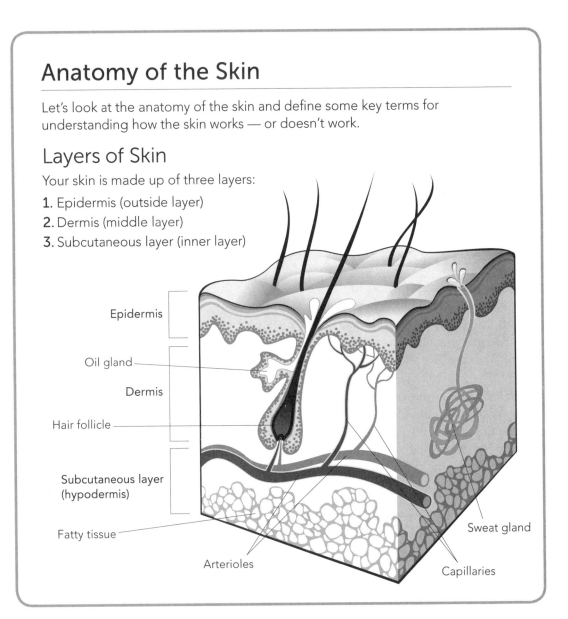

Epidermis

Oil gland

Dermis

Hair follicle

Subcutaneous layer (hypodermis)

Fatty tissue

Arterioles

Sweat gland

Capillaries

Epidermis

The epidermis is the outer layer of skin. It is thinnest on the eyelids at .05 mm and the thickest on the palms and soles at 1.5 mm. The epidermis itself contains five layers, or strata, with the stratum basale at the bottom and the strata corneum at the top.

The column-shaped cells in the bottom layer push cells into higher layers. As the cells move into the higher layers, they flatten and die. The top layer of the epidermis, the stratum corneum, is made of flat, dead cells that shed about every 2 weeks.

Specialized Epidermal Cells

There are three types of specialized cells in the epidermis:

- Melanocyte cells produce pigment (melanin)
- Langerhans cells provide frontline immunity
- Merkel cells (exact function is not known)

Dermis

The dermis also varies in thickness and includes several kinds of elastic fibrous tissue:

- Collagen
- Elastin
- Reticular fibers

Collagen is a group of naturally occurring proteins found in animals, especially in the flesh and connective tissues. It is the most abundant protein in mammals, making up about 30% of the whole body's protein content. Collagen is mostly found in fibrous tissues, such as tendon, ligament, and skin.

Elastin is composed of protein fibers that allow the skin to stretch and then snap back to its original shape when relaxed.

Reticular fibers are also an elastic connective tissue composed of collagen. They hold up and support soft tissue, such as the liver, bone marrow, lymphatic system, and skin.

Layers of the Dermis

The dermis has two layers:

- Upper, papillary layer, containing a thin arrangement of collagen fibers
- Lower, thicker, reticular layer, made of thick collagen fibers arranged parallel to the surface of the skin

Specialized Dermal Cells

The dermis also contains many specialized cells:

- Hair follicles
- Sebaceous (oil) glands and apocrine (scent) glands
- Eccrine (sweat) glands
- Blood vessels and nerves course through this layer, transmitting sensations of pain, itch, and temperature
- Meissner's and Vater-Pacini corpuscles transmit the sensations of touch and pressure

New skin cells form at the bottom of the epidermis, and when they are ready, they move toward the outer layer. This trip takes about 4 weeks. This is good news because it means that with the right building materials you can create better skin cells in only 4 to 8 weeks. Did you realize that in the minute or so you took to read this chapter, you've shed about 40,000 dead skin cells off the surface of your skin? (It's enough to make you want to change the bed sheets pronto!)

Subcutaneous Tissue

The subcutaneous tissue is a layer of fat, connective tissue, larger blood vessels, and nerves that regulate the temperature of the skin and the body.

Skin Types

There are several skin types identified by dermatologists. Guidelines for treating these skin types are provided in Part 3.

Normal skin: Feels supple and looks hydrated. It is not overly sensitive and has even pigmentation. May occasionally get out of balance and have an oily T-zone (forehead, nose, chin), small breakouts, or dry patches.

Dry or mature skin: Has trouble staying hydrated, gets flaky, may peel, or feel tight and dry. May have premature aging or sun damage.

Very dry skin: Nothing seems to soothe this skin type except a thick barrier cream and dietary changes.

Oily or impure skin: Oily, especially in the T-zone, enlarged or blocked pores, poor circulation, blemishes.

Sensitive skin: Easily irritated by weather, skin-care products, and food allergies. Red, inflamed skin, blotchy, patches of dryness, includes rosacea and eczema.

Combination skin: Oily T-zone and normal cheeks. Prone to minor breakouts in T-zone, skin is slightly out of balance; use products that won't aggravate/block pores. Don't exfoliate, as it may spread pimples.

Skin Talk

You may express yourself through words and actions, but your body can also "talk." Yes, you've probably heard of body language, which involves your eyes and facial characteristics, but your body also "speaks" through feelings of pain and through energy output. Pain warns you when something is too hot for the skin; a headache could signal you're dehydrated; and back pain can indicate anything from poor posture to something as serious as cancer. Poor energy levels can mean just about anything, from nutritional deficiencies and poor posture to early warning of some disease states. Fatigue should never be masked by downing seven cups of coffee a day. It's essential that you learn to listen to the secret language of the body.

Q. What is your skin trying to tell you?

A. When you try to "read" your skin, it's like playing the game "hotter and colder." When you get further away from good health, your body will say "colder" by making your skin look bad (your energy levels may also suffer, your breath could smell bad, and so on). But as you get closer to good health, your skin will begin to look better and you will start to feel more alive. Your skin is saying, "You're getting warmer, keep going!" And when your skin looks awesome and you have no medical conditions, unexplainable fatigue, or mysterious pains, then you're obviously on the right track. You're hot! So stick with it!

Causes of Skin Problems

Your health is dependent on many different food and lifestyle factors. When health experts only look at one bit of research or one body organ as the solution for optimal health, it just seems a little crazy to me. It's the same with your skin — there isn't one solitary factor that can make you look gorgeous. This is why scientific studies can end up with inconclusive or negative results because they test a single theory or nutrient, such as vitamin E, to cure eczema, and then they find that it doesn't work.

Skin problems are rarely caused by a single nutrient deficiency. You can induce a solitary deficiency, such as vitamin B_1, during a scientific experiment, but in real life someone with poor nutrition or inadequate digestion will have a whole range of nutritional deficiencies. A single supplement will not fix their skin. A more holistic approach to health is necessary.

Poor skin health typically arises from a variety of minor imbalances, and the underlying cause of them needs to be addressed, not just masked with supplements or medications.

> Poor skin health typically arises from a variety of minor imbalances, and the underlying cause of them needs to be addressed, not just masked with supplements or medications.

Your skin is affected by a number of internal and external factors. If you have poor skin, several of these factors may be out of balance. How do you know which ones? Let's have a deeper look at genetics and diet, because our genes and our nutrition are most often blamed for bad skin. Throughout the book, I will talk about the other causes.

Genetics

According to the current research, the human body has between 24,000 and 25,000 genes. Your genes are what you inherited from your birth parents and they determine things like the color of your skin, if you have freckles or not, and how easily your skin tans when exposed to UV light. Each gene in your body is a segment of DNA that can signal instructions to your cells.

Scientists, medical experts, and nutritionists alike talk about how our genes play a role in our susceptibility to skin conditions and diseases. People talk about being blessed with "good" genes — they rarely get sick and can drink truckloads of chocolate milk without getting a single pimple. In the past I've cursed my "bad" genes whenever my skin has broken out in a red, peeling rash. Our genes have a lot to answer for, and there's no doubt that they can affect our skin. However, our genetic makeup can be altered by our diet in some cases.

Diet

You may have a genetic predisposition to getting eczema, psoriasis, dark circles under the eyes, and cellulite, but this does not mean you have to suffer with these conditions forever. A healthy diet and good lifestyle habits influence your genes every day. In fact, good nutrition can switch on a gene that is malfunctioning due to a vitamin deficiency. For example, a biotin deficiency (caused by frequently eating egg whites) disables the delta-6-desaturase enzyme reaction, affecting the FADS2 gene, and dermatitis or eczema can result. This is known as egg white injury, and is quickly reversed when biotin is added to the diet and raw eggs are removed from the diet.

Researchers have shown that our genetically determined biology may not have had enough time to catch up with the radical dietary changes that have occurred in the Western world over the past century. What does this mean for your health? Let's consider the diets of your ancestors.

Our genes have a lot to answer for, and there's no doubt that they can affect our skin. However, our genetic makeup can be altered by our diet in some cases.

Skin Health Factors

- Genetics
- Diet
- Stress
- Lack of sleep
- Exposure to environmental chemicals, cigarette smoke, and drugs
- Exposure to UV radiation from sunlight
- Liver health
- Bowel and digestive health
- Blood and lymph circulation

It's more than likely that your ancestors spent much of the day looking for food and making sure they had adequate shelter. Food processing and soft drinks were unheard of, and artificial flavors and colors didn't exist. The traditional hunter-gatherers had diets that varied from region to region, but taking these differences into account, scientists have worked out the basic universal characteristics of primitive diets. It's estimated that our ancestors snacked on nuts, seeds, fruits, vegetables, and whole grains, and that they hunted for fish and chased after wild game.

Of course, your ancestral diet may have varied from this one, especially if you're of Inuit descent. You see, the traditional Inuit ate loads of seafood, so they consumed higher ratios of fat and omega-3 essential fatty acids. Grains weren't a staple part of their diet. Whatever your ancestry may be, today you no longer have to search for nuts or sprint after a wild pig. You simply drive to the shops and select from rows and rows of fresh and packaged foods.

> **Whatever your ancestry may be, today you no longer have to search for nuts or sprint after a wild pig.**

Processed Western or Traditional Diet

As a general rule, the more processed foods you eat, the less fresh and healthy foods you end up consuming.

You've got to admit that packaged foods and premade meals are a godsend at the end of a busy day when you're too exhausted to prepare fresh food. Modern convenience has its place in our society, but this expediency may come at a heavy price, and your skin could be the first thing to suffer.

Processed Western Diet

There's no argument that the modern Western diet varies greatly, but it often consists of the following foods and drinks:

- Farmed meats and processed meats such as ham, salami, and sausages
- Dairy products, such as full-fat and low-fat milk, cheese, and butter
- White bread, pastries, cakes, cookies, cereals, refined sugar, and syrups
- Refined cooking oils and margarine
- Coffee, tea, and alcohol

We also eat fruits, vegetables, fish, nuts, whole grains, and legumes.

Today, only a small number of traditional cultures continue to eat a natural diet that doesn't contain fast food, processed white flour, and sugar. These cultures are fascinating to study because they give us glaring examples of how diets can affect skin health.

Nutritional Changes

According to Loren Cordain and her colleagues, seven crucial nutritional changes naturally occurred when food processing procedures were introduced:

1. **Glycemic load increased.** Processed foods usually have a higher glycemic index (GI), which elevates your blood glucose (sugar) levels. This can damage blood vessels and lead to type 2 diabetes.

2. **Fatty acid balance changed.** Farmed animals don't get enough exercise, so they are practically devoid of omega-3 essential fatty acids and they have become higher in saturated fat.

3. **Macronutrient ratios changed.** Protein, carbohydrate, and fat intake have changed. More saturated fat and refined carbohydrates are being consumed.

4. **Micronutrients were restricted.** We now have fewer micronutrients in our diet. Processed foods, such as white

---

Did You Know?
....

Biological Catch-Up

In the *American Journal of Clinical Nutrition*, Loren Cordain and her colleagues say that our dietary changes began with the introduction of agriculture and animal farming about 10,000 years ago, but that this may have occurred too recently for our genetics to adapt. Our biological makeup hasn't had time to become accustomed to the barrage of chemical preservatives and artificial sweeteners, not to mention heavily processed foods, that are way too low in vitamins and minerals. Maybe many of us aren't victims of our genetic makeup after all — we're just confusing our poor little genes by eating foods that are unrecognizable to our bodies!

Many scientists now suspect that slow genetic adaptation to modern diets could be the reason diseases such as cancer, heart disease, and acne are found in modern societies. Population studies show that acne is rare or non-existent in traditional cultures that eat unprocessed foods.

---

bread and flour, have had most of their original vitamins and minerals removed.

5. **Acid–alkaline (pH) balance altered.** Western diets can cause low-grade metabolic acidosis that worsens with age. Having too much acid in the body can be detrimental to your health.

6. **Sodium-to-potassium ratio changed.** Higher intake of manufactured salt and lower fruit and vegetable consumption means there is less potassium in the modern Western diet. Researchers estimate there has been a 400% increase in salt ingestion, but we haven't increased our vegetable and fruit consumption at all; in fact, it has plummeted.

7. **Fiber content decreased.** Refined sugars, vegetable oils, alcohol, and dairy products are devoid of fiber, and refined grains contain much less fiber than whole-grain foods. The more nutrient-poor a flour product is, the whiter it looks.

Red Flag

Do not attempt to self-diagnose your skin condition. There are many different types of skin abnormalities and some may be serious, requiring medical attention. If you haven't had a doctor diagnose your skin condition, then be a smart cookie and see a specialist before starting the Healthy Skin Diet so you can be sure to read the information that is right for you.

Part 3

Eight Guidelines for Healthy Skin

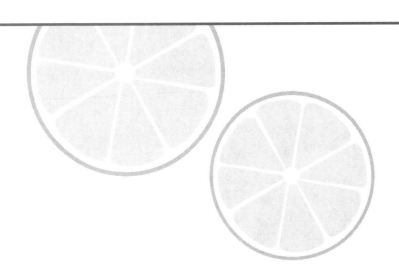

Developing healthy skin is not a mysterious phenomenon if you follow are willing to change your diet and lifestyle (sleep, exercise, routines). The Healthy Skin Diet presents eight specific guidelines for making these changes. Some people can have luminous skin by following only four guidelines, maybe five. To unlock the secret to beautiful skin, take one step at a time and see how good your skin looks week by week for 8 weeks and then assess if you need to continue all eight recommendations.

These guidelines are based on anti-aging research, so they are very specific for decreasing the appearance of wrinkles and premature aging. They can also eliminate undesirable skin conditions, such as contact dermatitis, hives, acne, psoriasis, eczema/dermatitis, rosacea, and dry skin, and they can reduce cellulite and other skin conditions.

Some people are born with beautiful skin; some people need to create it by following these guidelines. Expect to have great skin within 8 weeks.

> Some people are born with beautiful skin; some people need to create it by following these guidelines. Expect to have great skin within 8 weeks.

Guideline #1

· ·

Think Green and Friendly: Restoring Your pH Balance

For years I ignored the concept of balancing the body's pH with alkalizing foods. Now, when I look back, I feel so silly. Follow this simple guideline and you will quickly see and feel your health improving. You will know when it is working!

Your body has a natural acid and alkaline balance, which is measured by the traditional pH scale (pH literally means "potential of hydrogen"). For example, a pH of 1.0 is completely acid, a pH of 14 is all alkaline, and 7.0 is neutral. The pH of a substance is determined by how many hydrogen ions are in that substance. All acids in the body give off hydrogen ions as they dissolve in water.

If your blood pH becomes slightly acidic, your blood will burn holes in your blood vessels. In fact, if your blood pH was to vary by about one-tenth, your body's biomechanical functions would fail and you would die. To counter excess acid (acidosis) in your body, you need to "think green and friendly." Think green and friendly is not a mantra for a hippy commune but rather a first step toward achieving beautiful skin, involving "friendly" gut flora and "green" foods and drinks that have an alkaline, not an acidic, effect on the body.

> **Did You Know?**
> ·····························
> **pH 7.365**
> For the human body to remain alive and well, the blood needs to be slightly alkaline — at a pH of 7.365 to be precise. Some parts of your body need to be acidic, such as the stomach to enable digestion and the epidermis to enable protection from the environment. In general, your body's tissues and blood should be slightly alkaline.

How to test your pH balance

There are two ways you can find out how acidic you are:

1. First (and this is the more accurate way), your doctor can test your blood pH with a simple blood test. You need to ask for this test specifically because it is not a routine blood test. A healthy pH reading for your blood is between 7.35 and 7.45. As you can see, it is a very narrow range.

2. Second, you can test your saliva or urine pH with pH strips that you can purchase from your local pharmacy. These pH strips are made of litmus paper, which changes color when acidic or alkaline substances come into contact with it. Dr. Alex Guerrero, author of *In Balance for Life*, recommends testing the urine rather than saliva because the kidneys are one of the body's organs that eliminate acids. The urine test is not as accurate as a blood test, but it can reveal if you're acidic and you can do the test daily. This is useful because acid and base (alkalinity) levels fluctuate daily. When your body's pH is in balance, your urine pH will be between 7.0 and 7.5.

Q. How does the body balance pH?

A. The body, being the wise thing that it is, has many backup plans to ensure the blood's pH balance is maintained:

1. The body uses its alkaline mineral reserves to keep the blood pH at the correct level. If you keep eating an acidic diet and living an acidic lifestyle, these stores run out and your body needs to go to backup plan number 2…

2. Backup plan number 2 involves quickly removing excess acids from your blood and storing them safely in your fat cells. Unfortunately, overweight people who have heaps of acid stored in their fat usually have an incredibly difficult time losing weight because their body will do everything to avoid the influx of acid that would be released during weight loss. An acidic body holds onto excess weight, making healthy dieting extremely difficult.

3. After your body uses up its alkaline reserves and has stored acids in your fat, what happens next? Backup plan number 3: your body takes alkaline minerals, such as calcium, from your bones. This is one of the reasons why people get osteoporosis and shrink as they get older. Their acidic lifestyle is threatening to disrupt their blood pH and the body is protecting the blood by leeching calcium from their bones. Unfortunately, the modern Western diet is excessively acidic, which affects not only our bones but also our skin.

Acidosis and Skin Health

Excessive acid, or acidosis, can damage cells in your body, including in your skin. An acid-producing lifestyle can reduce the amount and quality of collagen and elastin being produced, so you can end up with premature aging and wrinkles. Good-quality collagen and elastin are essential for youthful-looking skin. Too many acids in the body can also cause demineralization, which can lead to dry and cracked skin, fingernails that split easily, and thin, brittle hair.

Demineralization

When you have an acidic system, your body will eventually tire of shunting calcium away from your bones and storing acid in your fat. If you're a thin person with limited fat cells, you are in a worse predicament than an overweight person. Where is your acid being stored? As you can imagine, skinny people can get sick very, very quickly. This means that Skinny-Minnies need to be extra healthy to feel great and have beautiful skin.

Red Blood Cell Damage

Having an overly acidic system can damage your red blood cells so they alter in shape, clump together, and die prematurely. Your red blood cells should look like round, flat discs — a bit like red Frisbees or a throat lozenge — floating freely through your blood plasma. They should also have a negative charge on the outside and a positive charge on the inside.

When your red blood cells are negatively charged on the outside, as they should be, they cannot clump together. They repel. Unfortunately, when acid strips some of your red blood cells of their negative charge, they start attracting each other and they form clumps. Your red blood cells should not clump together unless you've cut yourself and the blood flow needs to be stopped from escaping. Otherwise your blood needs to flow without clotting.

Did You Know?

Lack of Oxygen

Your skin is usually the first thing to suffer when red blood cell health is poor. Your red blood cells carry oxygen to your skin, but when they are sticky and bulky, they cannot give your outer layer a quick and efficient supply of oxygen. Your skin may also look dull and possibly even pasty or grayish from low oxygen supply. You can also feel very lethargic if your blood is sluggish with damaged red blood cells that aren't supplying enough oxygen. No wonder people often wake up tired after 8 hours of sleep and need a coffee pick-me-up!

Acidosis Questionnaire

Common Symptoms of Acidosis

Fill out this questionnaire to see if your body is showing any signs of acidosis. Check off any symptoms you experience on a regular basis (three or more times a week).

- ☐ Chronic fatigue syndrome
- ☐ Fatigue or weakness after eating meals
- ☐ Colds and flu, low immunity
- ☐ Poor circulation, cold hands/feet
- ☐ Low blood pressure
- ☐ Burning sensation during urination
- ☐ Kidney stones
- ☐ Excessive urination
- ☐ Headaches
- ☐ Pallor, dull complexion
- ☐ Gastrointestinal problems: abdominal pains, cramps, acid reflux, diarrhea, gas, ulcers
- ☐ Agitation, nervousness, anxiety, depression
- ☐ Lack of ambition, lack of joy
- ☐ Dental problems: bleeding or inflamed gums, cavities
- ☐ Cracked lips, loose teeth, tooth sensitivity
- ☐ Muscle cramps or spasms, tension in neck and shoulders
- ☐ Joint pain, arthritis-like pain
- ☐ Nail and hair problems: brittle hair, hair loss, split nails
- ☐ Allergies, runny nose, chronic bronchitis
- ☐ Vaginal discharge, *Candida albicans*
- ☐ Skin problems: dry skin, eczema, acne, hives, itchy skin, red and patchy skin
- ☐ Osteoporosis, brittle bones
- ☐ Insomnia, restless sleep

If you have checked off four or more symptoms, you may have too much acid in your body. Cross-check this by doing a pH urine test for 5 days in a row (to get a more accurate average). Do the urine test first thing in the morning, on rising. If this test confirms the results of the questionnaire, be sure to consult with your doctor.

Causes of Excess Acidity

- Acid-forming foods
- Caffeine
- Alcohol
- Smoking
- Chemicals
- Medications
- Constipation
- Dehydration
- Parasites (worms)
- Yeast and fungal infections
- Stress

Q. My dad has alkalosis, not acidosis. What is it?

A. Alkalosis is the opposite of acidosis. The blood is overly alkaline. Alkalosis is rare; however, it is most commonly caused by alkalizing drugs, such as ulcer and antiheartburn medications. Alkalosis can also be caused by chronic vomiting, diarrhea, and hyperventilation. Breathing is one of the ways in which the body expels acids, so breathing in a rapid, anxious manner can result in alkalosis. Symptoms of alkalosis include overstimulation of the nervous system, resulting in tetany (muscle spasms), cramps, and extreme nervousness.

Acid-Forming Foods

There are many types of acid-producing foods, but the most common ones come from animal products. These foods don't seem acidic before you pop them in your mouth. While they contain some acids, they also form acids once they are digested. Acid-forming foods are fine in moderation, but when your body is continually trying to counteract an acidic state, acid can become poison to your system.

You can probably guess most of the common acid-forming foods because they are also the usual offending foods that already have bad reputations, such as sugar, white flour products, foods high in saturated fats and damaged (trans) fats, meat, dairy, soft drinks, chips, and alcohol. What you may find surprising is that when you chomp on a piece of fruit, it creates acid during digestion. This is because most

> Acid-forming foods are fine in moderation, but when your body is continually trying to counteract an acidic state, acid can become poison to your system.

Acid-Forming Foods

WORST OFFENDERS Avoid eating excessive amounts of these foods. Eat them in moderation.	MILDER ALTERNATIVES Substitute these milder acidic foods for high-acid foods.
Meat, Fish, and Alternatives	
Pork, beef, processed meats	Chicken, eggs, lamb
Fish: herring, salmon, mackerel, carp	Fish: flounder, sole, trout
Shellfish: crayfish, shrimp, lobster	Shellfish: oysters
Dairy Products	
Yellow cheeses	Soft cheeses
Yogurt sweetened with fruit, sugar, or artificial sweetener	Plain organic yogurt
Legumes, Nuts, and Seeds	
Chickpeas, soybeans	Kidney beans, lentils, navy beans, peas
Peanuts, hazelnuts, pecans, pistachios, walnuts	Cashews, pine nuts
Sunflower seeds	Sesame seeds
Grains	
Millet, white rice, white flour products, white/yeast breads	Whole-grain breads, whole wheat, amaranth, barley, brown rice, oats, quinoa, spelt
Vegetables and Fruit	
Commercially made tomato sauce, blackcurrants, kiwifruit, mandarins, nectarines, oranges, pineapple	Apples, apricots, blueberries, cherries, coconut, figs, grapes, mangoes, melon, pears , plums, pomegranates, strawberries, watermelon, most dried fruits
Fats and Sugars	
Hydrogenated fats, margarine, peanut and walnut oils	Cold-pressed oils
Artificial sweeteners, table sugar	
Condiments	
Vinegar, pickles, mustard, processed table salt	Organic mustard
Beverages	
Black tea, cocoa, coffee, milk, processed fruit juice, soft drinks (soda pop), tap water, liquor and spirits, wine	Carbonated mineral water, beer

fruits have a high sugar content. Yes, these are natural sugars, but they promote acidity — and they provide a quick and easy meal for thriving microbes.

Q. Must I avoid acid-forming foods entirely to develop healthy skin?

A. No! The foods and liquids that exert the strongest acid-producing effect can be enjoyed in moderation. When you are on the 8-week Healthy Skin Diet, these foods and beverages will be strictly limited to no more than three servings per day. Two servings is two glasses of alcohol or one coffee and salmon or chickpeas for dinner. Keep your animal protein servings small — about the size of the palm of your hand — especially if you're eating meat.

When eating at restaurants, you usually can't control the serving size of your meats, so choose less acidic protein, such as chicken, trout, lamb, kidney beans, or lentils. Acid-forming fruits are also fine in moderation — two servings per day or less. After all, fruit supplies plenty of cancer-protective phytochemicals, vitamins, and minerals, but it can also supply too many simple sugars that parasites thrive on. Two servings per day is equivalent to two apples or a small handful of blueberries and half a mango.

Alcohol

• •

If you have a severe skin condition, the best thing you can do for your skin is abstain from alcohol, at least until your complexion clears. Alcohol is very dehydrating and acidic and may slow down your progress to beautiful skin. Abstaining can be hard to do, especially if your job involves considerable socializing. Here are a few options so you don't have to ditch your social life completely while on the Healthy Skin Diet:

- Keep alcohol intake low.
- When socializing, have no more than two standard alcoholic drinks.
- Have at least four alcohol-free days per week.
- Make a rule to never drink alone or at home.

If you have eczema, psoriasis, or rosacea, I recommend avoiding alcohol altogether, but if you must have the occasional drop, your best choices would be low-chemical alcohol — which doesn't contain salicylates, amines, or MSG — such as vodka, gin, and whisky. Have them with mineral or soda water (not tonic water, cola, or lime cordials).

Q. Should I be drinking red wine to improve my health?

A. Scientists may say that red wine is packed full of healthy antioxidants, but they don't mention that red wine also contains sulfite preservatives that can cause serious allergic reactions, such as anaphylaxis (in very sensitive people) and skin reactions. For example, one glass of red wine can cause red flushing and rashes in sensitive individuals with rosacea. Drinking excessive amounts of alcohol can lead to skin disease. If you love your wine, drink the preservative-free kind during the 8-week program. If you want a dose of heart-protective antioxidants, eat red grapes, blueberries, and raspberries and drink green tea.

Did You Know?

If you smoke...
You probably already know that cigarette smoking can alter your physical appearance dramatically, and not for the better. Smokers with a history of heavy smoking are five times more likely to have wrinkles than non-smokers. Smoking decreases vitamin C levels in the body and it affects the body's ability to form healthy collagen in the skin. Try these strategies for quitting smoking:

1. Imagine yourself looking fit and healthy, with beautiful skin.
2. Enrol in a quit-smoking program today, or better still, decide to "choose health" instead of focusing on "not smoking."
3. Focus on what you want rather than what you're trying to avoid.
4. When you have a craving for a cigarette, take five slow, deep breaths and drink in the fresh air.
5. Gradually decrease how many ciggies you have and don't be too hard on yourself if you occasionally fail. Even if you have only a few less than usual, you are on your way to being healthier.

Exposure to Chemicals

You just need to reduce your chemical load so you can decrease the amount of acids you are ingesting or inhaling.

Another cause of acidosis involves exposure to acid-producing synthetic chemicals. You are bombarded with small (and not-so-small) doses of chemicals every day — when you walk beside a busy road, when you drink chlorinated tap water, and when you put on your favorite perfume or moisturizer — and these increase acid in the body.

But even though your environment is laced with thousands of synthetic chemicals, there is no need to ditch your life and become a chemical-phobic hermit. It is not essential to eat strictly organic food, and you don't even have to give up wearing makeup or polyester elastic-waist pants (unless they're out of fashion, which is nearly always). You just need to reduce your chemical load so you can decrease the amount of acids you are ingesting or inhaling.

Sources of Chemical Exposure

Avoid using these products if possible. Substitute with green products. Otherwise, use them in well-ventilated settings. For example, you can make your own cleaning products with safe ingredients, such as vinegar and baking soda, or check out biodegradable brands from your local health food shop.

Cleansers	Beauty Aids
Bleach, furniture polish, oven cleaners, window cleaners	Makeup, nail polish, perfumes, skin moisturizers and astringents
Pesticides	**Foods**
Ant traps, fly sprays, spider sprays	Fried foods, food additives (flavorings and colorings), processed, preserved, and packaged foods, foods sprayed with pesticides
Interior Decorating	
Carpets, cloth furniture, paints, plaster	

How to decrease your exposure to chemicals (and balance your pH)

1. Open windows daily to ventilate your home and car. Chemicals are emitted from carpets and furnishings, and if you use chemical cleaning products, the chemicals can accumulate in enclosed spaces, so open your windows and let in the fresh air.

2. Soak fruits and vegetables in water and vinegar to remove residual pesticides. If you cannot afford organic food, you can minimize chemical load by washing your fruits and vegetables in a bowl of water containing 2 tablespoons (30 mL) of vinegar. Soak vegetables in the water solution for 5 minutes and scrub hardy vegetables (you can't scrub leafy greens as they will bruise).

3. Check food labels. Avoid preservatives, artificial color, flavors, and flavor enhancers. Look for products with natural preservatives, such as vinegar. Vinegar is acid-producing but safer than chemical preservatives.

Did You Know?

Vinegar's Virtues

Vinegar helps to remove pesticides and it also kills bacteria. In the old days, before refrigerators were common, vinegar was used to wash moldy meat to kill the bacteria, which often prevented food poisoning. Apple cider vinegar is the best choice because it is alkalizing. White vinegar is the budget option.

Food Additives

Check food labels for these acid-forming chemicals and then avoid them when possible:

- Calcium propionate.
- Preserved dried fruits, preserved wines, and flavored drinks.
- Artificial sweeteners. Instead of table sugar and artificial sweeteners, use natural sweeteners, such as honey, raw sugar, or stevia. Stevia is a sugarless herb that is the lowest sweetener on the glycemic index with no questionable side effects.
- Aspartame and saccharine because they can cause adverse reactions.
- Yellow, blue, and red food coloring. You don't need fake-colored foods! There are natural alternatives everywhere — just check the labels.
- MSG in Chinese and Thai foods (at a restaurant, ask if the food contains MSG or any other flavor enhancers).
- Fried food, and you will automatically avoid BHA. At the fish and chips shop, order grilled fish, and if you must have fries, also grab a big green salad for a dose of alkalinity.
- Breads that are not labeled preservative-free.

Constipation

Being constipated on a regular basis can increase acidity in the body. Ideally, you should defecate every day, even twice a day. However, many people experience irregular bowel movements where they don't do "number two" for days. Although not ideal, it is okay if you only have one bowel movement every second day. If you're only going once every three days, or longer — once a week — then toxins from your feces are being reabsorbed by your body.

As you can imagine, this can lead to skin problems, such as acne and rashes, and health problems, such as arthritis, aching limbs, and fatigue. If you have constipation or any other bowel complaints, it is essential that you improve your bowel health immediately.

> If you have constipation or any other bowel complaints, it is essential that you improve your bowel health immediately.

Red Flags

You should tell your doctor if you experience abdominal pain or notice blood in your stools. Do not use black walnut or clove oil supplements as a digestive remedy during childhood, pregnancy, or when breastfeeding, because there is a lack of reliable information regarding their safety during these periods. If you've checked off three or more symptoms on the next page, consider seeing your doctor. These problems will need to be addressed before your skin health will improve.

Bowel Health Questionnaire

You may have other bowel problems that can affect your skin. Check off any symptoms you experience on a regular basis (three or more times a week or enough to disrupt your life) to help determine if you have a digestive problem:

☐ Foul-smelling gas or stools
☐ Excessive gas
☐ Excessive burping
☐ Bloating
☐ Food allergies, food sensitivities
☐ Abdominal discomfort or pain
☐ Fatigue after eating
☐ Premature aging
☐ Constipation and/or diarrhea
☐ Nausea
☐ Reflux
☐ Headaches

☐ Constant hunger
☐ Irregular bowel movements
☐ Skin blemishes or rashes
☐ Undigested food particles in your stools (other than seeds and corn, which are normal)
☐ Pellet-shaped stools
☐ Pale, hard-to-flush stools
☐ Irritable bowel syndrome
☐ Unexplained back/shoulder/ abdominal pain
☐ Blood in stools

How to prevent constipation

1. Avoid becoming overheated. Overheating can cause dehydration. In winter, use blankets rather than a duvet because they allow excess heat to escape as you sleep and they breathe better than duvets.
2. Drink 8 to 10 glasses of water each day plus 2 to 4 teaspoons (10 to 20 mL) of chlorophyll in water. Chlorophyll promotes bowel movements (see Green Water recipe on page 344).
3. For every glass of alcohol you drink, follow it with one glass of natural mineral water.
4. Add 1 to 2 tablespoons (15 to 30 mL) of flaxseed oil to your meals.
5. Take laxative herbs, such as dandelion root tea (see the recipe for Soy Dande' on page 345).
6. Eat foods that promote bowel movements, notably green leafy vegetables, papaya, coconut, cabbage, prunes, peas, black sesame seed, sweet potato, asparagus, figs, oat bran, wheat bran, and rice bran.
7. Eat a high-fiber diet with brown rice, whole grains, and lots of vegetables.
8. Make sure you don't have parasites.
9. Do the 3-Day Alkalizing Cleanse (see page 317).

3-Day Alkalizing Cleanse

The first 3 days of the Healthy Skin Diet involve a cleansing program. You will eat 95% alkali-forming foods and drinks, and only 5% acid-forming substances. This gives your body a major cleanse to decrease acidity. This cleansing program is fantastic for your bowels, your skin, and your whole body. There are two versions of the 3-Day Alkalizing Cleanse to choose from: one for cold or winter-like weather and the other for warmer conditions (see pages 320 and 318). It's important to do a cleanse that is appropriate.

Here are some of the unique features of this particular cleansing routine:

1. **Kills parasites:** If you were to plant a vegetable garden, ideally you would first prepare the soil and pull up the weeds so the veggies didn't have to compete for vital nutrients. It is the same with your body: preferably you should make your gastrointestinal tract undesirable for unhealthy parasites, yeasts, and fungi, worms and *Candida albicans* (fungus), and prime for good digestion and absorption so you get the most out of your new diet. The 3-Day Alkalizing Cleanse does this for you. This cleanse changes the acid–alkaline balance in your body, making the body more alkaline. Parasites die off during the first week of the program.

2. **No lethargy or hunger:** This cleanse program is different from traditional detoxification programs because it contains solid food, so you won't feel too hungry or lethargic (maybe just a little).

3. **Neutralizes free radicals:** This 3-day program also has specially designed alkali-forming foods and beauty-boosting nutrients, such as omega-3 fatty acids, selenium, vitamin C, vitamin E, and chlorophyll, to help neutralize the heavy load of free radicals during detoxification. This means that the 3-Day Alkalizing Cleanse shouldn't make you feel ill like a traditional detox might.

4. **Reduces symptoms:** This cleanse is especially good for reducing pimples, eczema, hives, premature aging and cellulite when combined with the 8-week program. However, if you have eczema/dermatitis and a salicylate sensitivity, you may initially have a worsening of symptoms. Don't worry: this is only a temporary salicylate reaction (possibly from the Green Water). Your body will stop being sensitive to salicylates as your acid levels reduce during the 8-week program.

Dehydration

You **need to** drink enough hydrating fluids to prevent dehydration. Dehydration is associated with increased acids in the body, constipation, dry skin, acne, blood pressure problems, headaches, moodiness, and lethargy. Dehydration also quickly increases the appearance of wrinkles. Drinking more fluids can be a challenge, however.

Water Prescription

How much water do we need to drink to prevent dehydration? Work out how much water your body requires using the following equation:

Your body weight in kilograms (kg) x 0.033 = how many liters of water to drink daily.

For example, if you weigh 75 kg: 75 x 0.033 = 2.47, so you would need approximately 2.5 liters (10 cups) of water per day for optimal health.

If using pounds, divide your body weight by 2, so body weight in pounds ÷ 2 = ounces of water to drink each day.

How to make drinking water more enjoyable

Some people do not like to drink water. If you count yourself among these, here are some tips:

1. Buy a water filter that attaches to your kitchen sink or buy a water filter jug.
2. Serve your water chilled with ice and a splash of real lime or lemon juice (they are alkalizing).
3. Drink natural mineral water.
4. Drink other hydrating beverages, such as herbal teas and fresh vegetable juices (keep fruit to a limit because it is mostly acid-forming).
5. Drink one to two glasses of water in between meals to leave your digestive tract well lubricated for digestion. This also prevents excessive thirst during meals (a sure sign you are not drinking enough water in between meals).
6. Don't drink too many liquids during mealtime because they can dilute digestive juices and prevent proper digestion.

Q. I know I have to hydrate my body, but do coffee and tea with milk count as fluids that are okay for my skin?

A. No, coffee and black tea with milk can't be counted as hydrating fluids because caffeine has a dehydrating effect on the body; however, caffeine may not be harmful to the skin in small doses. The best rule of thumb is NEVER have more than two cups of coffee or tea per day because caffeine triggers the stress response in the body, releasing cortisol. You don't want to overstimulate this hormone because it contributes to premature aging. Caffeine also causes the adrenal glands to work overtime, so it can cause puffy eyes and dark circles under the eyes. If you have eczema, rosacea, acne, cellulite, or psoriasis, I recommend avoiding caffeine or switching to decaf coffee because it is less likely to exacerbate your condition.

Guidelines for Tea and Coffee Drinking on the Healthy Skin Diet

1. Look for water-decaffeinated coffee as opposed to decaf that has been produced with chemicals. Weak, freshly brewed bean is healthier than instant coffee and decaf coffee because of their chemical additives.

2. As an alternative, drink dandelion tea once a day because it helps the liver safely eliminate skin-aging chemicals. It's caffeine-free and tastes great. Look for the Soy Dande' recipe on page 345.

3. Drink only one to two cups of coffee or tea per day.

4. Avoid soft drinks containing caffeine (cola and energy drinks).

5. Drink green tea twice a day because it has liver-detoxifying and antioxidant benefits (but remember that green tea also contains caffeine).

Q. How can I increase my water intake without needing to urinate more often?

A. Your body needs time to adapt to the extra water, so increase intake little by little so your body benefits without feeling waterlogged. If you are still going to the toilet too frequently, add liquid chlorophyll and a pinch of good-quality sea salt to your bottle of water. You may also want to check for chromium deficiency and supplement if necessary (see page 82). If you don't usually drink water, try to gradually increase water intake over the period of a week. A good indicator is to increase water consumption as your urine output increases.

Parasites

Bad microbes — parasites, fungi, and yeasts — thrive when good intestinal flora are absent.

Our gut is populated with all kinds of "good" and "bad" microscopic bacteria, or flora. Some bacteria, such as acidophilus, are beneficial to your health. They work by adhering to your gut wall and policing the bad bacteria and other microbes so they can't multiply. These good flora are essential for healthy skin, while other bad microbes cause skin problems.

Bad microbes — parasites, fungi, and yeasts — thrive when good intestinal flora are absent. An acidic lifestyle can create a desirable breeding ground for these microbes. You can't avoid picking up germs from unclean surfaces, contaminated people, and the great outdoors. Have you ever walked barefoot in public change rooms? Do your pets lick your face or sleep in your bed? Have you ever forgotten or just couldn't be bothered to wash your hands before eating lunch? Like most people, you probably have, but these actions can unfortunately lead to little wriggly health problems if you also have an overly acidic body.

Luckily, we have great health-care facilities in the Western world, so parasite treatments are readily available to us.

Did You Know?

WHO

The World Health Organization (WHO) states that parasitic infections, if left untreated, weaken your body's defense system (immunity) because of blood loss, anemia, malnutrition, and tissue and organ damage. Non-specific symptoms include fatigue, nausea, abdominal pains, and loss of appetite. Sometimes worms can be spotted in the feces. In addition, because worms need vitamin A to survive, they can cause a deficiency of this key vitamin. Vitamin A deficiency symptoms include rough and dry skin, frequent infections, bumpy skin, and poor sense of smell.

Q. What should I do if I have worms?

A. If you suspect you have parasites, you have a number of options. You may want to speak to your doctor and get a stool test done to confirm what sort of worms you have so you can use a specific drug treatment. Keep in mind that even with medical treatment, if your microbe problem is caused by an acidic lifestyle, your parasite problem can quickly come back to haunt you. A multifaceted approach is by far the most helpful option.

1. **Change the acid/alkaline environment:** The first step is to make their environment (your body) so undesirable that the parasites will stop multiplying and start dying. You can do this by alkalizing your body and by taking antiparasitic herbal and probiotic remedies.

2. **Supplement with probiotics:** The most effective supplement to take is probiotics so you have plenty of good microbes ready to take over as the undesirables die. You can take antiparasitic herbs for 10 days if you have a severe infestation, or you can simply follow the Healthy Skin Diet for 8 weeks with the simple addition of a probiotic supplement and garlic.

Parasite Questionnaire

Check off any symptoms you experience three or more times per week:

- ☐ General weakness
- ☐ Facial pallor
- ☐ Anemia
- ☐ Vitamin A deficiency
- ☐ Withered, yellow look
- ☐ Huge appetite (may cause weight gain) or loss of appetite (and weight loss)
- ☐ Nausea
- ☐ Muscle wasting
- ☐ Unexplained thinness
- ☐ Bluish specks in the whites of eyes
- ☐ White, coin-sized splotches on the face
- ☐ Anal itching (especially at night)
- ☐ Itchy ears
- ☐ Poor sleep
- ☐ Excessive nose picking
- ☐ Grinding teeth during sleep

- ☐ Cravings for sweets or dried foods
- ☐ Cravings for raw rice or dirt (usually kids)
- ☐ Cravings for charcoal or burned foods
- ☐ Abdominal pain
- ☐ Digestive complaints: diarrhea, gas, bloating, belching, constipation
- ☐ Irritable bowel syndrome
- ☐ Mucus in stools
- ☐ Gluten intolerance
- ☐ Low blood sugar (hypoglycemia)
- ☐ High blood sugar
- ☐ Allergies
- ☐ Skin rashes
- ☐ Acne
- ☐ Depression
- ☐ Moodiness
- ☐ Hyperactivity (in children)

If you have more than five of these symptoms, you could have a parasite problem. Be sure to visit your doctor to create a plan for ridding yourself of these unhealthy creatures.

Anti-Parasitic Foods and Herbs

Before using any anti-parasitic food or herb, consult with your doctor concerning dosage and safety. The foods and herbs listed here have a moderate anti-microbial effect.

Foods

There are plenty of other food sources that help to control microbes, including raw garlic, raw onion, cinnamon, cloves, radishes, and mustard. Other foods include avocado, coconut, sauerkraut, seaweed, raw honey, extra virgin olive oil, black pepper, capsicum (bell pepper) and ginger. Foods that promote good bowel flora include miso (Japanese fermented soy paste that can be used as a soup base) and chlorophyll-rich foods, such as dark green leafy vegetables and alfalfa greens.

How to prevent parasite infestations

- Avoid sugary foods — cakes, sweets, pastries, doughnuts, white flour desserts, dairy desserts, sugar in coffee/tea, dried fruits, and chocolate that contains sugar create a breeding ground for parasites in the body.
- Eat plenty of alkali-forming foods, such as leafy green vegetables, almonds, lemon, and avocado.
- Filter your drinking water with a filter jug or tap fitting.
- Wash your hands thoroughly before preparing and eating meals.
- Wash all fruits, vegetables, and meats with apple cider vinegar and water before use. Soak them for 5 minutes, as this will remove any pesticide residues and kill microbes.
- When traveling to foreign countries, only drink bottled water and eat thoroughly cooked foods (avoid uncooked salads, iced drinks, and ice).
- Avoid consuming raw fish, but continue eating wasabi. This green paste made from horseradish is a natural anti-parasitic, so consume it whenever you eat raw fish.
- Eat garlic every day. Have one small clove of garlic with every meal.
- Avoid constipation.
- Chew food thoroughly so your food can be digested properly. Parasites thrive in poorly digested foods.
- Drink Green Water daily (see the recipe on page 344).
- Take a probiotic supplement.

Herbs

Pau d'arco, allspice, basil, bay leaf, caraway, cumin, coriander, nutmeg, oregano, sage, rosemary, and thyme can help control unhealthy parasites.

Black Walnut Extract

The chief anti-parasitic compound in black walnuts is called juglone. Studies have found it to have a strong anti-parasitic, an anti-fungal, and a laxative effect, which is really handy because it not only kills pesky worms but also helps to flush them out.

Clove Oil

Clove oil contains the constituent eugenol, which can destroy parasite eggs, *Candida albicans*, yeasts, and bacteria, such as staphylococcus and E coli. Other extracts and oils that are effective for treating worms include thyme oil, grape seed extract, and garlic oil.

Pumpkin Seeds

Cucurbita, a major compound in pumpkin seeds, is anti-parasitic, making pumpkin seeds useful for eradicating tapeworm. Pumpkin seeds are a safe treatment for worm-infested children as long as they're old enough to chew the seeds. Eat a handful of pumpkin seeds daily.

Candida albicans

Candida albicans, **also** known as thrush, is a yeast infection found in the vagina in women and in the digestive tract of both sexes. It may also be present externally on the skin and as a toenail fungal infection, or tinea. Women are eight times more likely to suffer from a yeast infection than men, which may be due to higher antibiotic use, higher estrogen hormones in the body, and birth-control use.

CASE STUDY
Candida Cure

A 30-year-old woman came to our clinic suffering from skin rashes and vaginal itching (her doctor diagnosed *Candida albicans*). She reported insatiable cravings for sweet foods and frequent colds and flu, which were occasionally treated with antibiotics. Green Water, probiotics, and garlic were recommended to improve her gut flora, and she did the 3-Day Alkalizing Cleanse. She replaced sugary foods and white bread and rice with good-quality vegetables, protein, brown rice, and whole grains. She also did some light exercise and relaxation routines at the end of the day to restore her immune system. Her vaginal itching stopped 2 days later, and after 3 weeks her skin rash began to clear and her cravings stopped. Six weeks later, her skin rash was completely gone.

Candida Questionnaire

Circle Yes or No beside any lifestyle factors or symptoms. For questions such as "Do you crave alcohol," only circle Yes if you crave it regularly (three or more times per week):

Have you taken antibiotics for more than a month in the last 6 months? Yes / No

Have you taken the birth control pill for more than 2 years? Yes / No

Have you taken any cortisone-type drugs for more than 2 weeks? Yes / No

Do you have athlete's foot? Yes / No

Do you frequently crave sugar and bread? Yes / No

Do you frequently crave alcohol? Yes / No

Does cigarette smoke really bother you? Yes / No

Do you have unexplained fatigue? Yes / No

Do you often feel drained or spaced out? Yes / No

Do you frequently suffer from constipation or diarrhea? Yes / No

Do you have bloating, gas, or belching? Yes / No

Do you have a loss of sex drive? Yes / No

Do you have PMS or period cramps? Yes / No

Do you have frequent mood swings? Yes / No

Do you have frequent attacks of anxiety or crying? Yes / No

Are you shaking or irritable when hungry? Yes / No

Do you have an inability to concentrate? Yes / No

Do you have frequent headaches? Yes / No

Do you have food sensitivities and intolerances? Yes / No

Do you have excessive body odor not relieved by deodorant use? Yes / No

Do you have bad breath? Yes / No

Do perfumes, insecticides, and chemicals make you feel unwell?** Yes / No

Do you have rectal or nasal itching?** Yes / No

Do you have vaginal itching, burning, or creamy discharge?** Yes / No

If you answered yes to more than five symptoms, you may have *Candida albicans*. If you said yes to any of the symptoms marked by asterisks (**), you are highly likely to have this yeast infection. If you suspect you have candida, take a probiotic supplement and consume alkalizing foods and drinks. Your *Candida albicans* should magically disappear; if it does not improve within a week, see your doctor.

Alkali-Forming Foods

How do you "think green"? Green drinks that contain chlorophyll are the best way to create a good acid–alkaline balance in your body. Consume green drinks every day for the best results. Being vegetarian may also help, but only if your food choices are healthy ones. Some vegetarian diets include dairy products, processed white breads, and sugar-rich desserts, so they too can end up producing acidosis.

Chlorophyll

Chlorophyll is the name of the green pigment found in plants. It is formed as the plant's leaves capture sunlight in a process called photosynthesis. Chlorophyll is structurally very similar to our own blood. The only difference is that chlorophyll has the mineral magnesium at the center of its structure and we have iron. Magnesium and iron are both essential for our health and can be obtained by eating leafy greens, such as spinach and parsley.

Q. I hate vegetables. How can I create a good acid and alkaline balance in my body without eating them?

A. To be honest, I don't know if you can be healthy without consuming vegetables. Scientists have concluded without doubt that eating lots of vegetables decreases your risk of many diseases, such as cancer, heart disease, and strokes. A diet low in vegetables increases your risk of getting severe skin conditions, such as acne. Studies show that a high intake of fruits and vegetables lessens the damaging effects of sun exposure and protects against premature skin wrinkling. Scientists, nutritionists, and other health experts may argue about what a healthy diet is (and is not), but they all agree that a diet rich in vegetables has the strongest and most consistent association with disease prevention. Can you believe it? All of the health experts agree on something!

How to choose an effective liquid chlorophyll supplement

There are many types of green drinks and supplements available from health food shops; however, most of them taste unpleasant (such as wheat grass) or they don't have the correct alkalizing effect (such as spirulina, which is acid-producing). Barley grass is suitable. The best drink is plain liquid chlorophyll, which not only tastes pleasant but is also inexpensive (see the Green Water drink on page 344 in the recipe section).

Liquid chlorophyll is available from health food shops, online and from places where health products are sold. Look for the following:

- Choose a liquid chlorophyll that is preservative-free. Preservatives are acid-forming and can irritate the skin (especially if you have eczema). Other suitable ingredients in a chlorophyll supplement are spearmint oil, alfalfa extract, and vegetable oil. Lactic acid or ascorbic acid may be present in small quantities.

- Choose a supplement that is low strength. Look on the ingredient panel for a chlorophyll concentration of around 200 mg per 100 mL. I prefer to use and only recommend low-strength chlorophyll because it is not only very effective at treating skin conditions, it also has a more pleasant color and taste than higher-strength chlorophyll. High-strength liquid chlorophyll supplements (with 2000 mg per 100 mL) usually appear black, and as a result of the dense color, they may stain your teeth after regular use. If you wish to use high-strength chlorophyll, reduce the dosage and clean your teeth afterwards.

A chlorophyll drink made from a liquid chlorophyll supplement can give you an extra dose of vegetables daily. It can help to neutralize acids in the body so your blood is less likely to clump together and become sluggish and inefficient.

Chlorophyll drinks taken in the morning can also stimulate a bowel movement so they're a great way to prevent constipation and toxic buildup.

Probiotic Supplements

Probiotics are microbes and enzymes that enable digestion and counteract acidosis, *Candida albicans*, and parasites. Probiotics can be used therapeutically for treating digestive problems, poor immunity, eczema, and *Candida albicans*, but you need to know the specific strain that has been scientifically proven to

Alkalizing Foods

STRONGLY ALKALIZING FOODS	MILDLY ALKALIZING FOODS
Vegetables	
Alfalfa sprouts, beet greens, beets, broccoli, carrots, cucumber, dandelion greens, dark leafy greens, kale (raw), lentil sprouts, mung bean sprouts, spinach (raw), vegetable juice (freshly made), watercress, wheatgrass juice	Asparagus, bell peppers, Brussels sprouts, cabbage (white or red), carrots, cauliflower, eggplant, endive, garlic, green beans, leeks, lettuce, olives, onions, potatoes, radishes, shallots, squash, sweet potatoes, turnips, yams, zucchini
Fruits	
Grapefruit, lemons, limes, apple cider vinegar	Avocado, bananas (fresh and dried), dates, raisins, tomatoes (raw)
Legumes, Nuts and Seeds	
	Almonds, Brazil nuts, flax seeds
Dairy Products and Eggs	
	Butter (unheated), buttermilk (uncooked), egg yolk, whey (fresh)
Oils	
	Cold-pressed extra virgin olive oil (unheated), flaxseed oil
Herbs and Spices	
	Sea salt/Celtic salt (unrefined)
Beverages	
Chlorophyll, green drinks, wheat grass	Almond milk, herbal teas (not green tea, which is acidifying), natural mineral water (not carbonated), spring or filtered water

suit your needs. There are many strains of probiotics, notably *L. acidophilus* and *L. rhamnosus*. The benefits you get from probiotic supplements are strain-specific: they do not all work in the same manner. For example, the probiotic supplement that is good for treating irritable bowel syndrome may not be beneficial for eczema.

Probiotics for *Candida albicans* management:
- *L. acidophilus* LA5
- *L. rhamnosus* GG
- *L. acidophilus* strain NAS
- *L acidophilus* NCFM.36

Q. If alkalizing foods are so good for me, would I be even healthier if I ate 100% alkalizing foods and avoided all acidic foods?

A. No! You should not eat an all-alkalizing diet every day. While an alkalizing diet is beneficial as a cleanse for short periods, one week should be your maximum. People who eat salads and vegetables with no protein can end up feeling unwell and may get sallow-looking skin that has poor tone. In fact, many overweight people who have lost the extra pounds by eating nothing but salads end up with very saggy skin. This is often (but not always) caused by protein deficiency.

Aim to balance acidic foods with alkalizing foods. All of the recipes in the Healthy Skin Diet have a healthy ratio of alkalizing and acid-forming foods with approximately 50% alkalizing and 50% acid-forming foods within one meal. This allows you to enjoy many of your favorite foods, such as meat, breads, and the occasional sweet treat, without adverse effect on your skin.

Probiotics for digestive complaints:
- *L. rhamnosus* GG
- *L. johnsonii* La1, L. plantarum 299v
- *L. paracasei* Shirota
- *Propionibacterium freudenreichii* HA-101 and HA-102
- Eat sauerkraut

Probiotics for compromised immune system:
- *L. acidophilus* LA5
- *L. rhamnosus* GG.38

For adults, the general rule is to take one capsule two to three times per day on an empty stomach (in between meals or at least 15 minutes before meals), or according to the manufacturer's instructions. Probiotics should be ingested with room-temperature water or almond/rice/soy drink. Avoid having probiotics with excessively cold or hot drinks because they may damage the beneficial bacteria. For children's dosage, see Children's Clear Skin Program (page 263).

Did You Know?

Alkalizing Surprises

The alleged acidic fruit, the tomato, is actually alkalizing to the blood. And isn't lemon usually acidic? Yes, but only before consumption; once they have been digested, lemons and limes have an alkalizing effect that is beneficial for your blood. I guess you can't always judge a fruit by its bite! Butter is a better choice than margarine because butter is slightly alkalizing when it's unheated. Apple cider vinegar is super alkalizing, but other types of vinegar are highly acidic and should be avoided or limited.

Quick Tips for Restoring Your pH Balance

- Consume "green" drinks every day.
- Drink 8 to 10 glasses of filtered water per day (this includes having Green Water twice a day).
- Limit or avoid caffeine.
- Avoid alcohol if possible, or when socializing, drink no more than two standard alcoholic drinks. Have at least four alcohol-free days per week.
- Avoid smoking and passive smoking.
- Eat two servings of fruit and at least five servings of vegetables per day.
- Take a suitable probiotic supplement daily.
- Eat anti-parasitic food daily, such as garlic, onion, ginger, herbs, and spices.
- Eat dark green leafy vegetables every day. They are like gold! They increase your energy stores and create strong, healthy red blood cells. Have two handfuls of leafy greens per day.

pH-Balanced Recipes

Several excellent alkalizing and energizing recipes that you will find in the recipe section are listed here.

Beverages
Green Water
ACV Drink
Flaxseed Lemon Drink
Almond Milk
Anti-Aging Broth
Skin-Firming Drink

Salads
Spicy Green Papaya Salad
Sweet Raspberry, Avocado and
  Watercress Salad
Tabbouleh
Rich Mineral Salad
Roasted Sweet Potato Salad
Tasty Spinach Salad

Soups
Roasted Corn and Cauliflower Soup
Therapeutic Veggie Soup

Snacks
Avocado Salsa
Avocado Dip with Dipping Sticks
Avocado Beauty Snack

Breakfast
Flaxseed Lemon Drink plus a handful
  of almond and Brazil nuts
Designer Muesli
Gluten-Free Muesli with homemade
  Almond Milk

Guideline #2

· ·

Moisturize Your Skin from the Inside Out: Eating Great Fats

Imagine you've spent a lot of money on a brand new sports car. Now, you wouldn't go and fill it with the wrong octane of gasoline, would you? If your car's manufacturer said it needed premium unleaded for enhanced performance and mileage, you'd buy the good stuff so that the car ran as well as it could. So too with your body: eating the wrong types of fats can decrease your performance and leave you looking not so hot, but eating the right types can make your skin look fantastic. You see, certain fats are moisturizing to your skin. They moisturize you from the inside out. They're more effective than even the most luxurious skin cream.

That's the good news, but the not-so-good news is that Westerners like to eat the types of fat that decrease performance and mileage — the ones that can cause inflammation, dry skin, premature aging, and enhanced feelings of pain. They also increase your risk of heart disease, asthma, eczema, and acne.

Some fats are bad, many are good, and others are great, leading to beautiful, gorgeous, healthy skin and improved vitality. Broadly speaking, there are three kinds of dietary fats and three corresponding series of prostaglandins that make these fats bioavailable.

You see, certain fats are moisturizing to your skin. They moisturize you from the inside out. They're more effective than even the most luxurious skin cream.

Did You Know?
· · · · · · · · · · · · · · · · · ·

The Omega-3 to Omega-6 Ratio
The current Western diet is low in omega-3 EFAs and high in omega-6 EFAs, at a ratio of about 1 to 30. The ideal ratio is 1 to 4. To achieve this ratio, increase omega-3 and reduce intake of omega-6 EFAs. This is best accomplished by eating more fatty fish and fewer processed foods.

Q. **What is a fatty acid?**

A. Fatty acids are a component of animal and vegetable fats that are used as a fuel source in many tissues, particularly the heart and muscle. There are many specific types of fatty acids, and while the consumption of excessive fat in general is harmful, we do, in fact, benefit from the consumption of certain fatty acids, such as omega-3 and omega-6 fatty acids, found in fish and flaxseed oils.

Kinds of Fat

There are three basic kinds of fat — saturated, unsaturated, and trans, or cis, fat. Some are good for you, a few are not, and still others are essential for good health and healthy skin. Most foods contain a mix of the different kinds of fat. Butter, for example, is more than 50% saturated fat, almost 20% monosaturated, and under 5% polyunsaturated fat. Olive oil contains about 70% monounsaturated fat, with the remaining fats about 15% polyunsaturated and 15% saturated.

1. Saturated fats

These fats are found in animal products, such as fatty meats, butter, cream, full-fat cheese, whole milk, and chicken skin. A few plant foods, such as palm, cocoa butter, and coconut oil, are also high in saturated fat. Saturated fats should be restricted in your diet because they produce high levels of cholesterol, which can prematurely age the skin and increase the risk of acne and heart disease.

2. Unsaturated fats (monounsaturated and polyunsaturated fats)

These fats are found in flaxseed oil, evening primrose oil, fish oil, olive oil, and canola oil, as well as avocados, almonds, cashews, peanuts, and sesame seeds. There are two kinds of unsaturated fats: monosaturated and polyunsaturated.

Monosaturated fats are derived from oleic acid. They are considered to be healthy fats involved in regulation of cholesterol, increasing HDL "good" cholesterol and lowering "LDL" bad cholesterol.

Polyunsaturated fats (PUFAs) include several series of essential fatty acids, notably the omega-6 and omega-3 series. These fats cannot be produced by the body and must come from the food we eat. For this reason they are called "essential." These essential fatty acids include:

- Alpha-linolenic acid (ALA)
- Linolenic acid
- Arachidonic acid (AA)
- Dihomo-gamma-linolenic acid (DGLA)
- Eicosapentaenoic acid (EPA)
- Docosahexaenoic acid (DHA)
- Gamma-linolenic acid (GLA)

The omega series of essential fatty acids (EFAs) are composed of these acids. For example, omega-3 EFAs include alpha-linolenic acid (ALA), eicosapentaenoic acid (EPA), and docosahexaenoic acid (DHA). Fish oil and flaxseed oil are high in omega-3 fats. Omega-6 EFAs include gamma-linolenic acid (GLA). Evening primrose oil is high in these fats.

3. Trans fats

These fats may be found in fried foods, cookies and crackers, pastries, cakes, french fries and potato chips, and products containing shortening or hydrogenated vegetable oil. These fats should be avoided. Most food manufactures have stopped using trans fat in response to medical concerns about its safety.

Prostaglandins

The body uses EFAs for the production of prostaglandins (PGs), powerful, hormone-like chemicals that affect your hormones, your heart, your blood vessels, your cells, and your skin's appearance. The body produces more than 30 different types of prostaglandins, which are grouped into three families, or series — PG1, PG2, and PG3. Which series a prostaglandin falls into depends on what type of fat it is originally made from — polyunsaturated omega-3, polyunsaturated omega-6, or saturated fats. Each prostaglandin has a highly specific function. They are short-lived, so you need to keep supplying them with the "building materials" — the fats and their synergistic nutrients — required to make them.

Some prostaglandins help to prevent acne, heart disease, arthritis, asthma, hay fever, and sinusitis. Even if you do not have these medical problems, prostaglandins are still relevant to you.

Prostaglandin Street

Okay, so you still may be thinking, "Prosta what?" Prostaglandins can be a bit difficult to visualize, but just imagine your prostaglandin biochemical pathways as three parallel streets, like the ones on a road map. Imagine that Street 1 and Street 3 are the "good" streets that lead to smooth, clear lakes set in tropical surroundings and Street 2, the "bad" street stuck right in the middle, leads to the dump (a.k.a. bumpy skin, acne, and rashes).

PG Traffic

Now, you also have inner traffic that travels along these three streets. Imagine your inner traffic looks like yellow dump trucks bringing fats to add to either the clear lakes or the dump. If a dump truck is full of fat, which street do you want it to go down? Do you want the truck to dump out fats that may harm your health at the end of Street 2 or do you want it to go down Street 1 or 3 and dump out fats that will keep the lake looking lovely and smooth? I'm guessing you said Streets 1 and 3 and by now you may have pieced together that the dump down Street 2 is rough, like skin inflammation, and the smooth lake at the end of Streets 1 and 3 represents skin that is healthy and smooth.

Let's work our way up from series 1 to series 3 prostaglandins.

Prostaglandin (PG) Series

Prostaglandin Series 1	Prostaglandin Series 2	Prostaglandin Series 3
Good Fats	Bad Fats	Beautiful Fats
Polyunsaturated fats	Saturated fats	Polyunsaturated fats
GLA (gamma-linolenic acid)	AA (arachidonic acid)	EPA (eicosapentaenoic), DHA (docosahexaenoic acid)
Omega-6 EFAs	Leukotrienes and thromboxanes	Omega-3 EFAs
Street 1	Street 2	Street 3

Detours

Series 1 prostaglandins (Street 1) have been found to improve circulation, lower blood pressure, and decrease inflammatory responses, such as eczema, PMS, and arthritis-like pain — but only if the pathway (or "street") is unblocked.

Street 1 leads to the smooth, clear lake (and gorgeous, clear skin), but this doesn't always occur. Street 1 can be blocked by various dietary and lifestyle factors requiring a traffic diversion to be set up, like a roadworks detour that redirects your healthy omega-6 fats into the inflammation-making dump at the end of Street 2. It's very important to determine if your Street 1 is blocked, because all your omega-6 polyunsaturated fats may be diverting to inflammation-making Street 2 right now.

How Fats Make Good and Bad Prostaglandins

STREET 1
"The Good"

OMEGA–6
Vegetable cooking oils, margarine, nuts and seeds, canola and soy oils

Delta-6-desaturase NEEDS... biotin, B6, zinc and magnesium

GLA
Also supplied in borage oil, blackcurrant seed and evening primrose oil

DGLA

Prostaglandin Series 1
Inhibits inflammation and high blood pressure, promotes heart health, healthy skin, and prevents release of AA from cell membranes.

STREET 2
"The Bad"

Saturated fats
Dairy, meat, fried foods (trans fats), tropical seafood, eggs, high meat/protein diet

DETOUR
(if blockage then omega-6 slowly converts to AA...)

Arachidonic acid(AA)
(blocked by EPA & DHA)

Prostaglandin Series 2
Promotes inflammation, salt retention, heart disease, pain and fever, increases allergic reactions, asthma, arthritis, eczema, dermatitis, psoriasis, hay fever, dandruff and sinusitis.

STREET 3
"The Beautiful"

Omega-3
Flax seeds, flaxseed oil, walnuts, omega-3 eggs, fish, leafy greens

Enzyme reation delta-6-desaturase

EPA and DHA
Salmon, trout, sardines, herring, tuna oil, mackerel

Prostaglandin Series 3
Inhibits inflammation, decreases blood pressure, reduces pain and depression, prevents heart disease, promotes beautiful skin, and prevents release of AA.

Roadblocks

There are two enzymatic reactions that need to occur for your omega-6 oils to be converted to GLA and then into substances that make smooth, lovely skin. These reactions are called delta-6-desaturase and delta-5-desaturase. Delta-6-desaturase is a slow enzyme process that converts linolenic acid into essential fatty acids (ALA and EPA) and PG3. This conversion can be blocked by too much saturated fat in the diet from meat and dairy products, high stress, high glycemic index (high insulin), alcohol, and trans fats. D-6-d dysfunction can be genetic or occur as you age.

However, one or both of these enzymatic reactions may be genetically faulty or temporarily blocked by:

- Chronic stress and anxiety
- High insulin responses (from high-GI foods)
- Trans fats

> Your genetics play a part in your body's response to omega-6 fats, but even with genetic blockage, you can fix the problem with dietary modifications.

Your genetics play a part in your body's response to omega-6 fats, but even with genetic blockage, you can fix the problem with dietary modifications. Through client feedback I have also found that drinking Green Water daily can prevent omega-6 blockage signs from occurring; this may be due to liquid chlorophyll's high magnesium content or its alkalizing effect.

Roadworkers

There are also six nutrients, enthusiastic roadworkers, who can work on fixing delta-5 and -6 reactions. They can remove the roadblocks that prevent you from building good-quality skin.

1. Vitamin B_6
2. Biotin
3. Zinc
4. Magnesium
5. Vitamin B_3
6. Vitamin C

For healthy skin, supplement your diet with these nutrients.

Prostaglandin Series 1 (The Good)

Prostaglandin series 1 are made from a polyunsaturated fat called linoleic acid, an omega-6 essential fatty acid. Omega-6 EFAs are not as famous as their cousin, omega-3 EFAs, perhaps because our Western diets are usually overflowing with omega-6 EFAs, found in corn oil, sesame, safflower, and sunflower seeds, canola, soybeans, walnuts, green pumpkin seeds (pepitas), borage oil,* evening primrose oil,* blackcurrant seed,* flax seeds, and green leafy vegetables.

The foods marked with an asterisk also contain GLA, which your body can more easily convert to silky smooth series 1 prostaglandins. There's no big buzz about their goodness because we're not usually deficient in it.

Omega-6 Questionnaire

Fill out the following questionnaire to see if you have any omega-6 blockage or deficiency signs. Check off any of the symptoms you experience on a regular basis (three or more times per week):

- ☐ Eczema-like skin eruptions
- ☐ Loss of hair
- ☐ Premature aging
- ☐ Behavioral disturbances, hyperactivity
- ☐ Kidney or liver degeneration*
- ☐ Excessive water loss through the skin (dry skin), combined with excess thirst*
- ☐ Frequent infections such as colds/flu/thrush
- ☐ Poor wound healing
- ☐ Sterility (in males)*
- ☐ Miscarriages*
- ☐ Arthritic-like pain*
- ☐ Period pain, PMS, breast pain during periods
- ☐ Breast/ovarian cysts*
- ☐ Heart and circulation problems*
- ☐ Growth retardation in childhood*

If you've checked off three or more symptoms, read the section called "Roadblocks"(page 60). If you (or your child) have any conditions that are marked above with an asterisk (*), you should speak to your doctor. These symptoms can also be caused by other factors.

Evening Primrose Oil

Evening primrose oil (EPO) is an omega-6 fat that increases skin hydration and enhances smoothness and resilience, especially when used in conjunction with omega-3 and the six key nutrients. If you have severe dry skin, premature aging and wrinkles, adult eczema, or premenstrual syndrome (PMS), an EPO supplement may help. Although EPO is not essential in the Healthy Skin Diet Anti-Eczema Program (see page 200), EPO should be used in conjunction with omega-3 foods or supplements.

Q. How much EPO should I take for good skin health?

A. Always have a daily dose of omega-3 from foods, such as ground flax seeds or flaxseed oil and oily fish, such as salmon, sardines, trout, herring, and mackerel. The EPA made from these foods has been shown to help EPO relieve inflammation.

Some sources recommend that adults should take 5000 to 6000 mg of EPO per day, in divided doses (this equates to approximately 500 to 600 mg of GLA at the end of the day). Check the information panel on your supplement container to see how many grams are in each capsule. If each capsule contains 1000 mg of evening primrose oil, you will need to take two capsules with breakfast, two with lunch and two with dinner. Have EPO supplements with liquid, and for best results have EPO with a protein-containing meal.

EPO Caution

Be aware that EPO can make symptoms worse in a select few people. This reaction usually means they have an omega-3 deficiency that prevents series 3 prostaglandins from being made in the body. EPO actually increases AA in the body, but this does not occur if you have omega-3 and EPA at the same time (for the relationship between omega-3 and EPA, see page 66). Avoid taking EPO if you are on phenothiazine drug therapy for schizophrenia. EPO can make drugs, such as chlorpromazine and trifluoperperazine, less effective. If you're on any medications, see your doctor before using EPO.

> **Q.** I've been taking two capsules of evening primrose oil a day, but my skin is still extremely dry. What am I doing wrong?
>
> **A.** The dosage may be too low. If you have severely dry skin that is aging fast and crying out for moisture, try evening primrose oil in therapeutic doses. Consult with your doctor for the safe dosage. I've never seen anything work so quickly and so dramatically at reversing dry skin and some signs of aging. However, it can cause pimples (as EPO also increases arachidonic acid in the body). To prevent this from happening, always use EPO in conjunction with omega-3 EFAs, such as fish oil.

Protaglandin Series 2 (The Bad)

You've met The Good, but have you heard about The Bad? You may have these troublemakers living on your street… thugs who may be vandalizing your body right now. They can cause skin inflammation, constrict blood vessels, trigger asthma attacks, and increase feelings of pain. They're nasty fellas. These vandals are called leukotrienes and thromboxanes, which are derived from saturated fats. It is important to reduce saturated fat intake, so you will need to temporarily avoid dairy products and reduce your meat intake. Leukotrienes are implicated in asthma attacks, atopic eczema/dermatitis, psoriasis, arthritis, and heart disease (atherosclerotic plaques). Thromboxanes are wanted for questioning for excessive constriction of blood vessels and blood platelet aggregation, which can lead to cardiovascular disease and pre-eclampsia during pregnancy.

Leukotrienes and Thromboxanes

Leukotrienes and thromboxanes are made from arachidonic acid (AA), which comes from saturated fats. I call these fats "The Bad," but they're not all strictly bad. Saturated fats are all right when eaten in moderation and if they are "policed" with foods that prevent the bad prostaglandins from being made, as you can see in the Q & A, "How can I stop 'The Bad' PGs from damaging my skin?" (below). Your body can also make AA from omega-6 EFAs (polyunsaturated cooking oils, margarine, nuts, and seeds).

Sources of Arachidonic Acid

It is best to limit these foods because of their poor quality or extra-high saturated fat content. They contain damaged (trans) fats that behave like saturated fats in the body.

- Animal products (food with eyes): fatty beef, veal, liver, and offal; chicken and turkey skin; fatty lamb and pork; cheap hamburger patties (unless you make your own lean patties)
- Egg, especially the yolk
- Tropical seafood
- Dairy products (milk, cream, cheese and ice cream), many desserts; and deep-fried foods and margarine

Q. How can I stop the "The Bad" PGs from damaging my skin?

A. Certain foods can help to protect against the damaging effects of bad fats on your skin.

- Carotenes (from brightly colored fruit and vegetables, such as carrots)
- Flavonoids (from high fruit and vegetable intake)
- Garlic
- Ginger
- Omega-3 EPA (salmon, trout, sardines, herring, mackerel, and fish oil supplements)
- Onion
- Selenium
- Turmeric
- Vitamin E

Q. If I need to reduce or avoid saturated fats found in dairy products in order to manage series 2 prostaglandins, won't my calcium levels fall?

A. Yes and no. Dairy products can cause inflammation in sensitive individuals. The fastest way to clear up acne, eczema, cellulite, and age-related skin conditions is to remove milk and other dairy products from your diet. For this reason, The Healthy Skin Diet is dairy-free. To compensate for the loss of this source of calcium, you need to get calcium from other food sources. Calcium supplementation may also be necessary if you are pregnant, breastfeeding, over the age of 40, or a child.

- Children with skin complaints should have 500 mg of calcium daily for the duration of the Healthy Skin Diet.
- Adults with skin problems should have 800 mg of calcium per day for the duration of the Healthy Skin Diet. Pregnant and breastfeeding women may need 1000 mg of calcium daily.

Note that calcium competes with skin-repairing nutrients, such as zinc and copper. Too much calcium can cause iron deficiency so do not have calcium intake in excess of 1000 mg per day until your skin condition improves. After your child's skin condition clears up, administer 800 to 1000 mg of calcium per day.

Did You Know?

EPA from Omega-3
Scientists have found that therapeutic amounts of EPA can inhibit the substances that cause inflammation and blood vessel constriction, so it might be worthwhile whipping up a salmon stir-fry tonight. Make sure you include plenty of red onions, garlic, ginger, and greens. Or you could make a delicious trout or chickpea curry with turmeric, onion, garlic, ginger, and carrots.

The fastest way to clear up acne, eczema, cellulite, and age-related skin conditions is to remove milk and other dairy products from your diet. For this reason, The Healthy Skin Diet is dairy-free.

Non-Dairy Sources of Calcium

Food Item	Serving Size	Available Calcium
Fish		
Rainbow trout, cooked	8 oz (255 g)	219 mg
Salmon (pink), cooked (Tinned salmon with bones has a higher calcium content)	8 oz (255 g)	543 mg
Sardines w/bones	1¼ oz (37 g)	111 mg
Snapper, baked	3 oz (85 g)	34 mg
Beans, Legumes, Nuts, and Seeds		
Carob powder	2 tbsp (30 mL)	56 mg
Kidney beans, canned	1 cup (250 mL)	138 mg
Navy beans	1 cup (250 mL)	130 mg
Refried beans	1 cup (250 mL)	155 mg
Soy milk, fortified	1 cup (250 mL)	300 mg
Soy flour	1 cup (250 mL)	180 mg
Soybeans, cooked	½ cup (125 mL)	90 mg
Tahini	1 tbsp (15 mL)	192 mg
Vegetables		
Broccoli, cooked	1 cup (250 mL)	90 mg
Collards, cooked	1 cup (250 mL)	150 mg
Yellow beans	1 cup (250 mL)	110 mg

Omega-3 converts to eico-sapentaenoic acid (EPA), which decreases inflammation and improves skin moisture.

Prostaglandins Series 3 (The Beautiful)

Prostaglandin Series 3 derive from omega-3 EFA, the beautiful fat. Let's look at why it is so beautiful. Omega-3 is beneficial in a number of ways. Omega-3 converts to eicosapentaenoic acid (EPA), which decreases inflammation and improves skin moisture. Omega-3 also helps to normalize blood pressure, which is beneficial for cardiovascular health, and it can reduce your risk of certain cancers. Omega-3 fatty acids are also beneficial in treating high blood pressure,* high triglycerides, and sticky platelets*; fluid retention*; mental deterioration*; slow metabolism*; retina/eye problems — inflammation/ischemia; risk of premature birth/low birth weight; Crohn's disease; asthma (however, current evidence is inconsistent); risk of stroke* (risk may decrease by 43%); risk of death by heart disease* (risk may decrease by up to 38% if fish is eaten weekly). Conversely, a deficiency of omega-3 in the diet can cause long-term problems.

Caution

Fish oil and flaxseed oil naturally thin the blood, so avoid taking supplemental omega-3 if you are a hemophiliac, undergoing surgery, or taking blood-thinning medications, such as aspirin. If diarrhea occurs from flaxseed oil, reduce the dosage.

Omega-3 Questionnaire

Check off any of the following symptoms you have experienced during your lifetime and still experience to determine if you have an omega-3 deficiency:

- [ ] General weakness
- [ ] Growth impairment in childhood*
- [ ] Poor vision (wear glasses)
- [ ] Learning difficulties
- [ ] Poor coordination
- [ ] Behavioral changes*
- [ ] Hyperactivity
- [ ] Tingling sensations in arms/legs*
- [ ] Dry skin

If you have checked off three or more symptoms, you may have a deficiency in omega-3 EFAs. However, please keep in mind that these symptoms can also be caused by other factors. If you or your child has any condition marked with an asterisk (*), you should let your doctor know. You can also check to see if you have any conditions that may be helped by adding omega-3 foods to your diet. Deficiency symptoms may take up to 12 weeks to reverse.

Omega-3 Food Sources

Did You Know?
....

Preparing Fish
According to Udo Erasmus, author of *Fats That Heal, Fats That Kill*, in order to get the most health benefit from eating fish, choose fresh fish, avoid frying, and eat the fish skin because it contains much of the beneficial oil. The top tip is to steam fish whole so the oils are not destroyed by oxygen, light, and high temperature. After you have eaten oily deep-sea fish, it takes 2 to 3 weeks for the EPA and DHA to be usable in the body.

If you suspect you need to increase your omega-3 intake, eat oily fish two to three times a week and use freshly ground flax seeds or fish oil supplements on the days you don't eat fish. Take approximately 2000 mg of EPA/DHA per day for a therapeutic effect.

Omega-3 fatty acids are abundant in cold water fish, such as sardines, trout, salmon, mackerel, and herring. Flaxseed oil and ground flax seeds contain around 50% omega-3, and lesser amounts are found in fresh walnuts and green leafy vegetables. There are high amounts in flax seeds and flaxseed oil, and lesser amounts in soybeans, wheat germ, walnuts, blackcurrant seed oil, brown and red algae, and dark green leafy vegetables. Note that the omega-3 amount equates to less EPA/DHA content than the therapeutic amount in some foods.

Tips for Storing Flaxseed Oil

Flaxseed oil goes rancid very easily. To solve this problem, try these strategies:

- Only buy refrigerated flaxseed oil.
- Choose a product that is packaged in dark glass (not plastic).
- To keep it fresh, always refrigerate the oil and use within 5 weeks.
- Store in the freezer to keep it fresh for longer.
- Because heat damages flaxseed oil, never heat it or add it to hot food. Whole flax seeds are more heat-resistant.

Avoid the following omega-3 (EPA and DHA) sources

Some sources of omega-3 fatty acids should be avoided:

- White bread with added omega-3: Liquid, invisible omega-3 goes rancid when it is baked. It's best to choose whole-grain bread where you can see whole flax seeds.
- Omega-3 margarines: You are better off having natural butter, fresh avocado, or extra virgin olive oil and leaving your omega-3 intake to more natural sources.

Omega-3 Food Sources

Food Item	Serving Size	Omega-3 Content
Fish		
Halibut, baked	4 oz (113 g)	620 mg
Herring	3½ oz (100 g)	1710–1810 mg
Mackerel, cooked	3½ oz (100 g)	340–1570 mg
Salmon, Atlantic, cooked	3½ oz (100 g)	1090–1830 mg
Salmon, cooked	4 oz (113 g)	2000 mg
Sardines	3½ oz (100 g)	980–1700 mg
Scallops, cooked	4 oz (113 g)	100 mg
Trout, rainbow, cooked	3½ oz (100 g)	840–980 mg
Tuna, fresh, cooked	3½ oz (100 g)	240–1280 mg
Tuna, canned in water, drained	3½ oz (100 g)	260–730 mg
Vegetables		
Broccoli, steamed	1 cup (250 mL)	200 mg
Cabbage, cooked	1 cup (250 mL)	170 mg
Cauliflower, cooked	1 cup (250 mL)	210 mg
Collard greens, cooked	1 cup (250 mL)	180 mg
Squash, cooked	1 cup (250 mL)	340 mg
Beans, legumes, nuts, and seeds		
Soy-flaxseed bread	2 slices	180 mg
Soybeans, cooked	1 cup (250 mL)	700 mg
Tofu	4 oz (113 g)	360 mg
Walnuts	¼ cup (60 mL)	2200 mg
Oils		
Flaxseed oil	1 tbsp (15 mL)	7200 mg
Flax seeds, ground	1 tbsp (15 mL)	1800 mg
Eggs		
Omega-3-fortified eggs	2	1114 mg
Spices		
Cloves, ground	2 tbsp (30 mL)	200 mg
Mustard seeds	2 tsp (10 mL)	200 mg
Supplements		
Omega-3 (EPA and DHA capsules)	1 capsule	300–500 mg

Note: The range of omega-3 content varies according to the region fish is sourced from, quality of storage, if fish skin was left intact and cooking method.

You should eat high-quality protein as a complement to taking an omega-3 supplement because this is how lipids occur in nature. Good-quality protein includes free-range eggs, antibiotic-free chicken, oily fish, seafood, lean meat, beans, and lentils. Eating protein with your oil supplements guarantees better absorption. If you experience negative digestive symptoms after taking fish oil, improve your digestion (as suggested in the previous chapter) and resume taking the fish oil 2 weeks later.

- Pre-ground flax seeds and FSA (a mixture of ground flax seeds, sunflower seeds, and almonds) that are not refrigerated (they may be rancid even if shopkeeper's store it in the fridge).
- Packaged walnuts: If they taste bitter or unpleasant, do not eat them, especially if you are pregnant. Walnuts should taste mild and be pleasant to eat.

Q. Should I supplement my diet with omega-3 (EPA/DHA) to improve the quality of my skin?

A. There are two answers here, one if you are trying to avoid omega-3 deficiency and one if you are using omega-3 therapeutically.

1. **Deficiency:** To avoid deficiency, your EPA/DHA dosage from foods and supplements should be 600 mg per day in divided doses — for example, take two capsules with breakfast, two with lunch, and two with dinner. On the days you eat fresh omega-3-rich fish, you can skip taking an omega-3 supplement. Also take 1 to 2 tablespoons (15 to 30 mL) of flaxseed oil per day (50% is omega-3).

2. **Therapy:** However, if you're an adult with acne, dandruff, dry skin, cellulite, eczema, psoriasis, rosacea, or wrinkles and premature aging, the therapeutic dosage is between 2000 and 4000 mg EPA/DHA (2000 mg equals approximately six capsules per day). To check how much is included in a capsule, read the label on the container. If a product says 180 mg of DHA and 120 mg of EPA per capsule, then there is a total of 300 mg of EPA/DHA in each capsule. Likewise, 300 mg x 6 capsules equals 1800 mg of EPA/DHA. You should also eat foods high in omega-3, such as dark leafy vegetable greens, flaxseed oil, and ground flax seeds). For children's dosage information, see the Children's Clear Skin Program (page 263).

Q. Is olive oil good for me?

A. Yes. Your humble bottle of olive oil is rich in omega-9 fats. Although omega-9 fatty acids are not essential like omega-3 and omega-6 EFAs (so you won't keel over if you don't have it), this fragrant oil has many health benefits, especially the cold-pressed extra virgin variety. Extra virgin olive oil contains a phenolic antioxidant called hydroxytyrosol. This little compound is wonderful at protecting your DNA against deadly mutations. Extra virgin olive oil also contains an unusually high amount of squalene, which has antioxidant properties that can reduce your risk of cancer.

Did You Know?

Barbecuing with Olive Oil

When you barbecue or brown (or burn) meats, the charcoaled portion is full of cancer-promoting substances, and scientists are now calling barbecued meats "carcinogenic." This sounds bad; however, scientists tested fried hamburger patties and discovered that cooking meat with extra virgin olive oil reduces the amount of cancer-promoting compounds. So extra virgin olive oil can make your barbecued meats a little bit healthier! Keep in mind that extra virgin olive oil can be damaged if it's cooked on high heat, and you'll know it's forming trans fats if your oiled pan starts to smoke. Don't skimp on quality by buying plain "olive oil" as it won't protect your barbecued meats in quite the same way as extra virgin olive oil. This is because most processed oils have lost all the health goodies, including phenols and vitamin E, during the refining process.

Quick Tips for Moisturizing Your Skin from the Inside

Recipes

Omega-3-rich recipes in the recipe section of this book include Marinated Whole Steamed Trout; Salmon Steaks with Peas and Mash; Rainbow Trout with Honey-Roasted Vegetables; Creamy Tuna and Mushroom Mornay; Smoked Salmon and Eggs; and Smoked Salmon and Avocado on Toast.

The right fats can literally moisturize your skin from the inside out. Good fats include evening primrose oil (GLA), while the great fats are omega-3 (EPA and DHA in fish and flax seeds). To increase your consumption of the good and beautiful great fats and to avoid the bad fats, follow these guidelines:

- Eat deep sea, oily fish at least twice a week — and I don't mean a piddly little can of tuna either, I mean the fresh stuff that's packed full of EPA and DHA. Trout and sardines are the best choices because they promote less acid production than the other omega-3-rich fish. You may need to visit your local fish shop.
- Eat ground flax seeds and flaxseed oil on a regular basis. If you don't eat fish or you want to have some fish-free days, have 1 to 2 tablespoons (15 to 30 mL) of ground flax seeds per day or 1 to 2 tablespoons of flaxseed oil (flaxseed oil contains more omega-3 than the ground seeds). For example, add 2 tablespoons (30 mL) of flax seeds to your breakfast cereal or use flaxseed oil in one of the healthy skin drinks in the recipe section, such as the Skin-Firming Drink, Berry Beauty Smoothie, Flaxseed Lemon Drink, and Pear Flaxseed Drink for Sensitive Skin. Flaxseed oil is a fantastic addition to homemade salad dressings.
- To get the most out of your high-omega-3 diet, reduce the amount of saturated fats you eat.
- When cooking meat, use a bit of extra virgin olive oil to grease the hot plate or pan and after cooking use a paper towel to blot away excess oil and fat from the meat. One cooking-savvy scientist also suggests that we add rosemary extract to our bottle of extra virgin olive oil to help retain its anticancer properties during storage.
- Limit sugary, processed foods, saturated fats, dairy, and stress as they are The Bad (not so good for gorgeous, hydrated-looking skin).
- Eat red meat less than twice a week, and protein servings should be no bigger than the size of the palm of your hand (thickness-wise too).
- Avoid dairy products for the duration of the Healthy Skin Diet.
- For therapeutic effect, consume 2000 mg of EPA/DHA per day.
- Eat omega-3-fortified eggs that are free-range or organic (rather than battery/caged chicken eggs).

Guideline #3

Eat Less: Controlling Your Carbs and Protein

I must confess I have not followed this principle until recently. In fact, I did the complete opposite. I previously ate three whopping big main meals a day and had lots of snacks in between. My partner used to say, "You never stop eating!" I used to recommend that patients eat lots of small meals throughout the day. This principle was designed to speed up their metabolism so they could eat heaps of food and burn it off quicker, the well-worn theory being: if you never give your body the chance to be hungry, it will store less fat because there's no need for it to save fat if your body never experiences a hint of famine.

It is true; this method does speed up your metabolism. However, this popular nutritionist's theory is flawed. The problem with eating lots of meals to speed up your metabolism is that it also seems to speed up the aging process. Scientists are discovering that the old rules of thumb "eat more and live

Did You Know?

Calorie Restriction Caution

If you already eat like a sparrow, do not cut your meals by a further 30%. If you suffer from anorexia or bulimia, or only eat one small meal a day, you are doing yourself no favors: you will accelerate wrinkles and you could also get very sick. Please don't mistake calorie restriction with starvation. Starvation or severe calorie restriction harms your appearance and your health.

Q. What is a calorie?

A. By definition, a calorie is the energy it takes to raise the temperature of 1 gram of water 1 degree Celsius. Calories are the food energy that fuel your body much like gasoline fuels your car. Just to exist, we need about 1200 calories to keep the body running at idle. Add another 1000 calories to enable the body to move. If you eat more calories than your body requires each day, you will typically gain weight. If you burn more calories than you consume or eat less, you should lose weight. The Healthy Skin Diet recommends eating 30% less food, which promotes better skin health and should result in weight loss. If you already know how to calorie count, go ahead. However, you should not count calories for more than a month (or at all!). It is a slow and arduous way to prepare food. In fact, it may put you off having a healthy lifestyle because it takes the fun out of mealtimes.

longer" or "snack all day and look younger" are not true. No wonder my skin was aging rapidly; I was eating enough for two people! However, there are hundreds of scientific studies that have produced the same results over and over again: eat less and live longer; eat less and delay the onset of aging; eat less and reduce your risk of cancer. The aim of the Healthy Skin Diet is to reduce how much you eat by 30%.

I just don't have the willpower to exercise and say no to desserts. How do I stop sabotaging my weight loss routine?

CASE STUDY

A 25-year-old woman came to our clinic because she was concerned about her infertility, irregular periods, fatigue, and pimples around the chin area. Her periods consisted of occasional spotting and no menses for about 10 weeks. Her diet for the past 17 weeks had consisted of an egg white omelet or a protein shake for breakfast, fish or chicken with salad for lunch, and red meat and vegetables for dinner, occasional fruit, protein bars, and coffee. She later confessed to being on a high-protein, low-carb diet. She was taken off this diet and put on the Healthy Skin Diet. After a week, her energy levels improved, and 6 weeks later her periods returned to normal and her pimples cleared.

How to reduce calories

1. Use a standard-sized dinner plate and fill half the plate with salad or cooked vegetables. The other half of your plate is for a small serving of protein (about the size and thickness of the palm of your hand), as well as a small serving of whole-grain carbohydrates. Don't overstuff this side of your plate!
2. If you're an active male, consume slightly more calories, but never eat more than what can comfortably fit on a standard-sized dinner plate.
3. Avoid going back for second helpings.
4. If you want to lose weight, skip dessert.
5. If you're having a heavier meal, such as pasta and meat, serve up a plate of food (dinner-plate-sized) and remove 30%, or approximately one-third, of your meal (this isn't quite 30%, but it is easy to calculate). You can add a side salad if you need more food to satisfy your hunger, but don't have any more bolognese.
6. Have approximately three dinner plates of food per day (minus the 30% or with 50% of the plate consisting of vegetables).
7. Make sure there are lots of greens on your plate because they are the most anti-aging of all the veggies and they ensure your body is less acidic and more alkaline.

Melatonin Effect

Eating less has been shown to increase the production of anti-aging hormones, specifically melatonin. Melatonin is a hormone secreted by the pineal gland in the brain and released during sleep. According to scientists, melatonin exerts an antioxidant effect that helps to protect against DNA damage. This is important because your DNA gives instructions to your skin cells, and damaged DNA can lead to age-related skin damage. Melatonin also stimulates production of an anti-aging substance called glutathione peroxidase. There is also evidence that melatonin helps to strengthen the immune system and decrease feelings of stress.

Did You Know?

Decreasing Melatonin Levels

Children naturally have high levels of melatonin. However (and this is the bad news), as you age, your body's ability to produce melatonin plummets. In fact, many scientists believe that a decline in nighttime levels of melatonin not only occurs with age but also contributes to the physical symptoms of aging, such as wrinkles and changes in pigmentation.

Melatonin Deficiency

When your body does not produce enough melatonin, the following can occur:

- Onset of aging
- Difficulty falling asleep at night
- Waking up after 8 hours of sleep feeling drowsy
- Irregular periods
- Early menopause

Did You Know?

Melatonin and Diet

A study published in the *Journal of Clinical Endocrinology & Metabolism* showed how melatonin levels can be manipulated by diet. Scientists did a 12-year study on rhesus monkeys because these mammals have a dramatic drop in melatonin secretions as they age, just like humans. Forty-four monkeys were put on a calorie-restricted diet and they ate 30% less food than the control group of 50 monkeys. The monkeys were categorized by age as either "old" or "adult." This long-term study and many others like it have shown that the animals eating smaller portions of food were the ones who ended up with fantastic melatonin levels. In fact, the old monkeys eating less produced remarkably more melatonin than the young monkeys who ate bigger meals.

You have to eat sensible amounts of food as a way of life to get a lowered risk of cancer or a significant melatonin boost and long-term anti-aging rewards.

Calorie Restriction

Animal studies have found that sensible calorie restriction not only improves melatonin production in aging animals, but also reduces body fat (but we knew that already); lowers blood glucose levels; and best of all, delays and greatly reduces age-related problems and the risk of cancer. And it is not just animal experiments that are showing dramatic results. Longer life and smoother skin in calorie-restricted humans has also been documented (see "The Village of Long Life" on page 92).

However, don't get all excited and put yourself on a 3-month calorie-restricted diet and then expect awesome melatonin levels and long life. You see, scientists have also noted that eating 30% less food for short periods of time, such as 2 to 3 months (the duration of most diets), does not improve your melatonin levels and it may only have a minor anti-cancer effect or none at all. They've found that you have to eat sensible amounts of food as a way of life to get a lowered risk of cancer or a significant melatonin boost and long-term anti-aging rewards.

Q. I'm overweight and look disgusting. How can I eat less?

A. If you have poor willpower and sabotage your health routine, it is a sign you have programmed yourself to fail. You can undo this with positive self-talk and self-confidence-building exercises (but they must be done daily and with enthusiasm). You also need to get an attitude of "I've had enough, I deserve more!" Then you'll be ready to pursue your health goals. If you're an overeater, also remember that food is not love. It's just fuel to give your body energy to live. Nothing more, nothing less. I know food can be a great comforter, but it is better to comfort yourself with reassuring words. Positive, comforting words said by yourself will not give you any negative side effects — you can't gain weight from self-praise. If you overeat, read the chapter entitled "How to Be Beautiful" (page 293) to find out how to prevent self-sabotage and poor willpower.

Carbohydrates

Now that you know you need to eat 30% less food, what types of foods should you be eating? Food is composed of three macronutrients — fat, carbohydrate, and protein. In the last section, good fats were identified, and here let's look at good-quality carbohydrates and proteins that have anti-aging qualities that promote healthy skin.

Q. What are carbohydrates and are they good for me?

A. Carbohydrates include sugars, starches, and certain kinds of fiber. Carbohydrates can make food taste sweet. They are the natural sugar found in fruit and the refined sugars added to junk food items, such as soft drinks and cakes. Carbohydrates are also the starchy parts of potatoes, bread, pasta, rice, and cereals. Vegetables and legumes also contain carbs. Dairy products contain milk sugar (lactose), which is a carbohydrate. Some carbohydrates are good for you and others (primarily processed white flour products) are giving carbs a bad name because they are not so good for you.

Did You Know?

Brain Fuel

Good-quality whole grains are essential for your health and vitality. Did you know that carbohydrate is the only source of fuel your brain can use? Your brain needs glucose that has been broken down from the carbohydrate portion of your food. Without a slow and continual supply of glucose, your intellectual ability suffers, you can't concentrate as effectively, and your body goes into survival mode. Your body then starts the arduous task of converting fats and protein into brain fuel. This makes you feel tired. If you have a good-quality carbohydrate meal, your brain function returns to normal. Carbs can be your friend if you eat them in moderation and pick the ones that are good for you.

Two Kinds of Carbs

This is probably familiar to you, but I want you to get to know the two types of carbs a bit better. These aren't the official names for the two categories; these are nicknames used to make it easier to remember carbohydrates' potential effects on your body. The first group is the "Hit and Run" carbs and the second is the "Commitment" carbs.

Hit and Run Carbs

> The Hit and Run carb is a lot like a con artist who offers you a moment of pleasure, then robs you blind while you're sleeping.

Now, the Hit and Run carb is here for a good time, not a long time. Take Mr Doughnut, for instance — he wants to give your taste buds a moment of pleasure you'll never forget. He'll happily supply your brain with a hit of energy that will make you feel great in an instant, then he'll quickly get "cold feet" and leave you to cope with an energy crash all by yourself. So you reach out for Mr Cake this time and hope that he'll be the one to make you feel satisfied; but yet another moment of pleasure comes and goes and now the energy he gave you is nowhere to be found (it's probably hiding on your thighs).

There is yet another problem with the Hit and Run carbs: although they supply you with a glucose hit, many of them are very low in nutrients, so your body cannot utilize their glucose gift properly. So Mr Doughnut and Mr Cake both end up making you pay for all the nutrient "extras" with your own vital body stores of vitamins and minerals. They steal your chromium (if you have any), which helps the glucose transfer into your cells. This produces a burst of energy, but your chromium stores are getting more and more depleted and the energy is short-lived. Yes, the Hit and Run carb is a lot like a con artist who offers you a moment of pleasure, then robs you blind while you're sleeping.

The Hit and Run carbs are the food and drink products that have a high glycemic index and don't supply enough nutrition for their utilization in the body.

The Hit and Run carbs aren't good for the skin because they "steal" many of the best nutrients that are needed for skin health. Eating Hit and Run carbs can lead to skin complaints such as pimples, rashes, and signs of premature aging.

Sources of Hit and Run Carbs

Have no more than one Hit and Run snack/item per day. This means having only one coffee or two weak ones per day, and ditch the white bread for "nice guy" whole-grain bread. Commit to choosing your carbs wisely!

- Bagels
- Cookies
- Cakes
- Candy
- Coffee
- Cookies and crackers
- Corn pasta, corn cakes
- Doughnuts
- Muffins, English muffins
- Pancake and biscuit mixes
- Pastries, waffles
- Potato chips, french fries
- Potato, especially mashed
- Pretzels, water crackers
- Rice/corn cakes, rice crackers (even the whole-grain ones)
- Sauces
- Scones
- Sports drinks
- Most white rice, especially jasmine rice
- White bread, Turkish bread
- Whole wheat bread
- Most breakfast cereals, including many corn and bran flake cereals
- Some breakfast bars

As you can see, this is not a complete list. There are too many processed and packaged foods to name them all; however, this will give you a good idea what to look out for.

What do high GI and low GI mean?

The Hit and Run carbs are largely derived from the research available in the book *The New Glucose Revolution*. The glycemic index, or GI, is a measure of how foods, specifically the carbohydrate content of food, affect your blood glucose levels (commonly called blood sugar). The fantastic research on the GI and glycemic load of foods has been beneficial to the advancement of our health. However, the Hit and Run list does not include some of the healthier high-GI foods, such as amaranth (97), dates (103), millet (71), parsnip (97), pumpkin (75), tapioca (70), watermelon (72), brown rice (66–80), because they supply an acceptable amount of goodness. (Yes, many of them bring along their own vitamins and minerals, so they offer more than just glucose).

- Low-GI foods fall in the range of 0–55
- Medium GI is 56–69
- High-GI foods are above 70

Q. Why are high-GI foods so bad for me?

A. High-GI foods can be bad for you if you eat them every day or in excessive amounts. High-GI foods give your pancreas a lot of work to do and, like all overworked organs (and people!), it can eventually malfunction. Over time, your pancreas may begin to make mistakes in measuring how much insulin it needs to release. This is not so disastrous at first… your silly old pancreas starts dumping out too much insulin — or too many "orders" — causing your blood sugar levels to drop so low that your brain is suddenly left without fuel. So you're left feeling lethargic. You may also feel confused and irritable and have weakened muscles. These are all signs of hypoglycemia, and in extreme cases where blood sugar levels drop dangerously low, loss of consciousness can result (hopefully you'll have a good-quality whole-grain snack before this happens).

If your pancreas is healthy, it will respond to the changes in blood sugar levels by promptly releasing insulin into your bloodstream. If your pancreas is tired from making too many insulin orders (from you eating Hit and Run carbs for too many years), then it may begin to make mistakes and you can end up with blood sugar disorders, such as hypoglycemia and type 2 diabetes.

CASE STUDY

A 27-year-old woman came to me suffering from recurring muscle weakness, mental fogginess, insatiable thirst not relieved by water, pimples on her forehead, lethargy soon after eating (to the point of needing to lie down), and frequent colds and flu. I advised her to see a doctor for a glucose tolerance test, which showed she had hypoglycemia (her blood sugar level dropped dramatically within 30 minutes of the glucose test). The woman was prescribed a chromium supplement that contained B vitamins and magnesium. She was put on the Healthy Skin Diet. One week after commencing the new regimen, her lethargy after meals ceased and thirst decreased. She had clear skin by the fifth week.

Commitment Carbs

You've met the Hit and Run carbs, so now I'd like to introduce you to the Commitment carbs. Mr Commitment carb has a lot to offer: he's a strong, good-looking, and dependable guy with a healthy nutrient account. And he likes to take it slow. A Commitment carb, such as Dr Soy and Flaxseed, takes his time because he can't be digested quickly and as a result he offers slow-release glucose for sustained energy. Your brain will just adore him!

You may recognize the Commitment carb, as he often has a tough exterior — he's not all white and fluffy with no substance like Mr Hit and Run. The Commitment carb regularly comes with his own edible packaging, and he may be naturally sweet and delicious. He's your fruits and vegetables, he's your whole-grain breads and some of the more natural low-GI products available at your local supermarket.

Whole-grain carbohydrates supply slow-release glucose, for greater mental clarity and sustained energy. Whole grains are also Commitment carbs because they supply their own carbohydrate-processing nutrients, such as the B group vitamins and chromium (so they're less likely to rob your supplies). However, be warned: product advertising regarding "whole grains" can be misleading. A cereal or bread product may claim to contain healthy whole grains, but if you can't see the grainy bits, it is not whole-grain — it's whole wheat.

> **Whole grains are also Commitment carbs because they supply their own carbohydrate-processing nutrients, such as the B group vitamins and chromium (so they're less likely to rob your supplies).**

Sources of Commitment Carbs

- Most fruits, especially cherries, berries, and apples
- Most vegetables
- Almonds
- Avocado
- Basmati rice
- Beans
- Brazil nuts (and other nuts)
- Carob
- Honey
- Hummus
- Lentils, chickpeas
- Rolled oats
- Seeds, flax seeds
- Soy milk
- Stevia (a natural sweetener)
- Sushi
- Tomato-based pasta sauces
- Whole wheat pasta
- Whole grains

Zero GI

Commitment carbs keep your brain stimulated and supply slow-release fuel so you feel good for longer. Most high-protein foods, such as meat, seafood, and eggs, have a GI rating of 0 because they contain little or no carbohydrates.

Glycemic index of common grains

The best grains to include in your diet include whole-grain breads (with a GI rating of 43–49), soy and flaxseed breads (36–50), whole-grain sourdough breads (48–54), rolled oats (42) (not instant oats), muesli (34–56), oat bran (55), pearl barley (25), brown rice (66–80), basmati rice (58), whole-grain rye, buckwheat (54) (not a true grain; gluten-free; rich in flavonoids), and millet (because it is alkalizing).

Q. I've heard that chromium is good for my skin. Should I take it as a supplement?

A Maybe… This little mineral is so important for your health and well-being because it is the key to getting glucose into your cells. A nutritional deficiency in chromium may contribute to fatigue associated with low blood sugar as well as the opposite: high blood sugar and type 2 diabetes. If you have chromium deficiency signs, you should take this supplement immediately because it is difficult to reverse the deficiency with diet alone.

Chromium Deficiency Questionnaire

Check off any symptoms you experience on a regular basis (at least three times per week):

- ☐ Dizziness and irritability after several hours without food
- ☐ Acne and pimples
- ☐ Anxiety
- ☐ Desire for frequent meals
- ☐ Cravings for sweets and carbohydrates
- ☐ Excessive hunger
- ☐ Excessive thirst
- ☐ Weakness in legs
- ☐ Fatigue
- ☐ Excessive sweating
- ☐ ADD, ADHD
- ☐ Depression

If you have three or more deficiency symptoms, take a chromium supplement for the duration of the Healthy Skin Diet (8 weeks), and if symptoms persist, see your doctor, because many of these symptoms relate to type 2 diabetes.

Good Sources of Chromium

Food Item	Serving Size	Chromium Content
Brewer's yeast	1 tbsp (15 mL)	Up to 60 mcg
Wheat bran/germ	1 oz (28 g)	32.5 mcg
Broccoli	1 cup (250 mL)	22 mg
Organic liver	3½ oz (100 g)	42 mcg
Raw onion	½ cup (125 mL)	12.4 mcg
Romaine lettuce	2 cups (500 mL)	15.6 mcg
Turkey meat	3½ oz (100 g)	10.4 mcg
Raw tomato	1 cup (250 mL)	9 mcg
Grape juice	1 cup (250 mL)	7.5 mcg
Cooked peas	1 cup (250 mL)	6 mcg
Dried garlic	1 tsp (5 mL)	3 mcg
Whole wheat English muffin	1	4 mcg

Q. How much chromium do I need?

A. Adults require 120 to 200 mcg of chromium per day, according to the US Food and Drug Administration. You should get this from a variety of sources, including supplementation and food intake. Adults who are showing chromium deficiency signs should supplement their diet with 60 to 200 mcg of chromium per day, especially when consuming carbohydrates. It is recommended that you take chromium with protein to help with its absorption. Those in the 12- to 15-year-old bracket who are showing chromium deficiency signs should take 30 to 50 mcg of chromium per day.

Did You Know?

Best Chromium

Among the various forms of chromium, use chromium picolinate because it is easier for the body to absorb. I've found that not all chromium supplements have measurable benefits; however, I have consistently seen positive results from a chromium supplement that contains a combination of chromium picolinate, chromic chloride, vitamins B_1, B_2, B_3 (nicotinamide), B_5, B_6, B_{12}, vitamin C, vitamin D-3, folic acid, magnesium, manganese, and zinc.

Chromium Caution

Do not take more than 250 mcg of chromium per day, as exceedingly high doses may inhibit insulin production. If you have insulin-dependent diabetes, seek advice from your doctor before supplementing with chromium, as it alters blood sugar levels, which could be dangerous if combined with insulin drug therapy (insulin would need to be reduced if you were taking chromium, but do this only with your doctor's supervision as this could be dangerous).

CASE STUDY

A 70-year-old woman presented to me with elevated blood glucose levels (a reading of 6.3, which is bordering on high). She had been told by her doctor that she needed regular monitoring with blood tests every 4 months to see if these high readings were a precursor to type 2 diabetes. However, I recommended she take a chromium supplement, which she took two or three times per day with food, for 4 months. Her diet stayed basically the same (as she ate vegetables and whole-grain bread already), but minus cakes and cookies at morning snack time, and she stopped putting sugar in her coffee. Her doctor retested her blood sugar level 4 months later and her reading had dropped to 5.8 and was now within the normal range. Her doctor was amazed. Her twin sister also had slightly elevated blood glucose, and she took the same chromium supplement. Three months later, the twin's blood glucose levels had also dropped 0.5. The twin sister had not changed her diet in any way.

Gluten

Gluten is a protein found in grains such as wheat, rye, oats, spelt, and barley. It is quite a useful protein because it provides elasticity and strength to bread dough, so it helps bread to rise nicely. However, gluten can be hard to digest for some people, especially if you were born with celiac disease.

Celiac (pronounced seel-ee-ak) disease is a medical condition where gluten damages the lining of your intestines. If this occurs, it makes it difficult for your body to absorb nutrients, so you may experience nutritional deficiencies as

Celiac Disease Questionnaire

Check off any of the following symptoms you experience three or more times per week:

Common adult symptoms
- ☐ Fatigue, muscle weakness
- ☐ Anemia that doesn't respond to treatment
- ☐ Stomach bloating, cramping, flatulence
- ☐ Diarrhea or constipation
- ☐ Nausea, vomiting
- ☐ Unexplained weight loss

Less common adult symptoms
- ☐ Easy bruising
- ☐ Ulcerations of mouth
- ☐ Infertility, miscarriages
- ☐ Muscle spasms
- ☐ Dermatitis herpetiformis
- ☐ Altered mental alertness
- ☐ Bone and joint pains

Common symptoms for children
- ☐ Stomach bloating, pain, flatulence
- ☐ Nausea, vomiting
- ☐ Diarrhea or constipation
- ☐ Large, bulky, foul-smelling stools
- ☐ Poor weight gain
- ☐ Weight loss in older children
- ☐ Tiredness, irritability
- ☐ Anemia

If you have three or more symptoms, you should speak to your doctor about further testing for celiac disease. If your results for celiac disease come back negative, first celebrate and then check for gluten intolerance by taking gluten-containing foods out of your diet for 1 to 2 months (during the Healthy Skin Diet). Gluten-free recipes are included in the recipe section of this book. If a gluten-free diet alleviates symptoms, check to see if the negative reactions return after you resume eating wheat breads and pasta.

Gluten intolerance can cause a skin condition called dermatitis herpetiformis, which has all sorts of annoying symptoms, such as blistering skin, itchy rash, small lumps like insect bites, and pink scaly patches of skin, or it may appear like hives.

well as bloating and skin rashes. If you have celiac disease, eating something containing gluten, such as a humble sandwich, could leave you feeling anything from mildly tired and bloated to violently ill.

Gluten intolerance can cause a skin condition called dermatitis herpetiformis, which has all sorts of annoying symptoms, such as blistering skin, itchy rash, small lumps like insect bites, and pink scaly patches of skin, or it may appear like hives.

Q. I've heard gluten is bad for your health. Should I avoid wheat and other gluten-containing products?

A. Not necessarily. You shouldn't need to avoid gluten-containing products unless you have celiac disease or symptoms associated with gluten intolerance (see the questionnaire on page 85). If you had digestive symptoms that improve after taking gluten out of your diet, this would be a sign of gluten intolerance and you should continue to eat gluten-free. Gluten-free grains include rice, corn, amaranth, buckwheat, millet, and quinoa.

Protein

• •

> **Protein is necessary for wound healing and vital for healthy skin.**

Protein is essential for your health. It is the major building material for muscles, blood, hair, nails, and internal organs, such as the brain. Protein is necessary for wound healing and vital for healthy skin. Skin sags when you are protein deficient. If your diet lacks sufficient "complete" protein, your body robs it from your muscles and other tissues. This can leave you with a poorly toned body, thin and brittle hair, and skin conditions that are slow to heal.

When protein is digested properly, it is broken down into amino acids that the body uses to keep us looking and feeling good. There are approximately 22 amino acids needed by the body. Your body can make all but nine of these — these nine are called essential amino acids. It is your job to make sure you get these nine amino acids from your diet by eating protein every day.

If you eat too much protein, the excess will either be converted to energy or stored in the body as fat. However, protein will only be converted to energy if there are no carbohydrates or fats available (your body's preferred energy source is carbs).

Make sure you consume some sort of protein every day — preferably in two of your main meals. If you suffer from eczema, dermatitis, arthritis, asthma, or heart disease, decrease your meat intake to once a week for the duration of the Healthy Skin Diet. If you're pregnant or breastfeeding, avoid fish high in mercury, and consult with a nutritionist about protein intake (as you will need to increase it).

Kinds of Amino Acids

Non-Essential Amino Acids
Your body produces these amino acids:

- Alanine (from pyruvic acid)
- Arginine (from glutamic acid)
- Asparagine (from aspartic acid)
- Aspartic acid (from oxaloacetic acid)
- Cysteine
- Glutamic acid (from oxoglutaric acid)
- Glutamine (from glutamic acid)
- Glycine (from serine and threonine)
- Proline (from glutamic acid)
- Serine (from glucose)
- Tyrosine (from phenylalanine)

Essential Amino Acids
Your body cannot produce these amino acids. They must come from your diet, specifically from protein:

- Arginine
- Isoleucine
- Histidine
- Leucine
- Methionine
- Lysine
- Phenylalanine
- Tryptophan
- Threonine
- Valine

Protein Deficiency Questionnaire

Check off any symptom you experience on a regular basis (three or more times per week):

- ☐ Slow wound healing
- ☐ Edema (swollen hands/feet/ abdomen)
- ☐ Wasting/shrinking muscle mass
- ☐ Sagging skin
- ☐ Anemia
- ☐ Poor digestion
- ☐ Fatty liver (diagnosed by a doctor)
- ☐ Hair loss (not including hereditary baldness)

If you have checked off more than three symptoms, you may not be eating enough protein or you may not be digesting your food properly. If you have poor digestion, you can refer back to Guideline #1 , which is designed to improve your gastrointestinal health. If these problems persist, consult with your doctor.

Q. How much protein do I need to eat to support the Healthy Skin Diet?

A. Your basic source of food protein should come from fish, eggs, lean meats, legumes, and seeds. Between 2¼ and 3½ oz (65 and 100 g) of cooked chicken will provide you with sufficient daily protein, as will two small lean pork chops, two slices of roast meat, or half a breast. A 3- to 4-oz (80 to 120 g) serving of fish or two eggs will also give you enough protein. One cup (250 mL) of lentils, beans, chickpeas, split peas, or soybeans served with a carbohydrate will provide your daily protein needs, as will ⅓ cup (75 mL) of almonds served with breakfast cereal.

You need to be aware of the quality of protein you are choosing. Not all proteins have the same potential for improving your skin health, and not all proteins are safe. Carefully avoid animal sources of protein that have been injected with antibiotics to increase weight and been preserved with nitrites. Consider more vegetable and grain sources.

Did You Know?

Portions and Servings

As a general guide when eating protein, eat a portion the size and thickness of the palm of your hand. Have a maximum of two servings of red meat (lean lamb, beef, organic liver) per week and a maximum of two servings of white meat (such as skinless chicken) per week. Eat two to three servings of seafood (at least one serving of omega-3-rich fish) per week, and daily servings of vegetarian combined protein.

Safe Sources of Animal Protein

Meat is the primary source of protein in the diet, but not all sources are safe. Be an informed consumer of animal protein.

Chicken

Antibiotics are routinely added to the feed of caged and free-range chickens. They are partly used to prevent infections spreading (as the chickens are often in small, cramped cages or barns) and also to speed up a chicken's growth. When you eat this chicken, some of the antibiotics may be passed on to you, and since antibiotics kill bacteria, they can destroy the healthy bacteria in your gut lining.

This may or may not be a problem for our health. However, routinely adding antibiotics to animal feed has long been criticized by doctors who believe that overuse of antibiotics is causing antibiotic-resistant bacteria strains that are detrimental to everyone's health. Organic poultry is raised free of antibiotics. Some free-range chickens are advertised as being "antibiotic-free" so they are the best choices if you are concerned.

Eggs

The quality of the eggs you choose is also important. Eggs from caged hens are often inferior because they have softer shells and paler yolks. Their shells are weaker because indoor-housed chickens fail to get vitamin D from sunshine and they don't get to roam around and peck in the grass and ingest mineral-rich soil. A paler yolk can indicate a poorer B vitamin content and bright orange yolks are often seen in omega-3-fortified eggs. Signs that you are buying good-quality eggs include tough shells, bright yellow yolks, and good egg white consistency (the whites should not be runny like water). Look for eggs that are free-range (or organic), antibiotic-free, and omega-3-enriched.

Red Meat

Red meat is allowed on the Healthy Skin Diet provided it is high-quality lean meat. Lamb (with all the fat cut off) is the best choice, as once digested it produces less acid than beef. Avoid ham that has been "smoked" with nitrate chemicals, and don't eat deli meats, because they are processed and usually contain preservatives. As a general guide when eating red meat, have a portion the size and thickness of the palm of your hand. Stick to a maximum of two servings of red meat per week (lean lamb or organic liver). Liver must be organic only because the liver is the animal's chemical processing organ, so it may be excessively high in pesticides if not organic.

Fish

Seafood, especially fish, is high in omega-3 fatty acids, protein, vitamins B_{12} and B_6, and it is low in saturated fats. Health authorities tell us to eat at least two servings of fish each week, and seafood lovers who consume high-omega-3 fish more than twice a week are less likely to suffer from eczema, psoriasis, heart disease, and depression.

Did You Know?

Fish Feeding Schedule

Health authorities suggest that if you eat a serving of high-mercury fish, avoid eating all seafood for at least 2 weeks afterwards to counterbalance the effects. Avoid larger fish with a high mercury content. The good news is you can safely enjoy omega-3-rich fish, such as salmon, trout, sardines, and herring, which are low in mercury, as is the case with hake, bream, shrimp, flounder, prawns, lobster, and oysters, to name a few. You can make a healthy snack with 3 oz (95 g) of canned tuna twice a week. Canned tuna is sourced from smaller-sized tuna.

Mercury Contamination

Some fish is high in mercury content and can therefore be harmful. Mercury occurs in nature, but it also leaks into our waterways from industrial pollution and ends up in our seafood, especially the larger fish that are higher up the food chain (they eat more food, thus digesting more mercury from the ocean or waterways).

Mercury poisoning occurs over the long term. Symptoms include irritability, headaches, and memory loss. Mercury toxicity can also cause infertility and miscarriages, so if you are planning to have a baby, it is best to avoid high-mercury fish. Unborn babies and small children are most at risk of mercury toxicity. Be aware of what you feed your children and avoid the fish listed if you are pregnant. There is a very handy wallet-sized card available from most doctors' offices specifically outlining the fish to avoid and the amounts you can have when pregnant.

Avoid these contaminated varieties of fish

- Barramundi
- Broadbill
- Gemfish
- King mackerel
- Ling
- Marlin
- Perch (orange roughy)
- Shark (flake)
- Snapper
- Swordfish
- Larger tuna (albacore, southern bluefin)

Complete Vegetarian Protein

Vegetarian meals can be made higher in protein by combining several different types of vegetarian protein to make one complete protein. If you are a meat eater, you need to get protein from a variety of sources, especially vegetarian protein, to keep your prostaglandins balanced. There is a simple rule to follow to make second-class vegetable protein complete:

Legumes/seeds/nuts	+	Grains	= Complete Protein
beans, green beans, peas, lentils	+	rice, oats, wheat, rye	
tofu, tempeh, seeds, pepitas	+	barley, corn, amaranth	
soy, almonds, Brazil nuts	+	millet	

Combining vegetarian protein: For example, if you eat a Thai dish of rice and vegetables, you may not get enough complete protein. However, if you include cashew nuts and snow peas, you increase the amount of usable protein in your meal. If you have oats for breakfast, add soy or almond milk and ground flax seeds to increase the protein content.

Anti-Aging Foods

Although eating less is a key guideline in the Healthy Skin Diet program, you do need to eat more protein-rich foods that promote healthy collagen formation and smooth skin. The word "collagen" comes from the Greek term *kolla*, which means "glue." Collagen is like the glue that keeps your skin together: if you cut your skin, collagen quickly repairs it with the help of a few other key nutrients. Collagen is an amazing protein structure in the skin that cross-links, so it is extra strong and durable — on a per weight basis, collagen is nearly as strong as steel!

Collagen is chiefly made from the amino acids glycine, proline, and lysine in roughly equal amounts. These amino acids are found in protein-containing foods, such as fish, eggs, meats, beans, nuts, and seeds. Lysine and proline also need co-factors vitamin C, iron, and manganese to form strong collagen in the skin, and zinc is also necessary for collagen formation. If you are deficient in vitamin C, iron, manganese, zinc, glycine, or hyaluronan, you increase your risk of premature aging. However, don't get bogged down with remembering the nutrient names, just know that the Healthy Skin Diet is specially designed to be rich in all of them!

> Although eating less is a key guideline in the Healthy Skin Diet program, you do need to eat more protein-rich foods that promote healthy collagen formation and smooth skin.

Q. What is hyaluronan?

A. Hyaluronan is found in collagen and elastin. It has even been called "the key to the fountain of youth" because studies have shown that hyaluronan can improve the appearance of wrinkles and assist with healing of scars, fractures, hernias, wounds, and damaged cartilage and ligaments. Formerly known as hyaluronic acid, this fluid cushions your important organs, chiefly the heart and skin, so it reduces the chance of damage to these areas. Hyaluronan is hydrophilic, which means it attracts water; it is also slippery, helping to lubricate your joints. Without hyaluronan, your body would ache as if you had arthritis. Low levels of hyaluronan are associated with premature aging, osteoarthritis, mitral valve prolapse, poor wound healing, and connective tissue irregularities, such as cellulite. Your genes play a role in how much hyaluronan your body produces. And smoking cigarettes decreases the amount of hyaluronan in your body.

The good news is that you can increase hyaluronan naturally by supplying its main building block, glucosamine, which you may have heard of because it's a famous nutrient for treating arthritic joints. Glucosamine works to normalize cartilage and restore joint function (at least partially). Magnesium is also needed to manufacture hyaluronan. Studies have shown that deficiencies in zinc and magnesium contribute to skin abnormalities. It's thought that people from traditional societies who age well do so because their traditional diet, rich in root vegetables, supplies plenty of magnesium and zinc for hyaluronan production.

Did You Know?

The Village of Long Life

A small Japanese village called Yuzurihara has been dubbed "the village of long life" because there are 10 times as many people living beyond the age of 85 as anywhere in America. Not only do they live longer, but they are also famous for their smooth skin, thick hair, and flexible joints. It is rare to find a villager who needs reading glasses, according to one of their local doctors, Dr Komori, who has written at least five books about Yuzurihara. He attributes the villagers' good health and great skin to their starchy-vegetable-based diet, which is low in calories and high in skin-cushioning hyaluronan. The local diet consists of root potatoes (similar to sweet potatoes), white potatoes, buckwheat noodles, millet, rice, red onions, sweetfish, and fermented soy, which is high in plant estrogens.

Brewing an Anti-Aging Broth

Broths have always been a great source of anti-aging protein, and they play a key role in the Healthy Skin Diet program. An anti-aging broth or stock contains many of the nutrients needed for healthy collagen production. But I'll be honest with you; this recipe is nothing new. For centuries, broths have been prescribed for all sorts of ailments involving the connective tissue (collagen and elastin), including problems with the skin, joints, digestive tract, lungs, muscles, and blood.

A well-made broth coats the gut lining, heals digestive complaints, and helps you to digest your food better. It is rich in glycine (one of the main amino acids needed for your body to make its own supply of anti-aging glutathione) and

How to make an anti-aging broth

The ingredients for a good broth are very inexpensive. You can use a leftover chicken carcass or fish bones or buy from your butcher a lamb neck and other bits that he usually discards or sells cheaply. Look for bones that have a little bit of meat, cartilage, and tendon left on them. You can add vegetable scraps, such as carrot or sweet potato peel. The vegetable skin is where most of the goodness is.

1. Start by boiling a pot of water and adding to the pot the vegetable scraps with the bones.

2. Add a decent splash of vinegar to the water. Vinegar is a weak acid that causes an acid–base chemical reaction; the minerals are the base and the vinegar is the acid that helps to draw the minerals right out of the bones.

3. Reduce the liquid. Simmer the bone and veggie liquid for a whole day, adding extra water if necessary, so plenty of collagen and nutrients are extracted. The longer it simmers, the richer the flavor and the more minerals and other goodies it accumulates. Skimping on the cooking period will result in a broth that is low in minerals and lacking that fabulous broth flavor.

4. After cooking, strain out the vegetables and bones.

5. Grab a bone to check out how brittle it has become — it is amazing to see how easily it crumbles in your fingertips from the loss of minerals.*

(*Maybe chicken osteoporosis is only interesting if you're a kitchen nerd, but if you want to look good, you'll be pleased to know that you've made a broth that is rich in calcium and phosphorus, magnesium, potassium, sulfate, and fluoride, so the broth is really good for your skin, bones, and teeth. See the recipe section for more information.)

sulfur, so it enhances liver detoxification and treats skin complaints, such as pimples and eczema. Broth also provides collagen, cartilage, connective-tissue-producing amino acids, chondroitin sulfate, and hyaluronan, which lubricate joints and are therefore also suitable for arthritis sufferers. Broth made with chicken meat and bones makes a more flavorful soup that contains cysteine. Cysteine reduces mucus in the body, so it offers relief when you've got the sniffles.

Eating Out

Eating healthy food is a lot easier when you follow a diet that offers healthy alternatives so that when you are out with friends at a café you can still order from the menu. Instead of having a sandwich made with white bread, choose whole-grain or sourdough bread (which has a GI of around 43). These breads are readily available in big-city cafés, but I have to admit, you might be hard-pressed finding whole-grain breads in small-town diners and rural cafés. If this is the case, order lean protein, such as tuna, skinless chicken, tofu, or lean beef, with your meal to lower the glycemic load of your meal. Or better still, order fish and salad when you're out and only eat carbs when you are at home so you can always have your healthy whole-grain foods.

Quick Tips for Eating Less for More Beautiful Skin

- Eating less food increases your nighttime melatonin levels, which promotes youthful skin and good-quality sleep. Aim to eat 30% fewer carbohydrates.
- For lunches and dinners, fill half your plate with salad or cooked vegetables that are low in calories. The other half of your plate is for a moderate serving of each of carbohydrate and protein.
- If you are eating a heavy meal (such as pasta and meat), only fill two-thirds of your plate, leaving one-third of your plate empty. Better still, only put the pasta on half your plate and have a large side salad.
- Eat approximately three (average-sized) dinner plates of food each day.

- Snack less. Have only one snack break per day (however, if you have low blood sugar or if you are pregnant, you will need two snack breaks per day). Have a supply of almonds and an apple on hand.
- Choose Commitment carbs, such as whole-grain breads, brown rice, and rolled oats.
- Eat protein every day, in two of your main meals. As a general guide when eating animal protein, eat a portion the size and thickness of the palm of your hand. If you are eating a vegetarian meal, you will need to eat double that amount in vegetarian (combined) protein. Vegetarian protein: beans/legumes/nuts/seeds + grains = complete protein.
- Eat less but don't starve yourself! Your food is your fuel, nothing more and nothing less.

Guideline #4

Be a Sleeping Beauty: Practicing Good Sleep Habits

The key guidelines for the Healthy Skin Diet focus on your eating habits, but other lifestyle habits affect your skin. Let's look at your sleeping habits before turning to exercise.

You may thrive on only a little sleep, you may suffer insomnia and toss and turn all night, or you might laze in bed all day and take this Sleeping Beauty guideline way too far, but I'm sure you will agree you feel better after a decent night's sleep. During sleep, your body releases a whole series of hormones that control some significant functions in your body and affect skin health. One of the most vital hormones triggered by sleep is melatonin, which is secreted by the pineal gland in the brain. Light suppresses the release of melatonin and darkness stimulates it, so sleeping at night in a darkened room increases your chances of optimal melatonin production. Melatonin is also made in tiny amounts during the day, but it is the "spike," or sharp increase, in melatonin during night sleep that is most beneficial.

> During sleep, your body releases a whole series of hormones that control some significant functions in your body and affect skin health.

Melatonin

• •

As mentioned in Guideline #3, melatonin is essential for good health because it sets your circadian rhythms so your body knows when to sleep, and it helps you wake up in the morning. Melatonin also influences female reproductive hormones and controls when menstruation begins and how long each period lasts. It even decides when your menopause should begin. Melatonin also helps to preserve your youthful good looks. Children naturally have high levels of melatonin, and as you age, your body's ability to produce melatonin plummets. When this happens, you experience the physical symptoms of aging, including increased wrinkles, difficulty falling asleep at night and waking up in the morning, feeling drowsy, and having irregular periods or early menopause.

Q. If melatonin inevitably decreases with age, why should getting enough sleep matter as you get older?

A. As I mentioned before, scientists have discovered a way to influence how much melatonin is released as you age. You can have good melatonin secretions at any age if you simply eat fewer calories and get a good night's sleep on a regular basis. For more on this subject, take another look at page 75.

Insomnia

• •

> Wound healing and skin cell renewal also happen at night, so you could be missing out on precious skin rejuvenation time.

Getting a great night's sleep so your body has a better chance of producing a nice big surge of melatonin is all very well, but what if you can't doze off in the first place? Insomnia can be a nightmare (literally) and can affect your appearance in many ways. Sallow skin, bags under the eyes, and tell-tale dark circles are just the beginning. Wound healing and skin cell renewal also happen at night, so you could be missing out on precious skin rejuvenation time.

Causes of Insomnia

What causes insomnia? Many things. If you're stressed about exams or fear you're not loved or live in an unsafe environment, then of course you're going to have trouble sleeping. Maybe you've simply trained yourself to be nocturnal or you go to bed feeling worried that it will be another sleepless night (yes, it will be). Substances can also affect your state — foods, drinks, and drugs — so be careful what you pop into your mouth.

Common Causes of Insomnia

- Worry, anxiety, and stress are probably the most common causes of insomnia — they all trigger your body's "fight or flight" nervous system, which releases adrenaline and cortisol. These hormones prevent sleep and give you more zest to either run away from or confront your crisis (even if it's an imaginary one!).
- Eating highly acidic foods, such as pork chops, and drinking alcohol leads to acid storage in body tissues that can cause poor sleep.
- Coffee, tea (including green tea), and cola soft drinks can also cause insomnia because caffeine triggers the release of adrenaline, which promotes alertness. Tea is less likely to cause problems.
- Over-the-counter cold and flu decongestants, corticosteroids, antidepressants, and bronchodilators used for asthma, as well as prescribed drugs and illegal narcotics, can interfere with sleep.
- Habits such as reading, working, or watching TV in bed train your subconscious mind to associate bedtime with activity rather than sleep.
- Pain, fever, and infections can make it difficult to sleep.
- Depression alters REM (rapid eye movement) sleep — about 40% of sufferers also have insomnia.
- Trauma, grief, and post-traumatic stress syndrome can affect your sleep.
- Sleep apnea (associated with snoring).
- Reflux also disrupts sleep.
- Changes in altitude and long flights lead to disrupted sleep patterns and result in jet lag.
- Eating a big meal before bed can lead to indigestion and poor sleep.

How to Improve Your Sleeping Habits

Adequate sleep is important for your skin's appearance. It's not just about nighttime sleep; you have to start your day right.

1. "Don't dine after nine" is a good rule to follow. Your body has difficulty digesting food during sleep, so you are more likely to wake up throughout the night.

2. Avoid foods and drinks that may inhibit sleep:
   - Foods and drinks that form acids in the body, such as fruit juice, spirits, wine, beer, soft drinks, chocolate, pork, and vinegar.
   - Spicy meals before bedtime.
   - Ice cream and other sweet desserts that increase acidity and mess up your nighttime blood sugar levels. You may initially fall asleep, but as your blood sugar levels change, you may wake up in the middle of the night and not be able to resume sleeping.
   - Too much food or alcohol. You may feel like you're sleeping heavily after a binge, but it will be poor-quality sleep, so you're more likely to wake up feeling lethargic.
   - Caffeine, which increases heart rate, breathing rate, speeds up the nervous system, affects blood sugar levels, and triggers the release of stomach acids.

3. Get a 10-minute dose of direct sunlight before 10 a.m. each day to help set your body clock. A great night's sleep begins in the morning when you wake up.

4. Choose a wake-up time and religiously stick to it (yes, even after a late night out) and then make sure you get 10 minutes of sunlight before 10 a.m. This will help to reset your body clock so you're more likely to wake up feeling refreshed.

5. Do some vigorous exercise daily, preferably in the morning. Don't exercise too close to bedtime.

6. Make sure you complete at least two tasks on that imaginary to-do list. If you're worried about something, such as paperwork or taxes, do at least part of it immediately and then schedule time each day to get it completed. Worry and stress can cause insomnia, so you need to show your subconscious mind that your problems are dealt with during the day. If you don't deal with them now, you will end up being haunted by them when you should be sleeping. Remember, a dynamic, active day equals a restful night's sleep.

> Worry and stress can cause insomnia, so you need to show your subconscious mind that your problems are dealt with during the day.

7. Have a nighttime ritual. Either have a warm bath 1 hour before bed or wash and steam your face (fill a basin with very warm water, wet your cloth, wring and hold over your face for 5 to 10 seconds. Repeat three times). When having a bath, add 1 cup (250 mL) of Epsom salts, as they contain magnesium, which relaxes your muscles.

8. Only use your bed for sleep or sex. Your bed is not an office, a movie theater, or a place to read adventure novels. Yes, I know it is nice to lie in bed and read, but if you can't sleep, you need to strengthen your (subconscious) association between bed and sleep, not bed and reading or bed and TV. Bed is for sleep!

9. Avoid coffee and other stimulants after 3 p.m.

10. Don't toss and turn in bed for too long. If you can't sleep and you are in insomniac hell, get out of bed. If you have been trying to relax, think peaceful thoughts and breathe calmly. If none of these strategies has worked, it is better to get out of bed than to struggle and get frustrated. Your frustration will only keep you awake.

11. If you get out of bed, this is not the time to catch up on emails, do paperwork, or watch TV. Turning on the lights at 2 a.m. and doing any of these is useful only if you want to train your body for shiftwork. If you don't do shiftwork, you don't want to associate 2 a.m. with activity. If you want to train your body to sleep properly, you need to get out of bed, keep the lights off, and go and sit in the dark in an upright position and concentrate on your breathing until you feel sleepy. Sounds hideous? Yes it is, especially if it is a chilly night and the heater's been switched off for hours. This is good. Your body will quickly associate nighttime wakefulness with being totally painful. Your body doesn't like pain, so it will do anything to avoid it. Eventually, your body will link comfort with sleeping in your cosy bed. But in the meantime: no pain, no gain. Keep the lights off, sit in the dark, focus on breathing in and breathing out, get sleepy, then go back to your deliciously cosy bed.

12. Never overstimulate yourself before bedtime. Sure, it's good to have a productive day, but don't overdo it too close to bedtime. Don't do vigorous exercise within 3 hours of bedtime, don't argue, don't watch tense or scary movies, don't read thrilling novels or watch exciting TV programs, as they can hype you up and this period before bed is the time to wind down and prepare for a restful night's sleep.

13. By the way… you are not an insomniac. Ban the "I" word if you're an insomniac — you get 8 hours sleep a night and you wake up refreshed. You are what you say you are. This may sound a bit wacky, but if you want to sleep 8 hours a night and wake up refreshed, then repeat it to yourself over and over again: "I sleep 8 hours a night and I wake up refreshed." If you have trouble saying this with a straight face, then try: "Wouldn't it be nice if I slept 8 hours a night and woke up refreshed?" And remember to ban the "I" word.

Guideline #5

• •

Sweat for 15 Minutes a Day: Exercising for Healthier Skin

Have you ever noticed what happens to a bucket of water when it has been left outside for a few weeks? It becomes mosquito-infested and putrid. Leave it for a bit longer and slime may appear around the edges. Debris falls in and slowly rots; some microbes die, while others excrete wastes, tainting the water. For water to be healthy, it needs to have a filtering system; it needs to move — down rivers, through crevices and springs, and past rocks. Movement is nature's filter; it cleans and renews and energizes.

> Lack of exercise can affect skin health.

It is a similar story with your body. If you are an active person, your lymphatic system and blood keep your body clean. This may not sound significant, but this flow keeps you alive and makes it harder for bacteria to proliferate. Your lymphatic system, unlike your heart, has no internal pump,

---

Q. What exactly is the lymphatic system?

A. The lymphatic system is made up of organs and tissues that produce, store, and transport white blood cells. These white blood cells are your immunity cells because they fight infections and disease. The lymphatic system includes the thymus, spleen, bone marrow, and lymph nodes. You may have noticed in the past when you've had an infection, two lumps in your neck (just below your jaw) swell up and feel tender or painful. These are lymph nodes.

There is also a network of thin tubes linking the entire lymphatic system. These tubes branch out like blood vessels into all the tissues of the body. This enables your white blood cells to travel wherever they're needed.

Movement from activities, such as power walking, running, cycling, and swimming, increases the circulation of your lymphatic fluids around the body, and as you probably already know, good circulation is vital for healthy skin. A pumping circulation is necessary to carry nutrients and oxygen to your skin so wounds can be repaired and new skin cells can be formed.

so without daily activity it will be sluggish and wastes will likely accumulate at a rapid rate. Dead cells and bacteria produce toxins, and these pile up to create an unhealthy internal environment — inside your body — as would rubbish on a footpath if the garbageworkers went on strike. In this way, lack of exercise can affect skin health.

Benefits of Exercise

You may be the type of person who doesn't worry about your risk of disease, especially if you are in your teens or 20s. And I agree. It is better to not worry about what-ifs, but that's no reason to get lazy now. So let's use the following positive benefits to motivate you to sweat.

- When you exercise, you release endorphins, which make you feel happy and relaxed. Runners can even experience "runner's high," which feels absolutely amazing.
- Exercise also gives you energy and increased vitality. Don't underestimate the value of having vitality. People with "spark" are more attractive to be around because they have more energy to give.
- Let's not forget that exercise is one of the best ways to keep your body looking trim, firm, and terrific. It also helps to prevent cellulite and gives your skin a healthy glow so you can look hot more often than not.

Did You Know?

Exercise Facts
Scientists have found that exercise can cut the risk of developing skin cancer (well it certainly did for the lab mice they tested). The mice were exposed to UVB radiation over a period of 16 weeks. The sun-baking mice who did not exercise developed skin cancer at a rapid rate, while the sun-loving mice who exercised developed fewer incidences of cancer or took much longer to develop skin cancer. However, you still should use sun protection, even if you exercise religiously, as exercise does not guarantee a cancer-free life. Moderate exercise burns up the body's fat stores, which leaves less fat available for inflammatory response (inflammation causes eczema, arthritis, and asthma).

- Moderate exercise decreases blood levels of arachidonic acid, an acid from meat and dairy that increases inflammation.
- Excess glucose in the blood can damage blood vessels (as seen in diabetes), and exercise reduces blood glucose levels.

Exercise Options

The kinds of activities you choose really depend on your abilities and tastes. For example, if you have a bad knee, you are not going to take up jogging. You may instead go to the gym and have a trainer design a program that won't irritate your injury, but will make you sweat all the same. If you love tennis, you can include it in your regimen, but also choose at least one other type of moderate- or high-impact exercise. Exercise can be categorized depending on how much sweat it produces and how much energy it burns.

Light Energy Burners

Light energy burners may not make you sweat enough to be beneficial, unless it is a hot day. Light energy burners include walking (average pace without stopping), golf, table tennis, stretching, 10-pin bowling, and a leisurely game of tennis.

Moderate Energy Burners

Moderate energy burners may promote sweating. These include fast walking, cycling, volleyball, cricket, horse riding, sailing, dancing, badminton, a moderately paced tennis game, Pilates, yoga, and aerobics. Household exercises include vigorous sweeping, scrubbing, vacuuming, pushing a wheelbarrow, building work/lifting, and clearing the garden. Slow swimming is also a moderate energy burner.

High Energy Burners

High energy burners make you sweat. These include fast walking uphill or carrying a load, soft-sand walking (knees up, fast paced), soft-sand running, sprints, fast-paced yoga such as astanga, interval training, gymnastics, tennis (fast paced), ice skating, rollerskating, fast cycling, football, basketball, rowing (moderate pace), jogging (at a pace of more than $4\frac{1}{2}$ miles/ 7 kilometers per hour), weight training, squash (moderate pace). High-energy-burning household activities include very heavy gardening, digging, chopping wood, very heavy building and lifting. Swimming (moderate pace) may not make you visibly sweat, but it still counts.

Q. I understand the value of exercising, but why sweat for only 15 minutes a day?

A. Exercise causes perspiration, which contains lysozyme, an enzyme that fights bacteria and flushes the nasty microbes from the surface of your skin. Sweating also assists with removing waste products from your body so toxic buildup does not occur. You can sweat for longer if you want to, but I've set a 15-minute minimum for each day because you only need to sweat briefly to improve your skin health. Besides, from a psychological point of view, 15 minutes is doable. It doesn't require you give up an hour or two of your day. If you are busy, you have no excuse. It is the time it takes to leisurely drink a cup of coffee; it's shorter than a TV sitcom; and briefer than a phone call to Mom (but just as important). Yes, the 15 minutes you spend sweating daily will give you so much more than a coffee or TV program ever will because sweat gives you your health.

Sweat Strategies for Busy People

- Do vigorous exercise around the house first thing in the morning to help with bowel movements and clearing toxic buildup. Try jumping jacks mixed with sprints.
- Take a sauna or a warm bath to promote sweating. They are also wonderfully relaxing.
- Swim in salt water to get your lymphatic fluid moving. Salt water is fantastic for healing blemishes and mild rashes (if you have sensitive skin, you can rinse off the salt water afterwards and then moisturize).
- Buy a digital clock and a skipping rope and skip for 20 minutes a day. If you need to rest, do so for no longer than 40 seconds each time.
- Buy an aerobics DVD or a professional yoga video.

How to exercise safely

- If you have injuries or any medical conditions, seek medical advice before taking up an exercise program.
- Before exercising, you should warm up with gentle stretching or walking.
- Avoid running on hard surfaces, such as concrete, which can hurt your back and knees. Run on softer surfaces like grass and sand. You should not experience sharp pain in any part of the body while exercising.
- Invest in a good-quality pair of sports shoes that are suitable for your activities.
- Take care when exercising. Injuries will stop your fitness routine in its tracks, so listen to your body to prevent making a silly mistake.
- Talk to a personal trainer or an expert in the sport you wish to do and ask about tips to prevent injury and techniques to help you excel. Learning from a fitness expert is much better than learning from your mistakes and injuries!
- Keep your exercise routine under 2 hours a day — too much exercise can age you prematurely and increase inflammation in the body.
- Find incidental ways to be active: walk up (or down) the escalators instead of standing still, take the stairs instead of the elevator, and park your car further away from your destination (especially if you are going to work and plan to be sitting down for much of the day).

Quick Tips for Exercising for Healthier Skin

1. Picture what you want. See yourself with beautiful skin and imagine how good you will look and feel.

2. Sweat for 15 minutes each day. You can sweat for longer if you want to, but don't exercise for more than 2 hours because overexercising can age you prematurely.

3. Exercise four to five times a week; the other days you can sweat in a sauna or a warm bath.

4. If you find yourself making excuses to skip exercising, remind yourself you don't have to feel like exercising, you just have to do it! And besides, you only have to do it for 15 minutes, so even the busiest person can fit it in.

Sweat Program

Your aim is to exercise four to five times a week — on the other days you can have a sauna, swim in salt water, or do a body scrub while having a relaxing, warm bath. Your exercise and sweat routine could be tailored any way you like: you could keep your routine the same and go jogging 5 days a week or you could spice it up with variety. The main thing is to just do it. Exercise on a regular basis. Grab your diary or planner and schedule in 15 minutes of sweating each day this week. Your aim is to sweat for 15 minutes daily, so you may need to exercise for 20 minutes to give yourself a chance to work up a sweat. Here is an example of an effective exercise routine:

Day of the Week	Planned Exercise	Incidental Exercise
Monday	Cardio workout: 20 minutes of walking, running, sprinting	Take the stairs at work.
Tuesday	Weight/strength training: 20–40 minutes of weight training, including core strength exercise for abdominal and back muscles	Walk up the escalators at the shops.
Wednesday	Deep breathing exercises: 5 to 10 minutes Warm bath: 20–30 minute warm bath to exfoliate your skin. You sweat in a warm bath!	Walk kids to school.
Thursday	Playing favorite sport: dancing, soccer, netball, surfing (with lots of paddling)	Park car further away from work.
Friday	Cardio workout: 10 minutes of jogging, 1-minute sprints, and 20 minutes brisk walking (or 30 minutes jogging with 1-minute sprints every 5 minutes)	Walk faster.
Saturday	Deep breathing exercises: 5 to 10 minutes Sauna: 15-minute sauna followed by a shower and moisturizer	Walk to local shop to get newspaper.
Sunday	Swimming: 20-minute swim (ocean or pool) plus dry skin brushing and a warm bath	Walk to the park.

If you are a busy parent and find it hard to leave home, then your exercise routine may look more like this:

Monday   20 minutes skipping in the backyard (aim to skip for at least 5 minutes before having a brief break of less than 40 seconds, then continue).

Tuesday   Jog around the house for 20 minutes non-stop.

continued…

Wednesday	Walk to the park or shops pushing the pram (at least 20 minutes non-stop).
Thursday	Relaxation day: do deep breathing exercises; have a warm bath and exfoliate your skin.
Friday	Follow a yoga or aerobics DVD in your living room.
Saturday	Go for a long walk with your partner or a friend.
Sunday	Warm bath.

The sweat-for-15-minutes program can be tailored any way you like so it suits your lifestyle. However, if you're truly unwell, rest, rest, rest. Then get back into your routine. A minor setback is never a reason to give up. You will find that you will recover faster if you give yourself a day to recuperate, and you will more than likely retain some of your previous fitness, so you won't have to start all over again.

5. Write a list of sports or activities you would like to try. If you hate exercise and can't think of something you would enjoy, ask yourself:

- What exercise might I enjoy if I was good at it?
- What sports would I like to be better at?
- I must exercise, so what should I try first?
- What can I do to make exercise more enjoyable? This is a great question — asking this will help you successfully start your program, and if you come up with some good solutions, you'll be more likely to stick to your new routine.

6. While it is fresh in your mind, do something proactive today. For example:

- Go to your local sports store and buy a skipping rope.
- Buy a yoga DVD and an exercise mat.
- Grab the phone directory or get on the Internet and look up your local sports centres, gyms, or yoga classes (whatever you have in mind).
- Make that first phone call. Inquire about joining fees, timetables, and personal trainers or coaches. If you can't afford a personal trainer every week, think about hiring one for three sessions only. That way you get an effective exercise program and they can monitor you a few times to make sure you're doing the movements correctly so you don't injure yourself. Then you can continue on your own.

- You could also get some friends together and form an exercise group. You may be able to negotiate a good deal with a personal trainer if you have enough people committed to getting fit.
- Go to your local park or beach early in the morning on weekends and see if there are any trainers conducting group sessions. This is a good way to pick an exercise coach because you get to see them in action (although always check their qualifications).
- Look for a personal trainer who is also a C.H.E.K exercise coach (trained in the methods of top exercise coach Paul Chek). These are highly specialized personal trainers who have extra knowledge and credentials in the field of health and exercise. They can also help you with postural correction, which is essential before you begin training. Bad posture will increase your risk of injury and make it more difficult to breathe deeply and perform well. Log on to the C.H.E.K website to look for a qualified coach in your local area: www.chekinstitute. com/prac.cfm (click on search and click on your country).
- If you're a new mom, you could inquire about group exercise classes especially designed for moms, where your child is minded as you exercise. Gyms often have childcare facilities that make it possible to exercise. Or simply put baby in the pram and walk to a hilly area; don't underestimate the sweat you'll produce as you push a stroller up a big hill.

7. After sweating, replace lost fluids straightaway. Have a glass of Green Water or mineral water and add a pinch of sea salt for instant hydration. See Guideline #1, page 42, for more information.

Guideline #6

Be a Hat Person: Avoiding UV Light Exposure

It is common knowledge that excess sun exposure can cause premature skin wrinkling, but I read so many alarming statistics about sun damage that during the middle of researching this guideline, I went out and bought a hat, even though I have always hated wearing them. I have effectively become a hat person and now I wear one practically every day.

Activity

Take a look at the skin on your bottom (I'm serious!). If you are in a public place, this may have to wait, or alternatively you can look at any part of your body that has not had sun exposure. Is the skin that has never been "sun kissed" in better condition than the sun-exposed areas?

Caution

This section is not designed to be prescriptive. Treatment for skin cancer should be prescribed by your doctor or skin care specialist.

Skin Cancer

Another concern with excess sun exposure, especially if you tend to get sunburned, is the increased risk of developing skin cancer, or melanoma. Melanoma is the most common type of cancer in the United States and the most dangerous, resulting in the majority of cancer deaths. However, through increased medical research and more public awareness from widespread media coverage, skin cancers are being detected earlier, so survival rates are remarkably high. This is great news.

> Melanoma is the most common type of cancer in the United States and the most dangerous, resulting in the majority of cancer deaths.

Alarming Skin Cancer Facts

- Approximately 1 million Americans are diagnosed with skin cancer each year, resulting in 1000 to 2000 deaths.
- More than 382,000 Australians are diagnosed with skin cancer each year; of these cases, approximately 8800 have dangerous melanomas and about 1400 die.
- In the United Kingdom approximately 68,000 people are diagnosed with skin cancer each year, even though the sun is not as harsh in this part of the world.

It's no surprise that people with pale skin who freckle and sunburn easily have a higher risk of developing skin cancer from UV radiation, but you may not know that people blessed with gorgeous chocolate skin (and truckloads of natural melanin protection) can still get skin cancer.

Ultraviolet Radiation

Ultraviolet (UV) radiation from the sun is the primary cause of skin cancer. UV rays are also produced by artificial tanning beds and sun lamps. UV radiation that reaches our atmosphere and us is made up of UVA and UVB rays: UVB rays are more likely to cause basal and squamous cell cancers as well as sunburn (FYI: As a reminder, the B in UVB stands for Burning). UVA rays penetrate deeper into the skin and promote free radicals that age your skin prematurely, but scientists also suspect that UVA can indirectly lead to melanoma. (FYI: As a reminder, the A in UVA stands for

Aging.) Note that sun beds, tanning booths, and sun lamps give out higher doses of UVA radiation, so they are not considered a safe alternative to sunbathing at the beach. The best tanning options are spray-on tans, tanning creams, or just loving yourself the way you are.

UV radiation is increased by reflective surfaces such as sand, water, snow, and ice, which is why it's easier to get sunburned during your annual holidays to the snow or beach. UV rays can also penetrate through windows, windshields, clouds, and thin clothing. A lifetime of sun exposure, with bouts of getting sunburned, increases your risk of skin cancer, but skin cancers sometimes appear in areas of the skin that are never exposed to UV light (yes, I mean that you can get skin cancers on your bottom). This indicates that UV exposure is not the sole cause of skin cancer. According to the latest research, diet, lifestyle, and genetics also play a role.

Caution

If you're currently taking Roaccutane, you may already know that it is absolutely vital to stay out of the sun or wear protective clothing, such as a wide-brimmed hat, because the skin becomes highly sensitive to light. If you are taking this drug and are concerned about the effects, then it is best to ask the advice of your doctor or specialist for more information.

Vitamin D Production

A little bit of sunlight is essential for your health. You need to have small exposures to sun on a regular basis so your skin can produce a form of vitamin D that helps your bones to stay strong. This is highlighted by the fact that children who are covered from head to toe with sunscreen and protective clothing can end up with rickets (causing deformed bones such as bowed legs). This is because their skin never gets a sensible dose of sun.

Minimum UV exposure is the key here: about 10 minutes of unfiltered sunshine directly on the skin will keep vitamin D deficiency away in healthy individuals. Get your 10 minutes of vitamin D–producing sun exposure during the morning or afternoon, outside the hours of 10 a.m. to 3 p.m., when the sun is not too harsh.

Skin Self-Examination

Early detection of skin cancer is essential. If you are lucky, someone else may notice a weird-looking spot on your body and mention it to you, but don't count on this happening. Take charge of your own health and regularly examine your skin for suspect moles and spots. You should also ask your partner (or your mom) to check your back, scalp, and other areas that can be difficult to self-monitor. Don't be shy: this could save your life!

The best time to examine your skin is after having a shower or bath and during the day when there is plenty of natural light. Use a full-length mirror and a hand-held one so you can see where your moles, birthmarks, and other spots are. Check how they look and feel. You may want to take photos of areas of the skin that have a large gathering of spots so you can record their appearance for future reference.

Check your skin from head to toe. Check your back, scalp, genitals, between your buttocks, between your toes, soles of your feet, toenails, and fingernails. Remember that the earlier you report suspect spots to your doctor, the more likely you will live a long and healthy life. Your doctor may do a biopsy to check if a spot is cancerous. You may also want to get a second opinion if you're concerned about the diagnosis. Don't be afraid to ask to be referred to a skin cancer specialist.

What to look for during the skin self-examination

- New skin spots, such as a new mole that looks different from the other moles, or a new red mole or dark-colored mole or a new flesh-colored, firm bump
- Flaky patch that may be slightly raised or a crusty sore that doesn't heal
- Small lump that is pale, red, or pearly in color
- Any spot that has changed in size, color, or shape over a period of weeks or months

How to decrease your risk of skin cancer

- Apply sunscreen and wear protective clothing and a hat (Remember the old slogan: slip, slop, slap).
- Keep out of the sun (as much as humanly possible) between 10 a.m. and 3 p.m. If you need to be out, seek shade when you can. UV levels are at their highest at this time, so avoid excess sun exposure during these hours.
- Eat small meals. Don't overeat throughout the day (or night) and never binge. Consume foods that are rich in antioxidants and essential fatty acids.
- If you're stressed, implement relaxation techniques, such as deep breathing exercises, into your daily routine.
- Exercise.
- Don't unnecessarily expose yourself to harsh chemicals because they create extra work for your body and chemicals can trigger mutations. To reduce your chemical load, use natural cleaning products and wash all fruits and vegetables before eating them (see Guideline #1).

Sunscreens

According to the scientific research, broad-spectrum sunscreens offer good protection against UVB rays and can decrease the incidence of certain skin cancers. However, sunscreen's ability to protect against free-radical damage caused by UVA rays seems to be limited. Even though sunscreens have their faults, they still play an important role in protecting your skin against premature aging. I've tested a lot of creams during my years of research and I've found that sunscreen is still the best topical treatment for minimizing wrinkles.

> Even though sunscreens have their faults, they still play an important role in protecting your skin against premature aging.

Clothing

A heavy cotton T-shirt and a wide-brimmed hat may not sound very sexy, but with a bit of styling you can look fab and also protect your delicate skin from cancerous spots. You also get bonus points because sun protection is your best defense against wrinkles and premature aging. Become a hat person today.

Activity

Buy hypo-allergenic sunscreen and a hat, and use them daily — when you look in the mirror at age 50, you will be very thankful that you did.

Did You Know?

Best Sunscreens

There are a lot of unnecessary chemicals in cheap sunscreens, so choose a hypoallergenic sunscreen formulated for babies or toddlers because they work just as well as the adult formulas and they are kinder to your skin. If you have uneven skin pigmentation, look for a sunscreen that has a high zinc oxide content (see Guideline #8). And always reapply sunscreen every 2 hours or after sweating or swimming.

Quick Tips for Avoiding UV light exposure

- Check your skin regularly for unusual spots, moles and freckles (or for any change to spots you already have) and get your skin checked by your doctor if you are unsure what to look for. You may want to check your skin on the first day of every month so you remember.
- Apply sunscreen, protective clothing and a hat if you're spending time in the sun.
- Try to keep out of the sun between 10:00 a.m. and 3:00 p.m.
- Avoid getting sunburnt at all costs — a tan is not worth sacrificing your precious skin or your life!
- Become a hat person and wear a hat when outdoors.
- Use a lightweight hypoallergenic sunscreen that is formulated for toddlers because they have fewer chemical additives.
- While it is important to avoid sunburn, remember that it is also essential for your health to have small daily doses of sunshine. Ten minutes of sun exposure a day is recommended for healthy vitamin D production.

Guideline #7

Relax: Making Peace with Your Body

When you relax, you feel good. You don't need a bunch of scientists to tell you this. However, if you want to get technical, relaxation is vital for your health in general because it stimulates the "rest and digest" part of your nervous system. This system, as the name suggests, allows you to have a good night's sleep and promotes good digestion. This is important for your skin health in particular because the nutrients extracted from your foods during digestion are necessary for skin repair and maintenance. If you have poor digestion, you will also have decreased absorption of fat-soluble vitamins, which leads to dry, cracked skin and skin conditions, such as eczema.

> If you have poor digestion, you will also have decreased absorption of fat-soluble vitamins, which leads to dry, cracked skin and skin conditions, such as eczema.

Did You Know?

Flight or Fight

Stress and similar states of mind, such as anxiety, worry, fear, and rage, all stimulate the "fight or flight" part of the nervous system while preventing the release of digestive juices and hormones, such as insulin. There's also a decrease in blood supply to your gut, liver, and kidneys. This can also occur if you are a chronic shallow breather or running a marathon (physical stress). Your body, during these states, releases adrenaline and increases blood pressure. Chronic stress can result in skin inflammation, constipation, insomnia, impotence, low sex drive, dry eyes, dry mouth, and digestive complaints, such as irritable bowel syndrome.

Stress

Stress is not easy to define because, as the saying goes, one person's stress is another's adventure. Whether your stress is justified or not, your body cannot tell the difference and experiences a cascade of hormonal changes to help it cope with the emergency. Is your body constantly in the fight or flight state?

Q. When I'm stressed, I always get dermatitis on my hands; they become red, raw, and peel, and it's really painful. Why does this occur?

A. Stress can affect the skin so dramatically because it causes the release of cortisol hormones, which are associated with dry skin and premature aging. Stress also blocks some key prostaglandins from being made. (See the discussion of prostaglandins on page 57). So you get red, hot inflammation in some form or another. Your genetic predisposition means this inflammation is expressed as dermatitis, while other people may get asthma, pimples, or psoriasis during times of great stress. Chronic stress not only leads to bad skin, it can also make you more vulnerable to serious illnesses.

Did You Know?

Good Stress

Let's clear up something before you read any further: a bit of stress is okay; in fact; it may even be good for you. A short burst of stress motivates you to study before exams and it can help you run away or fight if there is real danger. It is the regular or chronic stress that can be harmful to your skin and health in general. The solution is to switch off the stress response for a period of time each day. How do you do this? You make time to relax. It is not as simple as it appears. True relaxation is not just slumping on the couch and watching TV; you must also switch off your busy mind for a few moments.

Relaxation

If you want to have fabulous skin, the most important thing to do is relax.

If you want to have fabulous skin, the most important thing to do is relax. Listening to relaxing music, deep breathing and calm thoughts, having confidence in yourself, self-love, self-respect, and acceptance encourage relaxed feelings and can suppress the stress response. If you are the type of person who makes time to relax and re-energize, then it indicates you have a good level of self-love and respect for your health.

Effective ways to relax include having a warm bath, listening to relaxing music, and deep breathing exercises. Have as many relaxing moments as possible during your day.

The Stress Test

Complete the stress test below to see if you have any signs of chronic stress. (Circle yes or no.)

QUESTION	Yes	No
1. Do your shoulders rise up when you breathe in? (Stand in front of a mirror to check if you have shallow breathing.)	5	0
2. Is your sex drive currently lower than is normal for you?	5	0
3. Do you often feel lonely, anxious, misunderstood, or isolated?	5	0
4. Do you lash out at others or do you often get angry or upset if things go wrong?	5	0
5. Does your weight fluctuate because of stress?	5	0
6. Do you dislike yourself or suffer from low self-esteem?	10	0
7. Do you worry about your job, income, or debts or are you bothered by daily hassles (bad drivers, bank lineups, etc.)?	10	0
8. Are any of your relationships causing you stress?	10	0
9. Do you need to be around people to have fun, feel safe, or pass the time/does spending time alone make you anxious?	10	0
10. Do you have a psychological disorder or take any medications for stress-related problems?	15	0
11. Have you suffered a major loss recently that caused grief?	20	0
TOTAL SCORE:		
		/100

Score Card

50–100: If you scored between 50 and 100, you are likely to be highly stressed or have a decreased ability to relax. In this case, learning to calm your mind for a few moments daily would be a high priority for you.

20–50: If your score was between 20 and 50, you may experience moderate amounts of stress, and relaxation would be beneficial for your skin's health and your overall health.

0–20: If you scored less than 20, your stress levels are okay.

Have a warm bath and enjoy the sensations of the water. Play music that calms you, and breathe in a relaxed manner: in and out, in and out. Note, though, that a deep, tense breath will not make you relax. A calm, long breath will.

Relaxation Promotes Good Health

- Proper digestion
- Good sleep/wake cycles (circadian rhythms)
- Calm feelings
- Healthy sex drive
- Lower blood pressure
- Healthy skin

Activity

Have a warm bath tonight. For a relaxing bath, add 1 cup (250 mL) of Epsom salts, 1 teaspoon (5 mL) of oil, such as olive, coconut, or almond oil, and five drops of lavender essential oil. (Caution: oil makes bath surfaces slippery, so clean the bath with baking soda afterwards.)

CASE STUDY

I tend to be a workaholic (and I'm a recovering perfectionist) so I'm usually very busy. However, when I'm having one of those manic days and I hear myself saying, "I'll never make this deadline" (as I start to panic), I force myself to stop working. I effectively ban myself from continuing. I remind myself of this chapter (and the fact that a stressed person makes more mistakes and works less effectively), and I say to myself, "I'm not allowed to work until I calm down." Then I'll reluctantly move away from my desk and take a few deep, slow breaths. I'll also either go and make myself a cup of black tea or dandelion tea, or I'll go for a walk outside for 5 minutes. Quite often this is the time when I come up with a good idea or a solution to a problem.

Q. How could I possibly like myself when my skin is so disgusting?

A. When you greatly dislike your looks, whether it is your skin, your waistline, or a facial feature, you create an enormous amount of stress in your body. This is not good for you and it won't get you the skin you desire. You cannot hate yourself into having gorgeous skin! It's just not possible. However, you can choose to like yourself, imperfections and all, while you learn how to create gorgeous skin.

Making Peace with Your Body

Making peace with your body is the most important step to getting better-looking skin. When you accept yourself and praise yourself for your good qualities, then you will begin to realize you deserve better (better skin/job/lifestyle).
Another positive benefit of liking yourself, faults and all, is that your body releases endorphins that make you feel good. These chemicals are also released during exercise — it is often referred to as "runner's high" — and happiness, laughter, smiling, and warm hugs all cause the release of endorphins.

Did You Know?
....

Endorphins
When feel-good endorphins are floating around in your system, you are more likely to eat healthy food, exercise, and breathe deeply. These are all healing activities that are great for the skin. On the other hand, when you feel bad about your skin and berate yourself, you suppress the feel-good chemicals from being made in your body. As you deny yourself love and self-care, you deny yourself endorphin pleasure. You also block healing from occurring, so your skin conditions stay with you. It is a vicious cycle. If you focus on what you hate about yourself, such as your skin problems, then you inadvertently keep your skin looking bad. It's absurd to think you can hate yourself into having beautiful skin.

Activity

Right now: stand up and go over to a mirror (take this book with you) and look at your reflection. Focus on a part of your skin that you are not happy with, such as a pimple or wrinkles. Then tell yourself out loud (or in your head, if there are people nearby) the following: "My skin looks disgusting and I'm so ugly!" Say it again and put lots of emotion into it. Screw up your face, frown and cross your arms for extra effect: "My skin looks disgusting and I'm so ugly!"

Now how bad do you feel? I can guarantee you don't feel good. This is the feeling of stress chemicals flooding into your bloodstream. Did you also feel a sinking feeling in your chest area? Self-hate literally hurts your heart.

Now change your focus and look at a part of your body that has beautiful skin. Then stand up tall, smile a big warm smile and say with enthusiasm, "I have such beautiful skin!" Okay, I realize you may feel a bit silly doing this and it sounds like a sappy positive affirmation, but it is an exercise to teach you a very valuable lesson. Now say it again as if you mean it: "I have such beautiful skin, I'm so lucky!"

Now use your whole body to show your excitement; stand up tall and smile even wider: "My skin is so gorgeous, I'm so lucky!" How do you feel? If you did this activity with enthusiasm, then you have just created an endorphin rush that is good for your whole body. So what's the lesson? You do have control over how good you feel, even if only for a few fabulous seconds.

Eight Ways to Feel Good in an Instant

If you are experiencing stress, anxiety, or depression, it can be impossible to just "get happy." You can't simply tell yourself to cheer up and suddenly you are better. What if you have just gone bankrupt or your marriage has ended: how do you get an endorphin rush then? A long-term solution may be difficult to find, but there are plenty of short-term ways to make yourself feel good. You can create your own natural endorphins using the following eight strategies.

1. Practice Self-Compliments

If you feel uncomfortable about praising yourself for every little thing you do right, then this activity is the one for you. And if you're the type of person who thinks it is better to wait and hope that you will receive praise from someone else, this activity should wake you up from your delusions. In reality, it's no use waiting for someone else to lavish you with kind words. People may or may not oblige, but, quite frankly, expecting a compliment from others is like trying to control the weather. You can't turn on the rain by command or force a person to be nice to you. However, self-compliments are always reliable. You can make them exactly what you want to hear and they are available at a moment's notice.

I have such gorgeous skin!
I am so lucky!
I look so good in this dress!
My eyebrows are the best!
I am so caring and generous!
I am so clever and fine and one of a kind!

You get the message (and the endorphin rush).

If you have trouble praising yourself, begin by listing your strengths on a piece of paper and then read them out aloud, with enthusiasm. You need to put energy and emotion into your words so you can feel the rush of positive chemicals. Doing a bland old affirmation won't make you feel much better. It is the emotion you attach to the compliments that will release healing endorphins.

Activity

Grab a pen and piece of paper or your diary/planner and list your personal strengths. For example, if your sister is great at playing tennis and you are good at writing stories, don't pine about being a bad tennis player. Instead, praise your good fortune and talents as a writer. You may also be excellent at remembering song lyrics or people's names. List these traits and anything else you can think of. When you focus on your strengths and compliment yourself, it is impossible to feel anxious at the same time.

2. Listen to Your Favorite Music

Music can elevate your feelings in a split second. Play your favorite song, turn it up loud, and relax for a few minutes. Choose your music wisely, however. If you tend to be depressed and negative, you may naturally gravitate to sad ballads or thrash music that resonates with your mood. You want to rise above your negative feelings, so choose music that improves your feelings. If you have to do a task you find annoying, such as cleaning the house, then you can listen to music while you work to make the job more pleasant. You will have great company and a few extra endorphins to boost your energy.

Activity

Play your favorite CD today. Stand up and look for this CD (or your iPod) right now, and if you can't listen to a song right away, leave it in a prominent spot so you remember to listen later.

3. Engage in Your Favorite Hobby

Is there an activity that always makes you feel good? Whether it is painting, kicking a ball, window shopping, or designing shoes, you can elevate your mood with a positive activity that is either creative or involves movement. Steer clear of destructive hobbies like gambling, spending too much money, and binge drinking because they can lead to problems with your finances and your health. You don't want an even bigger reason to be stressed. Choose something fun. Take soccer lessons, round up some friends and do a fun form of exercise, or join a club.

4. Smile and Laugh a Lot

> Smiling and a good old belly laugh instantly release feel-good chemicals in your body.

Smiling and a good old belly laugh instantly release feel-good chemicals in your body — but how do you get more laughs into your day? The easiest way is to watch funny movies. Ditch the news, miss the dramas, and skip the cat fights caught on camera and divert your attention to comedies. Do this daily and laughing will become second nature. Smile when you are not laughing and you will continue to feel good. You don't

Activity

Pause from reading this book and smile for 30 seconds right now.

even have to find anything to smile about, as studies have found just the act of smiling a big, crinkle-eyed grin is enough to release endorphins. Smile and feel good in a flash.

5. Do Deep Breathing Exercises

Increase your oxygen intake in an instant with deep breathing exercises. Breathing exercises can also switch off your fight or flight nervous system and change your body into rest and digest mode without you having to suddenly change your view of the big, bad world. Learn how to relax with breathing exercises in the chapter on "Beauty Breathing."

6. Feel Grateful

Some people appear to have everything — money, fame, good looks, and a great house — but they are still not happy. I could name a few people in the tabloids right now who are rich and famous, but they are destroying their lives with drugs and alcohol, and the next stop will be rehab (again).

> **The quickest way to get health problems, bad skin, and low energy is to focus on what you don't have in your life. It encourages you to make bad choices.**

Why do people who appear to have everything still seem unhappy? According to happiness expert and motivational speaker Anthony Robbins, it's because they are not grateful. He says that when you are grateful, you feel rich. When you are ungrateful and looking at what's missing in your life, you feel poor and stressed and you end up doing crazy things to try to get that good feeling back. A prime example is resorting to drugs, binge drinking, and other addictions. The quickest way to get health problems, bad skin, and low energy is to focus on what you don't have in your life. It encourages you to make bad choices. When you put a spotlight on your problems, your negative feelings intensify and your judgment is clouded. It's okay to define a problem, but it's important to focus on a solution, or if there is nothing you can do to change a situation, then to look for the lesson or move on rather than dwelling on what you cannot change.

When you shift your focus and list all the things you are grateful for, your positive feelings are magnified. Now you are less likely to eat junk food or binge and you will be more likely to exercise and go to bed on time because you are more relaxed. It is not quite that simple, but this is a good start to being healthier and happier.

When you focus on the good things in your life and say a heartfelt thank you, it's impossible to feel bad in that moment. This may only make you feel good for 60 seconds, but that minute will be a beautiful one. Feel grateful for a few moments every day.

Activity

Grab your diary or planner and schedule in 5 minutes of gratitude each day. In fact, right now is a good time to list 10 things you're grateful for. Here are some questions to get you started:

- Are you grateful your home keeps you dry when it rains?
- Are you grateful you have a TV?
- Are you grateful for your loved ones? What are the specific things you appreciate about them?

Now read out what you have written, with emotion and intensity (as if you mean it), and you will get an endorphin rush. For example:

- I'm so grateful I have a roof over my head and I live in a beautiful house.
- I'm so lucky I get to eat delicious food.
- I am loved.
- I have a great family and I really appreciate everything they do. My mom is so wonderful because she is caring and kind, my dad loves me, and my sister is such a ray of sunshine.

You don't have to only be grateful for what has actually happened; you can also elevate you mood by imagining that what you want has already occurred. Have fun with it.

7. Observe Beauty

> Have you ever noticed how you feel when you appreciate a beautiful sunset or a pretty picture or anything you consider beautiful? You feel good.

Have you ever noticed how you feel when you appreciate a beautiful sunset or a pretty picture or anything you consider beautiful? You feel good. You can't help it because the appreciation of beauty causes a release of endorphins inside you.

On the other hand, if you view something you consider beautiful but then reject it or criticize it, you don't get any good feelings whatsoever. Say a beautiful woman (or man) walked into the room and you felt envious or threatened. You would instantly feel tense, on guard, or uncomfortable in some way as your body is flooded with stress hormones. You may call it fear, jealousy, or an inferiority complex, but they all cause the same internal disturbance. Jealousy is a quick way to suppress your good health and an instantaneous way to disregard your self-confidence!

If you want to feel good, don't reject beauty and the feel-good rush you receive from accepting it. Whether it is a beautiful person, a book, a painting, a view, or a trinket, just observe it for a moment and be thankful that there is so much beauty in the world. As you observe beauty and accept and appreciate it, you feel good. Read "How to Be Beautiful" (page 293) for more information.

8. Throw a Tantrum!

Anxiety can arise when you feel powerless. A quick remedy for feeling powerless is to throw a tantrum. This is usually more appropriate when you are alone. So take a moment to be by yourself and then stamp your feet and say to yourself, "I deserve better!" Look at the sky with determination and imagine you are yelling, "I deserve a promotion!" or "I deserve to be treated with love and respect!" A power "tantie" when enjoyed in private can stop an anxiety attack in its tracks simply because it feels good to say what you really want. Say it with conviction and you will feel much better.

> It feels good to say what you really want... Say it with conviction and you will feel much better.

While it may not be possible to feel good all the time, it is fun to indulge in endorphin-creating activities so you can at least feel fantastic sometimes. The eight ways to feel good in an instant really work. They are also scientifically valid, but you don't need a researcher to tell you that gratitude and listening to the right music elevate your mood, because when you do them you feel good. You can feel the endorphin rush. You may not say, "Oooh, that endorphin rush was nice," but it has still occurred.

Quick Tips for Relieving Stress

- Relax. Relaxation helps you to digest your food properly and sleep better at night.
- Make relaxation a priority. People who make relaxation time a priority are more likely to have great skin. If you are the type of person who makes time to relax and re-energize, it indicates you have a good level of self-love and respect for your health.
- Accept a bit of stress in your life. It can be a good motivator.
- Decrease your negative feelings about yourself.
- Compliment yourself often (no one else needs to know, so do it with enthusiasm).
- Listen to your favorite music. Make sure it is relaxing and elevates your mood.
- Enjoy your favorite hobbies once a week.
- Smile and laugh a lot. Watch funny movies or positive, uplifting TV programs.
- Do deep breathing exercises.
- Be grateful for everything you currently possess. This makes you feel fabulous, even if it is only for a moment.
- Appreciate beauty; don't attack it.
- To unwind after a long day at work, have a relaxing warm bath.

Guideline #8

● ●

Follow a Good Skin-Care Routine: Selecting Safe and Effective Beauty Aids

> You might be surprised to learn that many skin products contain ingredients that the scientific studies referred to in this chapter have deemed "harmful to our skin" or "not beneficial."

You wouldn't wash your car with a chemical cleaner that damaged your car's paint job, would you? So why would you want to wash your skin with a product containing ingredients that may damage your skin? You wouldn't? Well, you might be surprised to learn that many skin products, popular brand cleansers, commercial brand shampoos, bubble bath, and dish-washing liquids contain ingredients that the scientific studies referred to in this chapter have deemed "harmful to our skin" or "not beneficial." You may wonder why, if these ingredients are so bad for your skin, are they in your beauty creams in the first place? Because they are cheap and increase the "prettiness" of a product. They make a cream smell nice or feel silky, or they make it bubble and foam. Can you believe it? Many skin-care ingredients do nothing for your own gorgeousness!

The Name and Shame File

● ●

Before you find out what's good for your skin, let's first look at additives that you don't want on your delicate skin. If, after applying a skin-care product, your skin tingles, feels tight, or stings, it is being irritated.

> Scientific studies have shown over and over (and over) again that SLS penetrates the skin and damages the skin's protective barrier function.

Sodium Lauryl Sulfate (SLS)

Uses: A foaming detergent to make cleansing products bubble and an emulsifier that mixes oil and water so they don't separate.

Products: SLS is found in foaming toiletries, such as commercial toothpastes, shampoos, cleansers, hand wash, and bubble bath. This stuff seems to be in just about everything that foams!

Problems: Scientific studies have shown over and over (and over) again that SLS penetrates the skin and damages the skin's protective barrier function. This damage can be seen under a microscope for up to 4 weeks after the use of SLS (and 9 days by the naked eye). Products containing SLS create poor skin barrier function, causing excess water loss from the skin, making it easier for other chemicals, dust mites, and bacteria to penetrate the skin. SLS can cause reactions, such as rashes, dandruff, hair loss, and dry skin (and rebound oily skin and enlarged pores).

Avoid all sulfates. The following additives are similar versions of SLS, and although they are milder, they can still cause minor irritations:

- Sodium C14-16 olefin sulfate
- Sodium laureth (lauryl ether) sulfate (SLES)
- TEA-lauryl sulfate

Formaldehyde

Uses: This information covers formaldehyde and its derivatives imidazolidinyl urea and DMDM hydantoin. Cosmetic and skin-care preservative so the product has a longer shelf life.

Products: Found in shampoos, liquid hand soap, hair products such as gel, cosmetics, nail polish, and skin-care products such as body moisturizer.

Problems: DMDM hydantoin releases formaldehyde, which can irritate the skin and trigger allergic reactions, such as skin rashes and heart palpitations, and it may affect your breathing, according to the Mayo Clinic (the renowned non-profit medical and research center based in Minnesota). This additive can also aggravate asthma. DMDM hydantoin has caused birth defects in animal studies (keep in mind that this has not been proven in humans).

> DMDM hydantoin has caused birth defects in animal studies.

Mineral Oil

Uses: Acts as a barrier to lock in moisture.

Products: Mineral oil is found in cheap moisturizers and some baby oils.

Problems: It reportedly coats the skin like cling-wrap so your skin can't release toxins (Remember: the skin is a major organ for eliminating toxins). Mineral oil is a cheap skin-care ingredient that interferes with the skin's natural immunity barrier and may increase premature aging. However, mineral oil is a low-allergy oil that makes the skin feel softer (like most

> Mineral oil is a cheap skin-care ingredient that interferes with the skin's natural immunity barrier and may increase premature aging.

moisturizers do). Do not use if you have problem skin, and avoid use at night to allow your skin to effectively eliminate wastes. It is also not suitable for a baby's delicate skin.

Fragrance

Uses: To hide undesirable smells.

Products: There are as many as 4000 varieties of fragrance, many synthetic. Unspecified fragrance is found in moisturizers, deodorants, cleansers, hair conditioners, shampoos (including some baby shampoos), perfumes, cosmetics, and colognes.

Problems: May aggravate hand eczema and cause skin irritation or dermatitis of the face. Fragrance may also trigger dizziness and hyperpigmentation of the skin. Synthetic fragrance is not suitable for children's products because it may cause hyperactivity and irritation. If you suffer from skin pigmentation, then check to see if your skin cream or sunscreen contains "fragrance" or "parfum" because these ingredients can cause pigmentation.

Parabens

Uses: Methylparaben is a synthetic preservative/mold inhibiter.

Products: Includes methylparaben and its derivatives butyl-, ethyl-, and propylparaben. Parabens are used as a preservative in thousands of cosmetics, food, and pharmaceutical products. You'll see them on the ingredient list of exfoliating gels, cleansers, underarm deodorants, antiperspirants, cleansers, and moisturizers.

> Thousands of beauty products contain parabens and these parabens can be rapidly absorbed into the skin, especially since many cosmetic preparations contain penetration enhancers.

Problems: This preservative certainly wasn't added to your beauty products to help you look good. Methylparaben can trigger skin and mouth irritation. Parabens in general are infamous because they have been detected in breast tumors. Studies have shown that parabens can mimic the action of the female hormone estrogen and can drive the growth of human breast tumors. An editorial published in the *Journal of Applied Toxicology* brought up the point that little is known about the long-term side effects associated with low but consistent exposure to these estrogenic preservatives. We do know that estrogen can influence the growth of breast cancer, but it is unclear whether parabens, such as methylparaben, have anything to do with triggering cancer. The evidence looks coincidental at present.

But what experts do know is that thousands of beauty products contain parabens and these parabens can be rapidly absorbed into the skin, especially since many cosmetic preparations contain penetration enhancers. Scientists also agree that parabens in underarm deodorants and other cosmetics should be investigated further, as the findings in tumor samples seem to support the hypothesis that there may be a link between parabens in beauty products and breast cancer. Please note that there is no conclusive evidence that parabens are harmful to humans, but more research is underway.

Isopropyl Alcohol (Isopropanol)

Uses: An anti-bacterial solvent made from petroleum.

Products: Found in shaving creams and other men's skin-care products such as toners. Not a common ingredient these days, as irritation is common.

Problems: Drying and irritating to the skin, it strips your skin's natural acid mantle, making it vulnerable to bacteria and fungus. Can promote liver spots and pigmentation, and can irritate the eyes and skin.

DEA and MEA

Uses: An emulsifier used to mix oil and water in products and a foaming agent to make products lather when rubbed.

Products: Includes any ingredient with DEA or MEA in the name, such as "cocamide MEA." Some shampoos still contain lauramide DEA and cocamide DEA. MEA is common in many commercial products such as shampoos.

> Humans should not inhale MEA vapor because it is highly toxic.

Problems: DEA can cause contact allergies such as skin rashes, and this irritation can occur if a product has a 2% concentration of DEA. Many skin-care manufacturers have removed DEA from their products since negative reports (involving cancer) were published by the National Toxicology Program (NTP) in the United States way back in 1998; however, some still use DEA! According to the "Final Report on the Safety Assessment of Cocamide MEA," humans should not inhale MEA vapor because it is highly toxic. This means MEA shouldn't be used in aerosol products, but MEA is still found in many topical skin-care products. The report also recommended that "cocamide MEA should not be used as an ingredient in cosmetic products in which N-nitroso compounds are formed." But how do you know which products form N-nitroso compounds? You can only trust that the product's manufacturers have ensured their products are compatible with MEA and don't chemically interact to make toxic by-products. And if your beauty product contains MEA, then maybe you'd be wise to avoid using another product at the same time.

Q. Is it true that some skin-care ingredients are absorbed into the skin?

A. Unfortunately, yes! As mentioned earlier, many skin-care products, especially when applied as a patch or cream, contain penetration enhancers. Consider how nicotine patches work: you get a cigarette craving, so you place a clear patch on your arm and nicotine is absorbed through the skin, traveling via your bloodstream until it reaches the nicotine receptor sites on your cells. Your nicotine craving is killed, not by inhaling cigarette smoke, but from a patch located on the outside of your body. It is a similar story with birth control patches. A patch is placed on your skin, hormones are released into your bloodstream, this changes your hormonal balance, and pregnancy is prevented (in most cases). These patches also expose you to about 60% more estrogen than the traditional birth control pill, so they are very potent. So is it reasonable to suggest that skin-care ingredients can be absorbed into your body and influence your health? Yes, of course it is. Children are at higher risk of adverse effects from chemical products because they are small in weight and their bodies are developing at a rapid rate.

Activity

Check your current skin-care products — your moisturizers, cleanser, and even your shampoo and conditioner — and see if you can spot any questionable ingredients.

Fabulous Skin-Care Ingredients

You don't need synthetic ingredients that are infamous for causing skin irritations in your beauty products. There are many healthy alternatives available to protect you from the effects of artificial skin-care products.

Let's look in further detail at some ingredients that are a "must-have" in your skin-care products:

Almond Oil and Sweet Almond Oil

Uses: Anti-bacterial, contains fatty acids and triglycerides to moisturize the skin.

Benefits: Moisturizing, soothes irritation and dryness. Doesn't clog pores, so it is suitable for blemish-prone people.

Alpha Hydroxy Acid (AHA) and Beta Hydroxy Acid (BHA)

Uses: Exfoliates, has an anti-aging effect. For AHA, look for names such as glycolic acid, lactic acid, and malic acid (at least 8% concentration). For BHA, look for salicylic acid (at least 8% concentration). Most products sold in cosmetic department stores have only 4% or less AHA/BHA. You can get products containing more than 8% AHA and BHA from your pharmacy or doctor's office.

Benefits: AHA and BHA improve skin texture by thinning the stratum corneum (via a type of acid exfoliation). They also increase collagen synthesis within the dermis, and they don't damage the skin's barrier function.

Problems: They can make the skin temporarily peel, flake, and look inflamed.

Apple Cider Vinegar

Uses: Disinfectant and mildly acidic.

Benefits: The acid restores the skin's pH balance, does not strip the skin of its beneficial oils.

Beta Glucan

Uses: Antioxidant, anti-aging, moisturizing properties.

Benefits: Extracted from the fermentation process of yeast, it assists in the reduction of wrinkles and helps with skin repair.

Problems: It is a very expensive ingredient, and from what I can tell, scientific evidence is limited.

Blackcurrant Seed Oil

Uses: Anti-inflammatory and moisturizing properties.

Benefits: Contains gamma-linolenic acid (GLA), as in evening primrose oil, making it anti-inflammatory and suitable for reducing skin inflammation, redness, and irritation. A superb moisturizer.

Calendula

Uses: Anti-inflammatory, antiseptic, and astringent.

Benefits: Helps protect against bacteria, such as staphylococcus. Contains carotenoids. Reduces skin inflammation and helps with skin regeneration and healing. Useful for rashes, varicose veins, and bruising.

Carrot Seed Oil

Uses: Moisturizing properties, provides some free radical protection.

Benefits: Antioxidants help protect the skin from sun damage and premature wrinkles. Contains beta-carotene and provitamin A. Often used in natural sun-care products. Good for moisturizing aged skin.

Chamomile

Uses: Astringent, cleansing, anti-bacterial, anti-inflammatory.

Benefits: Contains fatty acids, flavonoids, quercetin, and rutin, which are anti-inflammatory. Calms irritated skin, controls excess oiliness and acne.

Coconut Oil

Uses: Moisturizing properties, anti-fungal, and anti-microbial.

Benefits: Contains capric acid, which is anti-fungal, and lauric acid, which is anti-microbial. Found in your skin's sebum. Protects the skin from microbes and dryness, a traditional and trusted moisturizer.

Evening Primrose Oil

Uses: Anti-inflammatory because it contains gamma-linolenic acid (GLA).

Benefits: Nourishing and rich in essential fatty acid, protects against free-radical damage to the skin.

Green Tea

Uses: Anti-inflammatory, anti-cancer, rich in antioxidants that protect against free-radical damage.

Benefits: Animal studies have found that when applied topically, green tea and green tea polyphenols can suppress some forms of UV-induced skin cancers. However, drinking the tea had an even stronger anti-cancer effect.

Problems: Some people are allergic to green tea.

Jojoba Oil

Uses: Humectant (protects skin from water loss), superior moisturizing properties.

Benefits: Hypoallergenic, contains wax esters and fatty acids. Restores skin's natural pH balance, won't block pores (non-comedogenic), similar to your skin's own sebum.

Lecithin (Derived from Soy)

Uses: A natural emulsifier and humectant with moisturizing properties.

Benefits: Attracts moisture to the skin and works like a detergent to disperse oil, so it allows oily ingredients to mix with water-soluble ingredients for a smoother-looking product.

Olive Oil (Extra Virgin)

Uses: Moisturizing properties. Contains phenolic compounds that protect against free-radical damage.

Benefits: The antioxidant hydroxytyrosol provides some protection against DNA damage and also contains high squalene concentration, vitamin E, and carotenes. Olive oil studies have found that topical application has an anti-cancer effect — it greatly reduces tumor frequency from UVB rays but doesn't eliminate risk of cancer from UVA rays.

Problems: Olive oil can be used on its own, straight from the bottle; however, it may leave oily patches on clothes if too much is used.

Rosehip Oil

Uses: Rich in antioxidants. Rosehips are the richest source of vitamin C. Also has a natural vitamin A derivative (trans-retionoic acid), lycopene, carotenoids, and essential fatty acids (EFAs).

Benefits: EFAs help to maintain collagen and elastin fibers, and may slightly improve appearance of fine lines and wrinkles.

Problems: Some rosehip oil products are bleached and colorless, so the carotenoids have been removed. Good-quality rosehip oil should be a rich amber color.*

Sea Buckthorn Berry Oil

Uses: Moisturizing properties, antioxidant protection. Traditionally, this oil was used for treatment of bruised and battered skin.

Benefits: High in antioxidants, such as vitamins A, C, and E. Anti-inflammatory. Unique 1:1 ratio of omega-3 and omega-6 oils. Omega-3 and omega-6 are essential for healthy skin and antioxidants protect the skin from oxidation caused by UV exposure. Contains 35% palmitoleic acid, a rare and valuable fatty acid that also happens to be a component of our skin's sebum; it supports cell tissues and wound healing, and protects against certain bacteria (known as gram-positive bacteria).

Shea Butter

Uses: An excellent moisturizer, especially for very dry skin.

Benefits: Contains fatty acids and natural UV factor. Moisturizes dry, damaged, and irritated skin, helps improve skin elasticity, healing of irritated skin and small wounds.

Problems: Not suitable for oily/acne-prone skin.

Vitamin A/Retinol

Uses: A natural preservative. Certain forms of vitamin A have a potent anti-aging effect. Look for names containing "retinol" and "tretinoin."

Benefits: Topical retinoids, such as tretinoin, have been proven to prevent and repair sun-induced skin damage, prevent loss of collagen, and stimulate new collagen formation.

Problems: Retinol and tretinoin can irritate the skin, making you look like a sunburn victim with inflamed, red raw skin for up to a week. You need to use sun protection daily after vitamin A use.

Vitamin C (Ascorbic Acid)

Uses: Natural preservative and antioxidant. Some forms of vitamin C have an anti-aging effect. Look for names such as L ascorbic acid (at least 10% to 15% concentration), ascorbyl palmitate, and magnesium ascorbyl palmitate.

Benefits: Increases elastin tissue growth and collagen production. Decreases UVA and UVB damage to the skin.

Problems: May cause skin irritation in sensitive skin. Skin may be more sensitive to light after use, so apply sunscreen daily.*

Vitamin E (d-Alpha Tocopherol)

Uses: Natural preservative and antioxidant.

Benefits: Helps protect your skin against sun damage and oxidation, protects against free-radical formation within your skin product. May improve circulation and aid new skin cell formation.

Problems: 100% vitamin E oil may cause browning of the skin if you use it over scars. Avoid synthetic vitamin E, which is identifiable by "dl" (dl-alpha tocopherol).

Xanthan Gum

Uses: A natural emulsifier used to keep the texture of a skin-care product uniform and prevent separation.

Benefits: A healthy alternative to chemical emulsifiers.

Sunscreen should play a starring role in your long-term quest for younger-looking skin. When going out in the sun, make sure you apply sunscreen to the parts of your body that age the fastest — your face, neck, décolletage, and hands. If choosing a non-zinc-based sunscreen, look for one that is formulated for children or toddlers because these products are more likely to be fragrance-free and lower in synthetic chemicals. And they are just as effective as adult sunscreens. Always reapply sunscreen every 2 hours or after sweating or swimming.

Zinc Oxide (in Sunscreens)

Uses: Zinc oxide is a sunscreen ingredient.

Benefits: Helps protect against sunburn, suitable for reducing skin pigmentation. Look for sunscreen that is "broad spectrum" with an SPF factor above 20 (SPF 20+) and high zinc oxide content (above 12%).

Problems: Sunscreen can make some skin types look pasty; if this occurs, you can use bronzer for a healthy glow. If you have very dry skin, zinc oxide may make your skin feel drier.*

(Thanks to cosmetic physician Dr Van Huynh-Park from Concept Cosmetic Medicine (Sydney), and Snezna Kerekovic from Bellaboo (teenage skin care) for supplying ingredient information as indicated by an asterisk.)

Caution

UVA rays from sun exposure and tanning beds penetrate the skin and cause free-radical damage that disrupts collagen and elastin fibers, which leads to wrinkles. Sunscreens don't adequately protect against UVA, so it is also necessary to wear a hat. For more information, see Guideline #6 (page 109).

CASE STUDY

I've always had very dry skin and was only prone to pimples during my teenage years. However, in my early 30s I bought a cleanser for oily skin by mistake. The first night I used the cleanser I noticed my skin felt tight and dry immediately afterwards, so I applied moisturizer (as usual) and pretty soon my skin felt okay. However, within a week of using the cleanser that was supposed to help oily skin, I had developed oily skin; I broke out in pimples and my pores became unusually large! My skin continued to feel unnaturally squeaky clean after cleansing. I threw away the product and bought a cleanser that didn't dry out my skin. My pores quickly returned to their normal size, but it took about a month for my skin to normalize and stop getting pimples.

Skin Types

You also need to consider what condition your skin is in before you choose a safe and effective beauty product. There are several problematic skin types that can change to a more normal condition if you eat the right foods and look after yourself mentally and physically.

Normal skin: Feels supple and looks hydrated. It is not overly sensitive and has even pigmentation. May occasionally get out of balance and have an oily T-zone (forehead, nose, chin), small breakouts, or dry patches.

Dry or mature skin: Has trouble staying hydrated, gets flaky, may peel or feel tight and dry. May have premature aging or sun damage. Super-dry skin requires a non-foaming cream cleanser, plus a heavier moisturizer or barrier cream to relieve discomfort, and regular exfoliation.

Very dry skin: Nothing seems to soothe this skin type except a thick barrier cream and dietary changes. Weekly exfoliation is also recommended.

Oily or impure skin: Oily, especially in the T-zone, enlarged or blocked pores, poor circulation, blemishes. Dietary changes are required to normalize skin. In the meantime, use lighter-textured products, nothing heavy.

Sensitive skin: Easily irritated by weather, skin-care products, and food allergies. Red, inflamed skin, blotchy, patches of dryness, includes rosacea and eczema. Super-sensitive skin conditions require a basic skin-care routine, with plain cleansers and creams that contain little or no essential oils or harsh chemicals. Exfoliation may not be suitable.

Combination skin: Oily T-zone and normal cheeks. Prone to minor breakouts in T-zone, skin is slightly out of balance; use products that won't aggravate/block pores. Don't exfoliate, as it may spread pimples.

Choosing and Using a Cleanser

A cleanser is a type of skin product that is used to dislodge dirt, pollution, and makeup. Some cleansers foam, others are thick and creamy with no bubbles, and some are soaps or soap-free bars. You apply the cleanser directly to your wet face using cotton balls or a damp cloth, wipe the cloth or cotton balls over your face and neck to remove residues, then wash off the remaining cleanser with water. Many cleansers are specifically formulated for oily skin and contain ingredients that strip the skin's natural oils. I call it the squeaky clean effect because your skin feels tight and dry after use. However, too much of your sebum is cleansed away with these products, which is not ideal because you want some sebum on your skin. Sebum is your skin's best friend because it helps to protect your body from invading bacteria, wind, and dry conditions.

If your skin feels tight and dry within a minute after cleansing, then the product is too harsh. You don't want that squeaky clean feeling. A good cleanser can remove dirt and pollution, and some excess oils, without stripping your skin of all its protective sebum.

Moisturizers

It's important to choose a moisturizer that is right for your current skin type. The only exception is if you have oily, impure, and acne-prone skin; then you may not need a moisturizer at all, or you could use a specific "normalizing" oil to help reduce excess sebum production. If you have extremely sensitive skin, choose a moisturizer with plainer ingredients, such as almond oil, and steer clear of too many essential oils. Dry and very dry or mature skin needs a heavier moisturizer, especially in winter. Before purchasing a moisturizer, check the full ingredient list and, if possible, test it on a patch of skin to see if any irritation occurs.

Q. I've had my favorite eyeshadows for years; in fact, I think they were originally my mother's from the 1990s. Are they still okay to use?

A. The answer is a big fat NO! Makeup deteriorates over time. Bacteria from your fingers can contaminate makeup products, and when you use them you may end up with adverse reactions, such as rashes and bacterially infected blemishes. Hand-me-down makeup, no matter how pretty it is, should never be used in different decades. As a general rule, makeup should be replaced within 3 years after leaving the factory.

Makeup

Makeup can also have a place in your skin-care routine (though perhaps not if you are a man). For those who want to use it, it can be useful to cover up a stray blemish, highlight your gorgeous features, or give the illusion of fabulous bone structure.

Activity

Wash your makeup brushes and sponges today. After that, wash your makeup brushes and other applicators at least once a week to remove bacteria that can cause skin infections. And avoid sharing makeup, especially eye makeup products, because you can spread bacterial infections.

Guide to Makeup "Use-By" and Expiration Dates

Once you have opened a product:

- Mascara can last for 3 to 6 months, but it is easily contaminated because of the pumping action of the brush, which can push bacteria to the bottom of the container.
- Moisturizer can last for 3 to 12 months.
- Foundation and concealer can last for 12 to 18 months.
- Powder, eyeliner, lipstick, and lip liner can last for about 2 years.
- Blusher and eyeshadow can last for 1 to 2 years.

When a product deteriorates, you may see a change in texture and consistency or it may smell off. Natural products that are free of chemical preservatives (they use natural preservatives such as herbs) generally don't last as long. However, these products usually have package information advising how long they will last after opening.

Skin-Care Routine

Here is an example of a simple skin-care regimen, suitable for most people. However, if you have acne, see the chapter on acne care, starting on page 147.

Morning

1. Wash hands with a gentle hand wash to remove any bacteria, then rinse off with water.
2. Fill a basin or large bowl with very warm water and splash your face four to six times. (If you cleansed your face the night before, then you don't strictly need to use a cleanser in the morning; in fact, I think it is better to avoid overcleaning your face so that your natural oils can work their magic. However, if you have oily and acne-prone skin, you'll need to cleanse now.) You can also cleanse while having a shower.
3. After patting your skin dry, add a small amount of moisturizer to your fingertips and pat it onto your skin, repeating if necessary until your entire face and neck is lightly covered with lotion. Use moisturizers sparingly. Blot skin with a tissue after applying if necessary.
4. If you're going out in the sun today, apply sunscreen after moisturizing.

Note: You may notice that I recommend patting the moisturizer onto your skin rather than rubbing. This will help you to use much less product (saving you money and reducing waste). It is also a more gentle way to handle the skin. This pressing motion helps to relax your facial muscles, which may reduce stress wrinkles.

Night

1. Wash your hands to remove any bacteria.
2. Fill a basin or bowl with warm water and rinse your face, splashing water onto your face and neck several times.
3. Apply your cleanser of choice — gently rub cleanser onto your face and neck.
4. Then wet two cotton balls or a soft exfoliating cloth and gently wipe off the cleanser, pollution, and makeup. Repeat if necessary.
5. Rinse the cleanser off thoroughly with warm water. If you have dry and flaky skin, then you may want to also exfoliate now (see "How to exfoliate your face" on page 142).
6. Apply a suitable moisturizer, using patting motions on the face and neck.

Exfoliating Your Skin

Exfoliating removes dead skin cells that tend to look flaky and dry so your skin will appear more smooth and hydrated. Your skin may be a little red afterwards, especially if you have sensitive skin, but this should only last about 5 minutes. It is not absolutely essential to exfoliate, but if you have dry skin, flaky skin, or wrinkles and premature aging, then a granulated cream or a quick scrub will leave your skin looking and feeling softer and smoother. However, you must take care not to use harsh exfoliators that can scratch the delicate skin on your face. This facial scratching may be visible and unattractive, so you really do need to exfoliate with care. Don't exfoliate your skin if you have acne or broken skin, such as wounds, bites, or rashes. Exfoliating may spread pimples.

> Exfoliating removes dead skin cells that tend to look flaky and dry so your skin will appear more smooth and hydrated.

Q. What is the best time to exfoliate and what equipment do I need?

A. The best time to exfoliate is at nighttime, before bed, so that any skin redness will subside during sleep and you'll wake up with fresh, hydrated-looking skin. Exfoliating scrubs are creams and gels that contain granules or beads. These microscopic beads polish the skin as you rub them in a circular motion on your face and body. Choose a facial exfoliator with spherical beads because they are the most gentle and effective. For the body, you can use mitts, natural body scrubs, or dry-skin brushing. Unfortunately, natural exfoliators can do the most damage because they use natural abrasives, such as crushed apricot kernels, which have sharp edges.

Did You Know?

You Must Know This!

Keep in mind that your skin-care routine should suit your lifestyle, your skin type, and your budget. Don't ever stress yourself by spending too much money on skin creams. Stress ages you prematurely, which negates any positive effects a miracle cream may have. And besides, you just can't look your best when you are having a panic attack about your finances.

How to exfoliate your face

1. Use a cream or gel containing gentle spherical beads.
2. After cleansing and rinsing your face with warm water, apply a pea-sized amount of exfoliator to your fingertips and softly rub in a circular motion onto your face and neck (use more exfoliator if necessary).
3. Rinse with warm water. Pat skin dry, then moisturize.
4. Use an exfoliator once or twice a week or whenever you skin develops flaky patches.

How to exfoliate your body

1. Have a quick shower.
2. Then spread a generous amount of scrub onto your damp skin and massage it with circular motions. Start at the feet and work your way up toward the heart (this is also how you use the exfoliator mitts).
3. Then exfoliate from your hands to your shoulders, your chest, and as much of your back as possible (a dry-skin brush is useful for exfoliating the back).
4. Rinse thoroughly with water by showering and then moisturize. Your body should feel deliciously soft!

An inexpensive way to exfoliate your body (but not your face) is to use exfoliating mitts or a dry-skin, long-handled body brush. If you are using an exfoliator mitt or glove (which feels rough, like Velcro), wet the mitt first, then apply a natural body wash or gel to the mitt, then exfoliate your damp skin and rinse off the body wash.

Quick Tips for Selecting and Applying Beauty Aids

- Establish a safe, gentle, and effective daily skin-care routine. Your skin type can change as your diet changes, so be prepared to alter your routine.
- Don't be fooled by product advertising. Check ingredient lists and test the product on your skin before purchasing it, if possible. Avoid harmful ingredients, such as sodium lauryl sulfate.
- Use products that include items from the list of "fabulous skin care ingredients."
- Don't fuss too much with your skin.

Review of the Eight Guidelines for Healthy Skin

I **hope you** enjoyed the Eight Guidelines for Healthy Skin. As you implement each guideline into your life, expect that you are creating beautiful skin. Remember, it takes 4 to 6 weeks for new skin cells to form and come to the surface, so it won't take very long to see positive results. Let's quickly recount the guidelines so you know the main points to remember. You may notice that I have excluded what to avoid doing. This is because you don't want to focus on what not to do; you only need to remember what you can do to create gorgeous skin and long-term health and vitality.

Guideline #1: Think Green and Friendly (Restoring Your pH Balance)

- Hydrate yourself with 8 to 10 glasses of fluids daily OR one to two bottles of Green Water.
- Eat alkalizing foods daily: salads, cooked and raw vegetables, avocado, almonds, banana, fresh lemon, lime, and apple cider vinegar.
- Eat two handfuls of dark green leafy vegetables every day.

Guideline #2: Moisturize Your Skin from the Inside Out (Eating Great Fats)

- Consume healthy fats, namely omega-3 (EPA and DHA) essential fatty acids from oily fish and flaxseed, and omega-6 (GLA) EFAs from evening primrose oil (EPO) and other foods.
- Eat fish two to three times per week (trout and sardines are the best choices because they are lower in acid).
- Take 1 to 2 tablespoons (15 to 30 mL) of ground flax seeds or flaxseed oil every day.
- Take 1 tablespoon (15 mL) of lecithin granules daily to help you digest the moisturizing oils properly.

- If you have dry skin, psoriasis, rosacea, dandruff, or wrinkles and premature aging, take an omega-3 fish oil supplement, or flaxseed oil if you are vegetarian.

Guideline #3: Eat Less (Controlling Your Carbs and Protein)

- Remember that sensible calorie restriction (no more than 30%) promotes youthful skin and good-quality sleep.
- Eat less, but don't starve yourself! Excessive dieting is bad for the skin, so be sensible and never skip a meal. Your food is your fuel, nothing more and nothing less, and if you choose mostly healthy foods and eat a sensible amount, your body will look and feel great.
- For lunches and dinners, fill half your plate with salad or vegetables because they are low in calories. The other half of your plate is reserved for carbohydrates and protein.
- Have approximately three average-sized dinner plates of food each day.
- Choose "Commitment carbs" — whole-grain breads, brown rice, rolled oats, and whole wheat pasta.
- Eat protein every day. As a general guide when eating animal protein, take a portion the size and thickness of the palm of your hand.
- Eat more foods that are great for the skin. From the recipe section of the book, these include Tasty Spinach Salad, Marinated Whole Steamed Trout, Anti-Aging Broth, Flaxseed Lemon Drink, and Skin-Firming Drink.

Guideline #4: Be a Sleeping Beauty (Practicing Good Sleep Habits)

- Remember that adequate sleep is essential for gorgeous skin.
- Get a 10-minute dose of direct sunlight in the morning (before 10 a.m.) to help set your body clock and boost your vitamin D levels.
- Have a nighttime ritual that signifies sleep: take a warm bath or use a warm face cloth, for example.

Guideline #5: Sweat for 15 Minutes a Day (Exercising for Healthier Skin)

- Aim to sweat for 15 minutes a day, but you can sweat for longer if you want to (keep exercise under 2 hours).

Guideline #6: Be a Hat Person (Avoiding UV Light Exposure)

- Wear a hat and apply sunscreen if you're spending time in the sun.

Guideline #7: Relax (Making Peace with Your Body)

- Make time to relax. A person who makes relaxation a priority for a few moments each day is more likely to have great skin.
- Make peace with your body by complimenting yourself often.

Guideline #8: Follow a Good Skin-Care Routine (Selecting Safe and Effective Beauty Aids)

- When choosing a beauty product, check the ingredient list and test the product on your skin.
- Establish a routine for safely cleansing and exfoliating your skin.

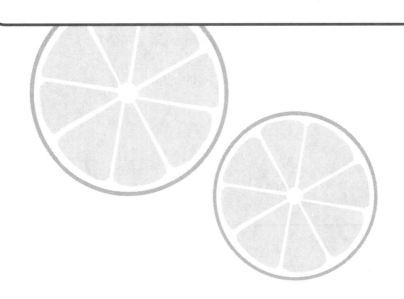

Part 4
Specialized Programs

Acne Care

Acne vulgaris can appear as tender red bumps, small white nodules, blackheads, and deep, painful, pus-filled cysts that can lead to scarring. The face, back, chest, and shoulders are the major problem spots. Sufferers can experience embarrassment, poor self-esteem, anxiety, and depression as a result of their appearance. Acne can be treated effectively with natural methods that are not only good for your entire body but also free of harmful side effects.

Did You Know?

Incidence and Prevalence

According to medical studies, acne has been clinically diagnosed in children as young as 4, and as many as 93% of students between age 16 and 18 can experience acne, with one in four of these students also having acne scars. However, acne is not just reserved for the young. In the United States, approximately 85% of 12- to 24-year-olds have acne.

Q. What causes acne?

A. I am sick of hearing, "There's no known cause for acne," "Acne is not caused by diet," and "Acne is caused by the sebaceous glands producing too much oil." The truth is, a lot is known about the causes of acne: acne can be caused by diet; some people do have breakouts after eating chocolate (or is it just me?); and the sebaceous glands are not the cause of acne — excess oil production is a symptom of something deeper happening in the body (or from something simple, such as using the wrong cleanser to wash your skin).

Let's look at the basic symptom of acne, without confusing it with the cause. Acne is inflammation of the skin's oil glands. When you have acne, the glands grow unnaturally large and produce too much sebum, which appears oily. This oily layer then mixes with the skin's natural bacteria and dead skin cells. This liquid becomes thicker, like pancake batter, blocking the skin's pores, which leads to acne.

Composition and Function of Sebum

Sebum is a mix of fats, proteins, cholesterol, salts, and pheromones (FYI: pheromones are your sexual attraction hormones, so you don't want to cleanse them away!).

- Sebum is your skin's best friend. It keeps the skin soft, prevents excessive water loss, and helps inhibit bacteria growth on the skin.
- Sebum coats the surface of your hair to prevent it from becoming dry and brittle.

Standard acne topical creams and cleansers treat the surface symptoms, such as bacterial infection and excess sebum, but remember that these symptoms are never the cause of your acne; they just have been triggered by something.

Did You Know?

Psychological Impact

Suffering from a serious skin condition can be depressing. It can cause social phobias, missed employment opportunities, and, if not treated, in very severe cases it can lead to suicidal tendencies. In the *Journal of Paediatrics and Child Health*, a study was conducted on 10,000 high school students in New Zealand and the results showed a strong link between severe skin problems and depression and suicide. The findings were very disturbing: one in three teenagers with severe acne had suicidal thoughts and more than one in ten had tried to kill themselves.

Assessment

Let's assess what may be contributing to your acne problem. Do you relate to any of the following factors that contribute to acne?

- Poor diet
- High dairy product consumption
- Hormonal changes
- Oral contraceptives
- Steroid medications
- Trauma and emotional stress
- Overuse of cosmetics
- Irritation from tight clothing
- Harsh cleansers and soaps

Drug Therapies

Many people turn to drug therapies to treat their acne. However, treating acne with medications is not only ineffective but also a potential health hazard with all sorts of side effects, including severe depression.

- Accutane (also known as Roaccutane and by the generic name isotretinoin) is often prescribed for chronic acne; however, the US Food and Drug Administration ranks it as one of the top 10 drugs that can cause depression and lead to suicide attempts.
- Antibiotics are often prescribed for acne vulgaris because they suppress acne-related bacterial infections (known as propionibacterium acnes). Antibiotics can become ineffective, however, due to emerging antibiotic-resistant strains. Antibiotics also wipe out the good gut bacteria that are necessary for a healthy gastrointestinal tract, and negative side effects, such as *Candida albicans* (a yeast infection), and future skin problems can result. So, as you can see, drugs are clearly not the answer.

Acne Management Program

The anti-acne program clears up blemished skin from the inside out. This program addresses the true causes of acne and goes beyond treating the surface symptoms by offering scientific ways to prevent your skin from breaking out. For your convenience, this whole program has been divided into five steps.

Step 1: Follow a Suitable Skin-Care Routine

If you have acne, you need an extra-gentle skin-care routine. You want to soothe the inflammation, minimize bacteria, and keep your skin clean without stripping all of its protective oils. Cleansing acne-prone skin offers some special challenges.

Moisturizing Acne-Prone Skin

If you are not using any medicated treatments for your acne and if your skin is excessively oily, you may not need a moisturizer at all. However, if you want to normalize your skin, a good moisturizer, with the right ingredients, can

---

Q. Should I use toners on my acne?

A. No. Do not you use toners on acne-prone skin. See Guideline #8 (page 138). In fact, never use toners on any skin problems.

How to cleanse acne-prone skin

First, choose the right cleansing product for you:

- Avoid using overly drying cleansers and soaps. If your face feels "squeaky clean" or overly dry immediately after cleansing, this product is wrong for you.

- Avoid irritating ingredients, such as sodium lauryl sulfate (unfortunately, this synthetic foaming agent is in most cleansers).

- Read Guideline #8 again for information on suitable cleansers and ingredients.

Second, follow this procedure:

1. Because unwashed hands may harbor bacteria, wash them clean before touching your face.

2. After washing your hands thoroughly, fill a small basin with warm water. Splash your face with water.

3. Apply to your fingertips one to two pea-sized drops of cleanser. Gently apply cleanser to your face and neck.

4. Use an exfoliating cleansing cloth (one specifically for acne) to remove the cleanser, or you can wet two cotton balls/pads, wring them out, and then gently wipe off the cleanser with them. You may need to repeat this process to remove makeup and excess oils.

5. Rinse your face with water at least six times to remove cleanser thoroughly.

6. Softly pat dry your skin with a clean towel.

help you do this. According to Dr. Rudolf Hauschka, acne sufferers can use a normalizing oil or skin product during the day and skip the moisturizer at night. Wearing no face product at night allows the skin to remove metabolic wastes as you sleep.

How to choose moisturizers for acne-prone skin

Look for moisturizers containing the following ingredients:

- Sweet almond oil
- Apricot kernel oil
- Chamomile
- Tea tree oil
- St John's wort (*Hypericum perforatum*)
- Vitamin E, d-alpha tocopherol
- Calendula
- Neem oil
- Jojoba oil
- Sea buckthorn berry oil
- Macadamia nut oil
- Alpha hydroxy acid (AHA)
- Beta hydroxy acid (BHA)

AHA and BHA have an exfoliating effect that helps to remove dead skin cells without damaging the skin (see Guideline #8, page 131).

How to apply moisturizer to acne-prone skin

1. If you have pimples or inflamed skin, after cleansing and drying your skin, apply a pea-sized amount of moisturizer to your fingertips.
2. Apply moisturizer to your acne-free skin first, to limit the risk of cross-contamination. Pat moisturizer lightly onto your skin.
3. Then apply it to the rest of your face and neck. Repeat the process if necessary.
4. If you have applied too much moisturizer, blot with a tissue (however, using the patting method should help prevent excess application of skin-care products and minimize the risk of blocking pores).

Q. Can I apply sunscreen on acne-prone skin?

A. This is a tough one … Applying sunscreen over acne or on acne-prone skin can often make it worse or cause new breakouts. If this is true for you, then I suggest you become a hat person. It is so important to protect your sensitive, acne-ravaged skin from UV rays; excess sun exposure may contribute to acne scarring.

Once your skin normalizes (after following the Healthy Skin Diet), you may find that you can use sunscreen without suffering any negative reactions. When you have acne, light moisturizers that also contain an SPF factor are less likely to trigger breakouts than sunscreen products. Do a patch test first.

Q. How come I always get a pimple just before I go out on a date and what can I do to clear it up quickly?

A. The universe seems to have a wacky unwritten law that states that you must get a pimple before a hot date, school dance, formal occasion, or much-anticipated night out. Special events can stir up stress chemicals in the body, which can trigger the appearance of a stray pimple or three. If this occurs, you may need to manage your stress a little better. The chapter on "Beauty Breathing" (page 281) provides techniques to help you relax without having to suddenly get a new perspective or change how you react to the world around you.

Salt Water Bath Remedies

If a pimple has already reared its ugly head, you could try the following salt water remedies:

1. Swim in salt water. Swimming in the ocean has a reputation for clearing up pimples. The natural salt water seems to initiate healing as if by magic. This is because salt water has mild anti-bacterial qualities and it is also alkaline, so it helps to normalize sebum production (your skin has an acid mantle, but your blood and tissues should be slightly alkaline). If possible, go for a swim in the ocean, dunking your whole body under the surface at

least three times. Do this at least twice a week, more often if it is convenient. Don't wash off the salt water for about half an hour after your swim, if at all. If you don't live near the sea, you can go swimming in a salt water pool or make your own salt water face bath at home (see below).

How to take a salt water face bath

1. Wash your hands and make sure your face is clean and free of makeup.
2. Then fill a bowl with warm water, add $\frac{1}{2}$ cup (125 mL) of natural sea salt, and mix until dissolved (to speed up the dissolving process, add the salt to a cup of boiling water, stir, and disperse in lukewarm water).
3. Splash your face with salt water or hold face under water, on and off, for a few seconds each time. This should take about 1 minute.
4. Then wash off salt with fresh water and moisturize. You can reuse this salt bath twice. To reheat it, just add some boiling water or briefly heat it up on your stove. Always test the temperature before use: it should be pleasant.

Step 2: Help Your Liver Remove Excess Hormones

Why aren't your skin's sebaceous glands behaving like normal glands? There are several reasons. One involves hormonal changes in the body. During puberty, a surge in hormones, such as androgenic, or sex, hormones, occurs. Boys and girls both have androgens, such as testosterone, but boys usually have more. These androgens tell your sebaceous glands how much oil to produce, and too many hormones give too many signals saying, "More oil, more oil!" Your oil glands grow bigger in order to fill the "more oil" command. As I said before, this excess oil then mixes with dead skin cells and bacteria, and this blocks your pores.

Did You Know?

Spot Treatments

Other quick spot treatments of blemishes include tea tree oil and products containing benzoyl peroxide or salicylic acid.

- **Tea tree oil:** Studies have found that topical use of tea tree oil (at 5% strength) can be an effective treatment for mild to moderate pimples (but not severe acne). Tea tree oil has anti-inflammatory and broad-spectrum anti-bacterial and anti-fungal properties. Dab a tiny amount directly onto your pimple and allow it to dry. Do not moisturize over the top.

- **Benzoyl peroxide (BP):** This strong chemical ingredient is used in commercial acne creams. BP works by destroying the bacteria associated with acne. It acts as an antiseptic and reduces the number of blocked pores. However, it is a very harsh ingredient that has temporary side effects, such as mild to major skin dryness, severe irritation, and redness.

- **Salicylic acid:** This mild acid ingredient is used in some over-the-counter acne treatments. It dissolves dead skin cells and helps to prevent clogged pores, whiteheads, and blackheads. When using salicylic acid, don't use any other medicated creams containing BP or sulfur. Salicylic acid may sting on application and cause redness and irritation.

- **Natural antiseptics:** Sweat and salt water can be just as effective as BP and salicylic acid (and kinder to your face) when managing acne symptoms.

Did You Know?

Hormone Regulation

Your hormones regulate most of your body functions — they dictate your growth cycles, sleep cycles, muscle production, and how much fat you store or burn up. Androgenic hormones trigger the development of sex organs. They can initiate sex drive and increase muscle and bone mass (which is a good thing), so your hormones aren't the enemy. Women can break out with pimples when menstruating because of a temporary increase in hormones. But if all teenagers get a surge in hormones, why do only some get acne? When the teenage body is overflowing with excess androgens, the liver should quickly deactivate and remove excess hormones from the blood. If your liver function is strong, you won't experience acne. However, if your liver is overworked from poor diet and not-so-good lifestyle habits, your blood stays loaded with toxins and hormones.

Adult Acne

Although hormone production should normalize by your early 20s, skin breakouts can still be experienced in adulthood. With adult acne, you have fewer androgenic hormones being released, but if your liver detoxification system is not efficient, higher amounts of hormones remain in the blood, sending out the "more oil" message to your oil glands. The liver's detoxification system slows down if it doesn't have enough of the right nutrients (helpers) to deactivate androgenic hormones. The right nutrients are supplied by healthy food, indicating that acne can be caused by poor diet, along with several other key factors.

Did You Know?

Anti-Acne Nutrients

According to specialists in liver detoxification pathways, there are several key nutrients needed to safely remove sex (androgenic) hormones from your system. They are essential fatty acids, especially omega-3 (DHA and EPA); zinc; magnesium; vitamin B complex (this includes B_1, B_2, B_3, B_5, B_6, biotin, folic acid, B_{12}); and calcium saccharate (formerly known as calcium d-glucurate), which helps to remove excess estrogens from the body. This is a specific type of calcium and other forms of calcium won't do the same task.

Liver-Cleansing Caution

Don't take a liver-cleansing supplement or high-dose vitamin A if you are pregnant or breastfeeding. If you are pregnant, take a multivitamin and mineral supplement that is specific for pregnancy. It should contain the liver nutrients zinc, magnesium, vitamin C, and B vitamins, including folic acid.

Detoxifying the Liver

You can remove excess hormones from your body with a good liver detoxification product. If you are over the age of 15, look for a liver detoxification or cleansing supplement that contains zinc, magnesium, chromium, glycine, taurine, vitamin A, vitamin C, selenium and B vitamins (B_1, B_2, B_3, B_5, B_6, biotin, folic acid, and B_{12}), milk thistle (St Mary's thistle, *Silybum marianum*). If you are female, also look for calcium saccharate in the ingredients list; however, this nutrient is not available in most supplements. Take a liver detoxification supplement for 2 to 4 weeks.

Step 3: Control Your Oil Production

Acne is synonymous with excess sebum, but you can literally control how much oil your skin produces when you ingest nutrients that alter your prostaglandins. Prostaglandins are a lot like project managers in the body — they transfer messages from your cells and they give these messages to your hormones so they can cause modifications in your body. Your prostaglandins alter sebaceous gland secretions so they control how much oil is produced in the skin. Prostaglandins regulate hormones, inflammation, pain, temperature, and fat metabolism. "Good" prostaglandins eliminate inflammation and promote clear skin, while "bad" prostaglandins can promote inflammation and excess oil production.

> "Good" prostaglandins eliminate inflammation and promote clear skin, while "bad" prostaglandins can promote inflammation and excess oil production.

Q. So how do I produce "good" prostaglandins to manage my hormones?

A. There are also good and bad project managers out there — you've probably heard at least one horror story about a bad builder who hired a dodgy plumber or botched the flooring on a home renovation. It's the same with your prostaglandins — some give out undesirable instructions to hormones, so inflammation and skin breakouts occur. So, no doubt, you want to hire the good prostaglandins to make your skin look as healthy as possible. You can do this simply by modifying your diet. Good prostaglandins are made when you eat very specific healthy foods and have a balanced life, which includes relaxation and learning how to cope with daily stress. Bad prostaglandins are manufactured by the body from foods containing saturated fats, especially fried foods that have damaged, or trans, fats. Stress, anxiety, and high glycemic index foods (such as pastries and other white flour products) also trigger a reaction that causes the production of "bad" prostaglandins (see Guideline #2 for more information).

Choosing Supplements to Manage Skin Oil Production

Although you should try to get all nutrients from good food sources, you may need to supplement your food with essential fatty acids, vitamins, and minerals.

Omega-3 essential fatty acids

It's not always possible to eat a perfect diet and be relaxed and stress-free, but you can begin to be healthy by eating the main ingredient for good prostaglandins — the essential fatty acid called omega-3. Omega-3 was discussed in more detail in Guideline #2, but here are the basics again:

- Unsaturated fatty acids, such as omega-3, are anti-inflammatory.
- Omega-3 provides anti-bacterial substances for healthy sebum production.
- Omega-3 has to be converted to EPA and DHA to make the good prostaglandins and beautiful skin.
- EPA and DHA are readily available in fish and fish oil supplements.

If you're eating fish, such as salmon, trout, or sardines, at least twice a week and adding flax seeds to your diet, then you should be getting enough omega-3 from your diet. Note that flasxeed oil can increase skin oil production, so avoid it if you have acne.

Zinc

> Oil gland activity is also regulated by zinc, so zinc supplement-ation is very specific for treating acne.

Zinc is another nutrient vital for acne-free skin. Zinc helps to convert the fats found in nuts and seeds (omega-6) into good prostaglandins. Zinc is needed to manufacture (and release) many hormones, including the sex hormones as well as insulin and growth hormones. Oil gland activity is also regulated by zinc, so zinc supplementation is very specific for treating acne.

Zinc is vital for teenagers. During your teenage years, you develop at a rapid rate, and this requires lots of zinc. Growth spurts can lead to zinc deficiency, which is bad news because the skin is the first to suffer when your body doesn't have enough of this mineral. The skin is low on the body's priority list when your zinc is depleted — what little zinc you have is used for more important jobs, such as DNA replication and fertility.

Zinc Deficiency Questionnaire

See if you have any signs of zinc deficiency by completing this zinc deficiency questionnaire. Check off any lifestyle habits or symptoms you experience on a regular basis (three or more times per week):

- ☐ Acne/pimples
- ☐ Stretch marks
- ☐ White, coated tongue
- ☐ White spots on fingernails
- ☐ Impotence
- ☐ Infertility
- ☐ Frequent infections
- ☐ "Frizzy" hair or hair loss
- ☐ Poor wound healing
- ☐ Poor sense of taste
- ☐ Poor sense of smell
- ☐ Testicular atrophy
- ☐ Drinking alcohol every week

Taste Test

If you checked off more than three symptoms, you may have a zinc deficiency. However, it's best to also do a zinc taste test to confirm if you have a true deficiency. Speak to a naturopathic doctor or nutritionist at your local health food shop about doing a zinc taste test. All you do is have a measured dose of liquid zinc and hold it in your mouth for a few seconds before swallowing it. Your taste buds will indicate the degree of need for zinc supplementation:

- If you have a deficiency, the mixture will taste pleasant, like water, or leave a furry feeling in the mouth.
- If you do not have a deficiency, the liquid will taste metallic or foul and you'll probably want to spit it out.

Causes of Zinc Deficiency

Zinc deficiency is very common and can be caused by:

- High calcium and salt intake. Canned food is high in salt and dairy products are rich in calcium, and too much of either can create a zinc deficiency. Zinc, sodium, and calcium compete with each other for absorption. Iron deficiency is also common from having too much dairy food, and copper deficiency can also occur.
- Alcoholic beverages. Zinc is needed to detoxify alcohol, so drinking alcoholic beverages is probably the fastest way to diminish zinc stores.
- Stress, coffee, tea, high-fiber diets, menstruation, and ejaculation (semen contains approximately 1 to 3 mg of zinc per ejaculation) all deplete zinc.

If you are deficient in zinc, you will need to use supplements.

- Adults (over the age of 15 years) who are suffering with acne require a supplement of 12 to 20 mg of zinc per day, plus zinc from food sources.
- Children between 9 and 15 years of age with acne should have 8 to 11 mg of zinc per day, plus food sources.
- Children 4 to 8 years with acne need to have 5 mg of zinc per day, plus zinc from food sources.

Note that fiber-rich foods and other supplements containing calcium, iron, and phosphorus can prevent zinc supplements from being adequately absorbed, so take your zinc supplement 2 hours apart from these substances. Take zinc for at least 2 months. Once your acne clears, stop taking the zinc supplement but continue to eat zinc-rich foods.

Did You Know?

Great Results

There is good scientific evidence that zinc supplementation is effective at eliminating acne. A group of scientists who treated acne sufferers with zinc oral supplementation found at the end of the 4-week study that, of the group who took zinc sulfate, 85% were acne-free. This is a great result!

Caution

Do not take zinc supplements if you have copper deficiency or if you are taking tetracycline (a drug for infections) because zinc competes for absorption with copper and may make your medical treatment less effective. Do not exceed the prescribed dosage.

Good Food Sources of Zinc

- Bran flakes
- Chickpeas
- Oysters (a serving of 6 medium oysters contains a whopping 76.4 mg of zinc)
- Roasted soybeans
- Rolled oats
- Red meat, such as liver
- Watercress salad
- Wheat germ

Dairy products

Milk and other dairy products are associated with acne outbreaks. Researchers from one particular study said that dairy consumption increased the risk of acne and this may have been due to the animal hormones and bioactive molecules found in milk products. Dairy products also contain small amounts of arachidonic acid (AA), which is the main building material for "bad" prostaglandins that increase

CASE STUDY

A patient visited our clinic complaining of always having a red, bumpy chin. The bumps looked like blind pimples, and they seemed to get worse when she was trying to eat what she thought was a healthy diet. I asked her what she was eating, and she told me that every day she was making fruit and protein smoothies using a quart (1 L) of low-fat milk and eating low-fat yogurt and cottage cheese with a salad and rye bread. I explained to her that her skin problem was likely linked to her dairy product consumption. Smoothie and milkshake addictions seem to go hand in hand with red chins. I looked for other signs of dairy sensitivity, specifically a runny nose (post-nasal drip), fatigue, fluid retention, and skin rashes. She confirmed experiencing these symptoms from time to time. I advised her to avoid dairy for at least 2 months during the Healthy Skin Diet (which is dairy-free). After her acne cleared up, she could resume eating dairy products in moderate amounts, eating one serving a day each of plain yogurt, milk in coffee/tea, and ricotta cheese on whole-grain bread. Plain yogurt that contains healthy live bacteria, such as acidophilus, is the best dairy option. She will also need to get her calcium from non-dairy sources, such as tahini, almonds, and dark green leafies, such as watercress. See Guideline #2 for a full list of non-dairy calcium sources.

Smoothie and
milkshake
addictions
seem to go
hand in hand
with red chins.
Removing dairy
from your diet,
for a minimum
of 2 months,
helps to
eliminate acne
quickly.

oil gland activity. Dairy is an acid-forming food group (see Guideline #1 for more information, and pay particular attention to this information because it is very relevant to your skin care). Dairy products also exert an insulin response, and foods that trigger excessive insulin are linked with acne and premature aging. Removing dairy from your diet, for a minimum of 2 months, helps to eliminate acne quickly.

Chromium

If you suffer from acne, you may be deficient in the mineral chromium. Chromium is essential for the metabolism of glucose; without chromium in your diet, you can end up with too much glucose floating around in your blood, and this may lead to skin breakouts and more serious conditions, such as type 2 diabetes and associated skin ulcers. For more information, see Guideline #3 and review the chromium deficiency questionnaire to see if you need a chromium supplement.

Vitamin A

Vitamin A is also important for healthy, acne-free skin because it helps to reduce oil production if your glands are overstimulated. However, scientific studies have shown that zinc is more effective than vitamin A supplementation in eliminating acne. Get your vitamin A or its precursor, beta-carotene, from your diet.

Activity

Control your oil gland production by supplementing with zinc for the duration of the Healthy Skin Diet (8 weeks). Commence taking these supplements after you have taken a liver detoxification supplement for 2 weeks. This is partly for the convenience of not taking too many supplements all at once, and also so you don't double up on zinc intake.

Step 4: Improve Your Bowel Health

If your gut is slow to remove waste products, your skin will have to help "put out the garbage," so to speak.

Bowel health is essential for clear skin. If your gut is slow to remove waste products, your skin will have to help "put out the garbage," so to speak. Remember, your skin is one of the body's major eliminatory organs, so you don't want it to have to compensate for poor waste elimination, constipation, or microbe overgrowth. Poor bowel health can also cause smelly gas, abdominal discomfort, bloating, and food allergies and sensitivities. It is very important to eat the right foods for good bowel health.

Choosing Foods for Good Bowel Health

1. **Eat insoluble fiber from fiber-rich carbohydrates and vegetables.** A high-fiber diet is essential for clearing up acne. Fiber binds to and removes toxins from the colon and promotes healthy bacteria in the gastrointestinal tract, also minimizing the bad bacteria and fungus that can cause undesirable skin conditions. Eat whole-grain products, such as brown rice, whole-grain bread, whole wheat pasta, dark green leafy vegetables, sweet potatoes, and other vegetables.

2. **Eat soluble fiber from apples and pears.** Apples and pears also contain pectin, which promotes healthy bowel movements and beneficial gut flora. Remember to drink plenty of water, exercise, and relax (and be confident) because stress causes all sorts of gastrointestinal disturbances, such as ulcers and irritable bowel syndrome.

3. **Drink a liquid chlorophyll supplement.** Liquid chlorophyll contains magnesium and chromium. This supplement helps to prevent constipation, deodorizes the body, and helps to cleanse the liver. Drink one bottle of Green Water daily. See Guideline #1 for more information about chlorophyll. Pay particular attention to the 3-Day Alkalizing Cleanse, because this cleansing program is great for improving acne. You also find out how to make pleasant-tasting Green Water in the recipe section.

Step 5: Exercise and Sweat

Although I am a nutritionist, I must say that you shouldn't rely solely on diet and supplements to make all your pimples disappear because true holistic health comes from having a balanced life. For fantastic skin and long-term health, I recommend that you also exercise and sweat. When done on a regular basis, exercise will change your health like nothing else and it will enable you to have clear skin without having to have a perfect diet.

For the value of exercise and sweat in treating acne, review Guideline #5. Remember that moderate exercise decreases skin inflammation, sweat is anti-bacterial, and exercise promotes healthy bowels and elimination of wastes.

> When done on a regular basis, exercise will change your health like nothing else and it will enable you to have clear skin without having to have a perfect diet.

Recipes for Acne Care

1. **To get more omega-3 in your diet:** Eat recipes with fish (salmon, trout, sardines, mackerel, herring) at least twice a week, and eat omega-3 rich eggs, walnuts, and flax seeds on a regular basis. Recipes include Salmon Steaks with Peas and Mash; Rainbow Trout with Honey-Roasted Vegetables; Salmon and Salad Sandwich; Marinated Whole Steamed Trout; and Salmon, Smoked Salmon and Eggs.

2. **If you don't eat fish** or you want to have some fish-free days, you can add 1 to 2 tablespoons (15 to 30 mL) of flax seeds to your food or use flaxseed oil in one of the skin drinks. Try Flaxseed Lemon Drink, Berry Beauty Smoothie, and B Muesli with flax seeds (many of these recipes are also high in B vitamins). Also eat lots of bright red and orange vegetables because they are rich in beta-carotene, which is converted to oil-reducing vitamin A.

3. **To get more zinc and magnesium in your diet:** Eat sardines on whole-grain bread for breakfast, pepitas and almonds for snacks, and a few oysters at your next social function. Remember that alcohol rapidly depletes zinc and magnesium, so it is best to avoid alcohol during the Healthy Skin Diet. Recipes to increase zinc and

magnesium intake include Roasted Sweet Potato Salad, Designer Muesli, Gluten-Free Muesli, and Vitamin E Muesli. Chlorophyll is rich in magnesium, so drink one to two bottles of Green Water per day.

4. **Swap dairy for other high-protein foods,** such as free-range chicken (antibiotic-free), free-range eggs, fish, beans and chickpeas, and small servings of red meat. Get your daily requirement of calcium from the Anti-Aging Broth, Almond Milk (naturally high in calcium), Calcium-Rich Smoothie, tahini spreads, sesame seeds, almonds, and dark green leafy vegetables, such as watercress. Try the Sweet Raspberry, Avocado and Watercress Salad.

5. **Remember to drink enough fluids** — water, Green Water, Spot-Free Skin Juice, herbal teas, fresh vegetable juices, mineral water with freshly squeezed lemon. Also do the 3-Day Alkalizing Cleanse and the Healthy Skin Diet.

Quick Review of the Acne Management Program

Step 1: Follow a suitable skin-care routine

- Make sure your skin-care products are suitable for your skin.
- Swim in the ocean or use a salt water face bath.

Step 2: Help your liver remove excess hormones

- Take a liver detoxification/cleansing supplement for 2 weeks.

Step 3: Control your oil production

- Avoid dairy products and decrease saturated fat intake (limit meat and butter, avoid pork and deli meats).
- Avoid fried foods, trans fats, and margarine. Use avocado, tahini, and extra virgin olive oil instead (in moderation).

- Increase omega-3 intake by eating salmon, trout, tuna, sardines, omega-3-fortified eggs, flaxseed oil, and flax seeds. Add lecithin granules to your diet so you digest and eliminate fats correctly.
- Take a zinc supplement during weeks 3 to 8 of the Healthy Skin Diet.

Step 4: Improve your bowel health

- Ditch the white bread, white flour, and white sugar and switch to whole-grain foods and honey or stevia (which can be bought in health food stores).
- Review the bowel health questionnaires in Guideline #1 and complete the 3-Day Alkalizing Cleanse (necessary for all acne sufferers).
- Think green! Eat salads every day (with either lunch or dinner) and have more fresh, fiber-rich vegetables, especially the bright red and orange ones. Ensure you have five servings of veggies and two servings of fruit every day.
- Drink one to two bottles of Green Water per day (6 cup/1.5 L bottles).

Step 5: Exercise and sweat

- Sweat every day and exercise 4 days a week. See Guideline #5 to help build a skin-health exercise routine.

Cellulite Care

The good news is that you don't have to worry about your cellulite dimples any longer because a solution is at hand.

Cellulite is a fancy name for dimpled skin that resembles the texture of orange peel (if you're lucky); however, if you are not so fortunate, you may look in the mirror some days and wonder who super-glued the cottage cheese to your behind. It's no practical joke, though. Having cellulite can cause distress. The good news is that you don't have to worry about your cellulite dimples any longer because a solution is at hand. You probably won't like the answer to your problem, however, because it's not a quick-fix miracle and it involves effort and patience. Lots of it. Read on if you want to know more.

Q. What exactly is cellulite?

A. Cellulite is found in the fatty layers of your skin, but it is not normal body fat, nor is it unique to overweight people. Even slim women can have cellulite. It looks like hail damage on your skin, typically on the thighs, hips, bottom, and stomach. It afflicts women more often than men because men have a genetic tendency for stronger connective tissue in the dermis layer. Unfortunately, women are more likely to have irregular connective tissue immediately below the skin, making them more prone to getting disorderly connective tissue fibers that lose flexibility and movement, similar to when an old bathing suit loses its elasticity and no longer fits snugly. This tissue weakness allows the fatty layer (the subcutaneous layer) just below the skin's deep dermis layer to protrude into the dermis, which makes the skin look lumpy.

Although cellulite occurs in varying degrees in as many as 85% of women, not all women get cellulite, and it is from these ladies that we can gain hope and also a bit of insight into how to avoid cellulite in the future. However, don't get me wrong: cellulite is not necessarily a bad thing. It's quite a common cosmetic condition that can naturally happen as you age. There's certainly nothing wrong with learning to love yourself, lumps, bumps, and all.

Anatomy of Cellulite

There are two internal factors that can cause the appearance of cellulite: irregular connective tissue in the dermis layer of the skin; and the intrusion of the fatty layer into the dermis, making skin appear lumpy.

Connective Tissue

You wouldn't want your liver to dislodge and squash an artery, blocking off your valuable blood supply, would you? Luckily you have connective tissue, which is a fibrous material that literally connects your muscles and organs to one another so they can't aimlessly move around the body. This cellular glue also helps bring nutrients to the tissues and gives tissues form and strength. Without good connective tissue, the skin becomes fragile and sags.

Connective tissue is where you find the famous beauty materials collagen and elastin: both provide the skin with strength, the ability to stretch, and the capacity to return to its original shape after extension (this is the ideal scenario). If the connective tissue doesn't return to its normal shape, it becomes irregular and cellulite can occur. Connective tissue can also tear if it hasn't been supplied with the right skin nutrients (such as the mineral zinc), causing stretch marks to appear.

Factors Involved in Poor Connective Tissue Quality

Stress: Stress burns up valuable nutrients that could have otherwise been used to repair connective tissue.

Environmental pollution: Toxins from pollution and cigarette smoke are absorbed into the body and can become lodged around connective tissues.

Poor diet: If you eat a poor diet that doesn't supply enough protein, connective tissue loses strength and your skin eventually sags. This is often seen when overweight people follow poorly designed diets that consist of nothing but salads and soups. Poor digestion can also hamper protein supply to the skin. If your body can't digest protein properly and "pluck" out the amino acids needed to make collagen and elastin, you will end up with connective tissue dysfunction.

Hormones: Fluctuating estrogen levels (the hormone that is generally higher in women) can also play a part in weakening connective tissue.

Genetics: The quality of your connective tissues is also a product of genetics. Some people are born with less or more high-quality connective tissue.

Intrusion into the Dermis

Another structural problem seen with cellulite is lumpiness caused by the fat layer pushing into the dermis, which can be caused by faulty fat cells. Inside your body, billions of tiny cells sit together, side by side, and layer by layer they form your skin and the rest of you. Your connective tissue keeps them all in place. Remember that when cellulite occurs, your fatty (subcutaneous) layer starts pushing into your skin layer, making it look bumpy — this fatty layer is mostly made up of fat cells. The health of your fat cells determines just how good your skin looks on the outside.

Leaky Cells

When your fat cells store chemicals and acids (toxins), they can get damaged and become leaky. Imagine a cell is like a balloon filled with water, and over time, wear and tear has caused little pin-prick holes to appear in the balloon membrane, causing fluid to seep into surrounding tissue.

If this leaked fluid builds up enough, you can see it: it is what we call fluid retention or edema. Swollen ankles, puffy eyelids, and cellulite all have "problem water" hanging out where it is not supposed to be. In the case of cellulite, the water may have been drawn there because the body wanted to use the fluid to dilute acids, or it may have been from leaky cells that cannot hold on to water. It is impossible to tell which is the case, so anti-cellulite treatment should involve addressing both of these issues.

Q. Why might my cell walls be leaking fluids?

A. Your cell membranes are largely made up of fats (lipids), but the types of fat used to build your cell walls will help determine how resistant they are to leakage. You choose what types of fats your cell membranes are built with every time you eat a meal: saturated fats from meat and dairy can make rigid cells and essential fatty acids from nuts, seeds, and fish oils contribute to more flexible, resilient cells.

Cell Repair

Cell membranes can be prone to damage if they are not continually repaired.

- **EFAs:** The best patching materials for leaky cells are EFAs, such as omega-3. EFAs also work to draw "problem water" from outside the cell back into the cell. This means EFAs help to keep fluid in the right place so you have hydrated cells and healthy-looking skin.

- **Lecithin:** Your cell membranes are also made up of lecithin (phosphatidylcholine). Lecithin sits in the cell walls and helps to determine what enters and leaves your cells. A shortage of lecithin equals faulty cell membranes that can leak fluids into your subcutaneous layer. Lecithin helps to break up cholesterol and promotes proper digestion of fats, it helps cleanse the liver, it maintains a healthy nervous system, and it promotes healthy weight loss. Your body doesn't produce enough lecithin of its own, so you need to eat foods that contain it (see Step 2, page 175).

Cellulite Management Program

• •

The management plan is your first step to feeling more comfortable in your skin. This section details topical treatments and camouflage ideas. The anti-cellulite program involves changes in diet and lifestyle that will improve and even eliminate your cellulite. In all, there are five steps to follow.

> To treat cellulite, you want to decrease your skin's waste burden, increase toxin removal, and improve local circulation.

Step 1: Use Massage Oils

Everybody loves a topical treatment, but most commercial cellulite creams are loaded with chemicals and additives, such as artificial fragrance, that contribute to your body's toxic load. To treat cellulite, you want to decrease your skin's waste burden, increase toxin removal, and improve local circulation. Massage oils — containing no artificial ingredients and with the addition of natural essential oils — specific for cellulite are your best option (see Guideline #8 for more information on artificial chemicals found in beauty products).

Choosing an Anti-Cellulite Oil

When choosing an anti-cellulite oil, look for these two ingredients:

Birch oil is extracted from the plant *Betula alba*. It contains salicylic acid and it is astringent, so it helps to tone the skin. Birch oil also improves circulation, increases toxin removal, and has a mild diuretic effect.

Rosemary oil increases circulation to the skin and assists with elimination of toxins. Do not use this oil on its own — it can be found in anti-cellulite massage oil formulas, or mix it in with almond and birch oil.

Caution

Do not use rosemary oil during pregnancy or if you have epilepsy or high blood pressure. Other suitable ingredients include apricot kernel oil, almond oil, jojoba seed oil, wheat germ oil, vitamin E, limonene, grapefruit extract, calendula/marigold, carrot oil, fennel extract, rosehip oil, and kelp/seaweed.

How to apply anti-cellulite oil

1. Have a shower or a bath as usual and then pat your skin dry.
2. To apply your anti-cellulite oil of choice, tip a small amount (about the size of a large coin) into the palm of your hand, then rub your hands together to warm the oil.
3. Apply the mixture where necessary (thighs, bottom, stomach, arms), using more oil as necessary.
4. Then give yourself a slow massage, working in a circular motion from the legs to the heart (to help your lymphatic system remove toxins).

Tip: Apply oil to affected skin twice a day. Ideally, use anti-cellulite oil in the morning and at night (it's not essential to bathe beforehand). Also remember to moisturize the rest of your skin with a suitable natural-based moisturizer (see Guideline #8).

Q. What are toxins?

A. "Toxin" is a general term for a substance that has no positive use in the body, such as chemicals from cleaning products, pesticides, artificial food additives, and the pollution you've inhaled. Toxins are also waste products generated by your cells. Your body has several ways of removing toxins, including the lymphatic and blood circulatory systems, sweating, and not forgetting the waste you dump when you go to the toilet. Toxins and hormones that can contribute to cellulite formation include: pesticide residues found on fruits and veggies; artificial additives, such as preservatives; pollution and cigarette smoke; excess hormones, such as estrogen; chemical cleaning products; and beauty products containing artificial chemicals.

Caution

Never use a cellulite cream or oil without the addition of exercise. Anti-cellulite products can mobilize toxins, and these chemicals may deposit somewhere else in the body if you don't exert yourself and sweat.

Reducing Your Toxic Load

Since cellulite can be caused by fluid and toxins becoming trapped in the subcutaneous layer of skin, you can help to reverse this accumulation by reducing your toxin load.

1. Swap those stinky chemical cleaners for natural ones.
2. Cut down on packaged goodies, such as potato chips, crackers, and cookies, and soft drinks.
3. Take a liver detoxification supplement to speed up toxin elimination in the body.

Q. I'm meeting my friends at the beach on the weekend and I need to know how I can hide my cellulite. Can you help me?

A. If you want to instantly make your skin look better, you can camouflage cellulite with fake tan products. Spray-on tans, applied by trained professionals, can give you a wonderful natural tan that lasts up to a week, but you can still use a home-applied fake tan bought from a pharmacist or department store. But I have to tell you that fake tans are full of chemicals that are readily absorbed into your skin. Chemicals can contribute to connective tissue damage and lead to cellulite, so you could make your skin condition worse with regular fake tan abuse. To be on the safe side, keep the tan-in-a-can use to a bare minimum. And after 5 days, when it starts to go patchy, have a good body exfoliator on hand.

If you're still panicking about being seen on the beach, you may want to try the following:

- Buy a gorgeous wrap or sarong that complements the color of your bathing suit.
- Buy a bathing suit that draws the eye toward your best assets.

A Model's Cellulite Treatment

It is claimed that this treatment is used by supermodels, but I haven't heard of anyone famous owning up to it. This remedy was often talked about within the modeling industry in the 1990s, but I have to warn you: it's only a temporary skin tightener and it may only work on the genetically blessed.

The natural compounds in coffee are said to marginally tighten the skin. Seaweed is also considered to have a toning effect when applied to the skin, which is why it's often an ingredient in anti-cellulite treatments and creams.

Ingredients
¼ cup (60 mL) warm used ground coffee (preferably organic) or organic instant coffee
¼ cup (60 mL) extra virgin olive oil (can infuse it with rosemary or birch oil)
4 soaked kombu (seaweed) strips
Plastic wrap

Method
1. Mix coffee and oil in a glass bowl.
2. Line the floor or shower with newspaper (some of the coffee mixture is bound to fall off).
3. Massage the mixture in a circular motion over cellulite-affected thighs for 1 minute.
4. Wrap the area with kombu.
5. Wash your hands and then apply plastic wrap around each affected area to hold the mixture in place. Leave on for 10 minutes and then have a shower to rinse off.

Repeat this once a day for at least 2 weeks, as results take 2 to 4 weeks to appear.

Self-Confidence

Self-confidence is very attractive, so take time to work on your self-esteem.

Self-confidence is very attractive, so take time to work on your self-esteem. In the meantime, you could go to the beach and pretend not to care what anyone else thinks. Basically, "Fake it till you make it." Walk tall, all the way to the water's edge, and enjoy the water, the sand, and the sunshine, just like everyone else. The more you step out of your comfort zone, the sooner you'll feel what it's like to be truly confident. And remember, you are so much more than just a pair of wobbly thighs! Remind yourself about your strengths and positive attributes, and then have fun at the beach, because you deserve to be there as much as anyone else.

Step 2: Consume Nutrients to Repair Tissues and Cells

Now let's get to work on the anti-cellulite program, creating healthy cells and improving connective tissue.

Nutrients for Healthy Cells

As you've read, your cells leak fluids when they don't have the right nutrients, such as omega-3 EFAs and lecithin, for maintenance and repair. You can get these nutrients, along with their little helpers (antioxidants), from the meals and special drink recipes of the Healthy Skin Diet, such as the Skin-Firming Drink, which has been specifically designed to reduce the appearance of cellulite. As mentioned earlier, omega-3 is found in oily fish (trout, sardines, salmon, tuna), as well as flax seeds, flaxseed oil, and in small amounts in dark green vegetables. Lecithin is found in egg yolk, liver, nuts, soy products, and corn. You can also buy soy lecithin granules.

Lecithin Dosage: Adults with cellulite should take 2000 to 4000 mg of lecithin per day. Note that 1 tablespoon (15 mL) of soy lecithin granules contains approximately 1700 mg of lecithin, so have $1\frac{1}{2}$ to 2 tablespoons (22 to 30 mL) of lecithin daily. Add lecithin granules to the Skin-Firming Drink or muesli.

Nutrients for Healthy Connective Tissues

Collagen and elastin are made up of amino acids, including glycine and proline and a substance called hyaluronic acid, which has recently been renamed hyaluronan. I discussed hyaluronan and its essential role in healthy skin in some detail in Guideline #3. Remember that its main building block is glucosamine, which normalizes cartilage and restores joint function. Magnesium is also needed to manufacture hyaluronan, and studies have shown that deficiencies in zinc and magnesium contribute to hyaluronan abnormalities. Supplements with glucosamine, glycine, proline, vitamin C, copper, manganese, magnesium, and zinc can help to restore elasticity and strength to connective tissue. These nutrients can be found in some glucosamine complex supplements, available in most health food shops.

Glucosamine Dosage: Adults should take 1200 mg (1.2 g) of glucosamine sulfate or glucosamine hydrochloride (HCL) per day, with either food or the Skin-Firming Drink. Make sure your glucosamine supplement also contains magnesium, zinc, vitamin C, copper, and manganese.

Step 3: Exercise and Improve Your Circulation

Your circulation plays an important role in having smooth, evenly textured skin. Circulation of blood is essential for health, but it is also the lymphatic circulation that will help to keep your skin looking fabulous. If you want to get rid of your cellulite, you must exercise. You don't have to like exercise or be good at it; you just need to set aside at least 15 minutes a day to get some good lymph-pumping movement. Some experts claim that exercise won't get rid of cellulite, but you just have to watch the Olympic Games and look at the average female athlete, with her firm, toned body, to know that exercise does a good job at preventing cellulite.

> **If you want to get rid of your cellulite, you must exercise.**

Caution

If you suffer from any kind of medical problem, such as a heart condition or diabetes, please have a chat with your doctor before trying to improve your circulation because some treatments, such as high-impact exercise and warm and cold water therapy, may not be suitable for you.

Boosting Your Circulation

There are several strategies you can use to boost your circulation. Make sure you exercise and move daily (see Guideline #5 for information and inspiration).

- Use dry-skin brushing (see Guideline #8).
- Take a shower and alternate from wonderfully warm water to chilly cold water, then exfoliate your skin with a granulated gel or cream
- Massage your skin with an exfoliation glove.
- Get a lymphatic massage from a qualified masseuse.
- Gently self-massage cellulite-prone areas with natural anti-cellulite oils.
- Do breathing exercises

Activity

For severe cellulite, I suggest doing heart-pumping activity for at least 15 minutes. (If you aren't able to do high-impact exercise, combine walking with other forms of exercise. Do 15 minutes of continuous high-impact exercise today, then over the following weeks work up to a 30- to 60-minute routine. A personal trainer could also work wonders for you!

Anti-Cellulite Exercises

The best anti-cellulite exercises include soft sand jogging, fast-paced soft sand walking (keeping your knees high), running, swimming, cycling, and running up lots and lots of stairs. Be warned: you'll miss your knees if you damage them, so remember to avoid movements that trigger sharp pain and be kind to your body by running on soft surfaces only, such as sand, grass, and carpet. Also wear good-quality running shoes during workouts.

One of the very best exercises to help you get rid of cellulite is sprinting. Sprinters have the most amazing bodies, and it is from them that we can gain inspiration to be cellulite-free. If you are a walker and are able to do so, combine walking with 30-second sprints every 5 minutes. For example, power walk for 5 minutes, then sprint as fast as you can for 30 seconds, then briskly walk for 5 minutes and again sprint as fast as you can for 30 seconds or more (up to 1 minute) and so on. Do this routine for at least 20 minutes. If you are a jogger, combine slow jogging with 30-second sprints in a similar manner to the walking routine.

> One of the very best exercises to help you get rid of cellulite is sprinting.

Step 4: Avoid Dairy Products and Sugar

Just as there are foods that strengthen connective tissue and cell walls for gorgeous skin, there are foods that can promote the onset of cellulite. The main offenders are dairy and sugar.

Avoiding Dairy Products

> Dairy products can increase your risk of cellulite because they are mucus-forming.

Dairy products can increase your risk of cellulite because they are mucus-forming. To demonstrate this, the next time you have a cold or flu, drink a glass of milk and see if you suddenly have an increase in phlegm or mucus production. Naturopathic doctors say that dairy products make your lymphatic fluid thicker, so it has a harder time traveling around your body. A sluggish lymphatic system can't remove cellular waste fast enough, so it builds up. These cellular toxins can be harmful if they are floating in your blood, so they are quickly relocated to be safely stored in your fat — especially on your lovely soft thighs.

Dairy also supplies saturated fat and arachidonic acid (AA), which your body can use to make rigid cell walls that are prone to leaking. I find that eliminating dairy products from the diet is essential to reducing the appearance of cellulite. This dietary change works better than any other treatment because it quickly enhances lymphatic health and it allows better absorption of other minerals, such as zinc, copper, and magnesium, which are essential for firm and toned skin.

Avoiding Sugar

Eating too much sugar can also increase your risk of cellulite. This occurs because sweets, junk foods, and processed white carbohydrates, such as white bread, pastries, and cakes, increase acid in the body and affect your blood sugar levels. This surge in glucose in the blood uses up lots of vitamin C and may cause low levels of this important antioxidant as a result. Excess glucose in the blood can also cause blood vessel damage, which may hamper circulation to cellulite-prone areas. Vitamin C is essential for strong, healthy blood vessels and low levels of vitamin C can lead to poor blood vessel strength and varicose veins, which are often associated with cellulite. Vitamin C is also important for cell membrane health and may help prevent leaky cells because of its role in recycling vitamin E.

> Eating too much sugar can also increase your risk of cellulite.

Foods and Drinks to Avoid if You Have Cellulite

- Dairy products. Milk, milkshakes, cheese, yogurt, ice cream, creamy spreads, and butter
- High glycemic index carbohydrates: pastries, cakes, doughnuts, cookies, crackers, granola bars, white bread, white rice (basmati is okay), sweets, white flour pancakes, and chips
- Soft drinks, diet soft drinks, fruit juice, and alcohol
- Margarine

For more information on non-dairy calcium-rich alternatives to dairy, see Guideline #3.

I had mild cellulite in my late teens... maybe it was because I must have been the laziest teenager on the planet. I hated exercise. I would sit in my room and write and draw all day, and I'd only take breaks to have milkshakes and mountains of toast made with white bread. I used to drink a quart (liter) of milk and eat a bowl of yogurt and ice cream every day. However, my dimply butt miraculously firmed up when I ditched the dairy. After I made dietary changes, I also had a lot more energy and my skin was less prone to rashes. Now that I'm older and I've had a baby, dietary changes alone are not enough. I also need to jog on soft sand several times a week and sweat and use massage oils to keep my skin firm.

Step 5: Promote Good Bowel Health

Good bowel health is essential for healthy-looking skin. Poor bowel health can result in constipation, allowing toxins from your feces to be reabsorbed by your body, which slowly poisons your whole system. If you have constipation or any other bowel complaints, it is essential that you seek treatment before your bowels harm your health. See Guideline #1 for more information about constipation and gut health.

Hydration

It is important to drink enough fluids each day to prevent dehydration and a sluggish lymphatic system. Dehydration can also damage your cells and cause constipation and poor bowel function. Cellulite can be impossible to get rid of in a select few people.

3-Day Alkalizing Cleanse

Cleanse your bowel on a regular basis. See page 317 for instructions.

Positive Attitude

Please never, ever dislike yourself because you have cellulite. Remember that it is your self-confidence that ultimately makes you attractive because you walk taller and give off an air of being relaxed and lovable. Other people adore being around someone who is confident and relaxed in their skin because it helps them to feel at ease too (don't underestimate this power). Self-hate and self-criticism can damage your self-confidence, ruin your motivation, and suppress your ability to make healthy improvements

Love the body you are in and focus on your best assets — the parts of your personality and your body that you love — and make them stand out with the right clothes and accessories. If you want to work on your cellulite, then go for it; you can get rid of dimpled skin one way or another, but don't hate yourself along the way, because it will be a slow and arduous mountain to climb if you do. Also remember that Olympic athletes don't get fit overnight; it takes time and effort for them to reach competition standard. Cellulite removal is kind of the same: you can't get rid of it overnight, or in a week or two. It takes time, effort, and truckloads of patience. Great results may be seen in 2 to 6 months, and earlier than this if your cellulite is mild.

> If you want to work on your cellulite, then go for it; you can get rid of dimpled skin one way or another, but don't hate yourself along the way, because it will be a slow and arduous mountain to climb if you do.

Recipes for Managing Cellulite

To reduce the appearance of cellulite from the inside out, try these recipes on a daily basis: Anti-Aging Broth (page 392): This broth is rich in glycine, calcium, magnesium, and natural collagen. Skin-Firming Drink (page 350): You will need to buy a powdered glucosamine supplement (one that contains some or all of the following: glucosamine sulfate, glucosamine hydrochloride, vitamin C, magnesium, copper, zinc and manganese).

To get more omega-3 and lecithin in your diet, try these recipes: Skin-Firming Drink; Flaxseed Lemon Drink; Salmon and Salad Sandwich; Perfect Poached Eggs; Egg Soldiers; Creamy Mayonnaise; Salmon Steaks with Peas and Mash; Rainbow Trout with Honey-Roasted Vegetables; Smoked Salmon and Eggs; and Tuna and Avocado Wrap.

To get more zinc in your diet: Eat fresh oysters when out socializing or try the recipes for Oysters with Dipping Sauce and Lamb Stir-Fry.

To get a good dose of magnesium: Green Water drink is the best choice. Drink one to two bottles of Green Water per day.

To increase the amount and variety of antioxidants in your diet: Buckwheat Crêpes (with the topping of your choice), Creamy Chickpea Curry with Brown Rice, Roasted Sweet Potato Salad, Designer Muesli, Vitamin E Muesli, Gluten-Free Muesli, and snack on a small handful of hazelnuts and pepitas. All of these recipes contain a rich variety of antioxidants.

Quick Review of the Cellulite Management Program

Step 1: Use massage oils

- Massage your skin using anti-cellulite oils containing all-natural ingredients.

Step 2: Consume nutrients to repair tissues and cells

- Eat healthy food rich in omega-3, lecithin, and antioxidants.
- Make the Skin-Firming Drink daily and have Anti-Aging Broth and Green Water.

Step 3: Exercise and improve your circulation

- Exercise and sweat daily.
- Improve your circulation in as many different ways as possible.

Step 4: Avoid dairy products and sugar

- Avoid dairy products for 2 months (while on the Healthy Skin Diet) and stop adding sugar to your food and drinks.

Step 5: Promote good bowel health

- Drink enough water.
- Avoid constipation

Cradle Cap Care

As you may already know, cradle cap is not a cute bonnet made to match that twin set and booties Grandma sent last Christmas. It is a skin condition that looks like a cap and consists of thick, yellow crusts and scales on your baby's sweet little head. Your baby might not even notice (or care) about this musty mop top, although it may become a tad itchy and affect your child's sleep.

Cradle Cap Management Program

Here is a simple management plan for you to follow in caring for your baby's skin condition. For more information on children's skin care, see the Children's Clear Skin Program (page 263).

Step 1: Use Natural and Gentle Skin Care

1. You will need to find a natural baby shampoo that is free of sodium lauryl sulfate. This is not so easy — you'd be surprised at how many commercial baby shampoos contain SLS or its close cousin, sodium laureth sulfate. Be suspicious if your children's products foam and bubble on cue! Also avoid brightly colored products containing synthetic dyes and fragrances. You might need to visit your local health food shop to find a decent gentle shampoo, although still check the ingredients, as some health food shops stock "natural" and "gentle" products that contain synthetic chemicals. Also avoid baby shampoos that contain diethanolamine (DEA) and triethanolamine (TEA), as they can cause skin irritations and your baby doesn't need a chemical cocktail on his or her delicate noggin.

> **Be suspicious if your children's products foam and bubble on cue!**

Babies don't need bubbly, colored bath products. They can be adequately cleaned with water and a soft cloth. There is a list of natural baby products on my website (see page 460 for the website address).

2. You should plan to shampoo your baby's hair and scalp often. Three times a week is ideal. Your baby does not need to be bathed every day. While shampooing, massage the head. Be gentle and thoughtful and your little one will just adore the extra attention.

3. Massaging your child's head with a natural oil will help take care of cradle cap. Rub a natural oil, such as olive oil or rosehip oil, into the cradle cap two to three times a week (you can do this when you are bathing your baby). Then loosen the crusts by brushing the scalp, in a circular motion, with a very soft toothbrush (or you can gently use a fine-tooth comb). Shampoo afterwards to remove some (not all) of the oil.

Suitable Moisturizing Ingredients

If your child's scalp needs moisturizing, gently massage the scalp with a suitable oil product that contains some of these ingredients:

- Calendula
- Extra virgin olive oil
- Rosehip oil
- Sweet almond oil*
- Vitamin E
- Apricot kernel oil
- Manuka oil
- Evening primrose oil
- Flaxseed oil

(*Caution: Sweet almond oil is a nut oil. Do not use it if you know your baby has a nut allergy or if there is a family history of nut allergy.)

Step 2: Feed Your Child Moisturizing Foods

Your child may need essential fatty acids, such as omega-3 fats, to moisturize the skin from the inside out. If you are bottle-feeding your baby, make sure the infant formula contains omega-3 (EPA and DHA) fatty acids. Omega-3 may also be written as alpha-linolenic acid. If you are breastfeeding your child, you can increase omega-3 in your own diet. Some of the essential fatty acids will end up in your breast milk and be passed on to your child. This will help to moisturize the skin from the inside out. Your child may need to have a probiotic supplement to enhance immune system development. See the Children's Clear Skin Program (page 263).

Quick Review of the Cradle Cap Management Program

Step 1: Use natural and gentle skin care products

- Only use gentle skin and bath products on your baby's delicate skin.
- Gently remove crusting and moisturize your baby's scalp.

Step 2: Feed your child moisturizing foods

- Choose an infant formula with added omega-3 (EPA and DHA), or if you are breastfeeding, you can consume omega-3 to increase the amount of essential fatty acids in your breast milk.
- Read the Children's Clear Skin Program for suitable supplements and dosages.

Dandruff Care

You look gorgeous in that black dress, but what's with the white flecks on your shoulders? On closer inspection of your scalp, it is dandruff, a combination of inflammation, flaking skin, lumps, and crusts. But don't freak out; just exchange your little black frock for a cream one and try not to scratch, because dandruff can be as itchy as an infestation of head lice.

Seborrheic dermatitis, the technical term for dandruff, can commonly occur on the scalp, face, and middle of the chest, but (if you are extra unlucky) it may manifest anywhere on the body. Dandruff can simply occur when you are run down, overworked, or stressed, and it can occur in conjunction with psoriasis. Anti-dandruff shampoos address none of these factors.

Factors That Trigger Dandruff

Aim to avoid these products and deficiencies so you don't trigger dandruff. Check off anything on this list that you suspect may have triggered your dandruff.

- ☐ Chemicals
- ☐ Climate (especially winter)
- ☐ Emotional or physical stress
- ☐ Fungal/yeast infection
- ☐ Psoriasis (dandruff can appear during or after psoriasis)
- ☐ Sodium lauryl sulfate (SLS)
- ☐ Excess use of hairspray or gel
- ☐ Hair dyes
- ☐ Excess sugar and starch in diet
- ☐ Infrequent shampooing
- ☐ Inadequate rinsing of hair after washing
- ☐ Overly dry scalp or excessively oily/greasy scalp
- ☐ Diets high in saturated fats
- ☐ Deficiency of essential fatty acids, especially omega-3

Dandruff Management Program

The dandruff management plan includes identifying possible triggers and applying topical treatments to eliminate dandruff as quickly as possible.

Step 1: Check Your Hair-Care Products

Maybe your shampoo is to blame? Sodium lauryl sulfate (SLS) is a synthetic detergent commonly added to commercial brand-name shampoos, liquid hand soaps, and cleansers to make them lather up nicely. SLS also adds the froth and bubbles to bath products. This lathering effect is what we have come to expect when using cleaning liquids, but the SLS additive is one of the most irritating chemicals found in hair and skin products today. SLS use can trigger inflammation, dandruff, and skin rashes and exacerbate existing scalp flaking. SLS also strips your scalp's natural sebum, which is supposed to protect your skin from invading fungus and bacteria.

> **The SLS additive is one of the most irritating chemicals found in hair and skin products today.**

Safe and Effective Shampoo Ingredients

There are a number of shampoo ingredients that are ideal if you have dandruff. They are anti-fungal, anti-microbial, and anti-inflammatory.

- Tea tree oil
- Licorice root
- Gotu kola
- Vitamin E
- Chamomile
- Calendula
- Manuka honey
- Panthenol (vitamin B_5)
- Olive leaf extract
- Citrus seed extract

Did You Know?

Tea Tree Oil and Citrus Seed Extract Cures

In a study of 126 patients with dandruff, 5% were given either 5% tea tree oil shampoo or a placebo shampoo. They were told to wash their hair daily, leaving the shampoo on for 3 minutes before rinsing. At the end of 4 weeks, scalp lesions were significantly lower and less itching was seen in the tea tree oil shampoo users. The cure rate was low, however, so use tea tree oil shampoo in conjunction with other remedies. Daily shampooing can help reduce the appearance of dandruff. Citrus seed extract/grape seed extract is a potent fungicide and antibiotic, inhibiting many different types of fungus, bacteria and parasites. Citrus seed is good for drying damp conditions, such as oily scalp. An oily scalp promotes fungus-related dandruff.

Activity

Review Guideline #6, taking note of the ingredients to avoid. Then look at the ingredient panel on your shampoo bottle: does it look like a chemical cocktail that only a biochemist could decipher? If so, get rid of your shampoo today and buy one with beneficial ingredients from a health food shop.

Anti-Dandruff Recipes and Home Remedies

Olive Oil Treatment

If your dandruff is of the dry variety or appeared in conjunction with psoriasis, this olive oil treatment can be very effective.

Ingredients/apparatus:
   ¼ cup (60 mL) extra virgin olive oil
   Plastic bag to cover hair

Method:
1. Put the oil into a glass and place the glass in a small tub of hot water to heat the oil. Do not make the oil too hot.
2. Wet your hair, shampoo it, and rinse.
3. Apply the oil to your scalp and massage with fingers.
4. Cover your hair with a plastic bag and leave the mixture on for 3 to 5 minutes.
5. Rinse with warm water.
6. Shampoo twice to remove excess oil, then use a gentle conditioner.
7. If your hair is still greasy, you might want to wash it again the next day.

Natural Anti-Fungal Treatment

This recipe is designed to exfoliate flakes, soothe dry skin, and balance the pH of your scalp so your head is not so appealing to fungi (ingredients for 1–2 treatments):

Ingredients/apparatus:
½ cup (125 mL) grape seed oil
2 tablespoons (30 mL) cornmeal
1 tablespoon (15 mL) apple cider vinegar
Plastic bag to cover hair

Method:
1. Mix the grape seed oil with the cornmeal and vinegar.
2. Stir well.
3. Rinse your hair with warm water and shampoo it with a gentle shampoo.
4. Rub a tablespoon (15 mL) of the oil mixture between your palms to warm the oil.
5. Apply to scalp. Rub in with your fingertips. Repeat until you have applied the mixture to your entire scalp.
6. Cover your hair with a plastic bag. Leave mixture on for ½ hour.
7. Rinse thoroughly and shampoo as normal.

Home Remedies from the Grapevine

If you are trying a home remedy from the grapevine, I recommend you try the vinegar remedies for at least 3 consecutive days and the oil treatments once or twice a week for a couple of weeks. Best results are likely to be seen after 1 to 2 weeks.

ACV (Apple Cider Vinegar) Remedy

If you don't mind briefly smelling like a salad, then this remedy could be for you. This will offer relief from itching and may even clear up your dandruff. This remedy may be best for oily dandruff caused by fungus.

1. Shampoo your hair.
2. Rinse scalp with quality apple cider vinegar.
3. Leave on for 3 minutes. For severe dandruff, leave on for 30 minutes before rinsing
4. Rinse off and apply conditioner if necessary.

White vinegar: See reader question opposite.

Wash your hair more often: If your flakes are mild, you may simply need to wash your hair more often, with an SLS-free shampoo, finishing with a suitable conditioner.

Olive Oil + Sunlight

This works brilliantly for psoriasis, and it can also work for dandruff related to psoriasis.

1. Shampoo your hair and apply extra virgin olive oil to your scalp.
2. Gently massage into your scalp.
3. Hop out of the shower (get dry and dressed).
4. Sit in direct sunlight for 5 to 10 minutes. See the psoriasis section (page 232) for more information.

Q. My scalp is so oily and itchy that it distracts me from my studies and I'm always scratching my head in class. I don't have a lot of money for expensive treatments. What can I do to stop this embarrassing itching?

A. Use white vinegar to treat oily dandruff and reduce scalp itching. This is the cheapie version of the ACV remedy. Fill a spray bottle with no-name brand white vinegar, spray onto scalp, and leave it to dry overnight. If there is no smell, you may not need to wash it out the next day. Or you can dilute $1/2$ cup (125 mL) of vinegar with $1/2$ cup (125 mL) of filtered water and apply to your scalp. This may sting a bit, but try to leave it on for half an hour before rinsing. Use this remedy for 3 days in a row for best results. If your itching continues, follow the whole dandruff management program.

Did You Know?

....

Medicated Shampoos

Some people love using medicated shampoos, but, unfortunately, the research suggests that your dandruff is likely to return time and time again when using medicated anti-dandruff shampoos as the only treatment. This is not surprising, because shampoos cannot eliminate the underlying cause of the dandruff. Don't get me wrong; anti-dandruff shampoos and home remedies are great for treating existing fungus and washing away scales, but you must fix up your lazy (sick, suppressed) immune system to win the war against dandruff. So let's move on to Step 2.

If your immune system fails to do its job, pityrosporum's offspring, cousins, aunts, and uncles take over your head and inflame your skin.

Step 2: Look After Your Immune System

Your immune system normally guards your skin from invading bacteria and yeasts, but when you are run down, stressed, or sick, your immune system can let its guard down. A common yeast called pityrosporum lives on your scalp. Pityrosporum yeasts can be found on everyone, but they only cause dandruff in approximately 20% of people. Your immune system ensures that this freeloader doesn't multiply or claim too much territory. If your immune system fails to do its job, pityrosporum's offspring, cousins, aunts, and uncles take over your head and inflame your skin.

Common dandruff treatments, such as medicated shampoos, work by killing these pesky fungi, but these treatments don't usually have a long-term beneficial effect because they don't address the underlying cause. What's more, not all dandruff is accompanied by pityrosporum. The first thing you need to do is assess your diet and lifestyle to see if you're pushing your immune system to its limits.

Strengthening Your Immune System

Follow these instructions for boosting your immunity.

1. Get plenty of rest and relaxation

Quality sleep is essential for a strong immune system. When you sleep, your body goes into repair mode and your immune system recharges its batteries. To have quality sleep, get to bed before 10.30 p.m. and get 8 hours of sleep (but no more than 8 hours because too much sleep can leave you feeling foggy). See Guideline #4 (page 95) for more information on sleep and skin.

2. Relax with breathing exercises

It can be hard to suddenly change from being stressed and anxious into a calm person, but you don't need to quit your life or get a lobotomy (just yet) to feel relaxed; you can simply take the first positive step by learning some breathing exercises. Good-quality breathing techniques instantly switch your nervous system from stressed fight or flight responses into rest and digest mode. Check out the chapter on beauty breathing (page 281).

Did You Know?

Chinese Damp

Why is stress, and its close cousins anxiety and worry, so bad for you and your dandruff? According to Chinese physiology, anxiety and worry can cause "damp" excess in the body, which promotes fungus overgrowth. Western health and science researchers may have different reasoning, but all health practitioners agree that chronic anxiety, worry, and stress are bad for your health.

Immune System Questionnaire

The first thing you need to do is assess your diet and lifestyle to see if you are pushing your immune system to its limits. Check any of the following habits that describes your diet and lifestyle habits:

- [ ] I eat sugar every day (a dash of sugar in coffee or tea, jam, cake, cookies, soft drinks, ice cream).
- [ ] I have sugar cravings.
- [ ] I crave dairy products/I eat a lot of dairy.
- [ ] I eat white bread, I crave processed carbohydrates.
- [ ] I avoid garlic and onions.
- [ ] I prefer not to exercise/I exercise less than twice a week.
- [ ] I'm stressed, anxious or a 'worry- wart' — life is tough for me!
- [ ] I often get less than 7 hours of sleep a night (three or more nights a week)..
- [ ] I take antibiotics when I'm sick (within the last 6 months).
- [ ] I'm on the birth control pill.
- [ ] I'm taking cortisone medicines.
- [ ] I drink alcohol more than twice a week or I binge drink.
- [ ] I have been exposed to a high dose of chemicals (pesticides, harsh cleaning products such as oven cleaner/bleach etc.).
- [ ] I know my diet should be better (it can't get any worse!).

If you checked off three or more diet and lifestyle factors that promote a poor immune system, you may have found the underlying cause of your dandruff. If your dandruff was triggered by chemical exposure or psoriasis, you should take a liver detoxification supplement for 2 weeks. See the chapter on psoriasis care for information on liver detoxification (page 237).

3. Ditch the stress addiction

You may fret about not getting enough sleep; you could agonize about losing that job; worry about what other people might think; lose sleep when other people gossip about you; and be concerned about bank queues, traffic, the safety of your family, or the state of the economy. Yes, these are all super good reasons to worry, but I'll give you one more: you are ruining your health! Being a worrier (the opposite of a warrior) will make your body's main defence system less effective, and this is bad for your whole body, not just your scalp's health.

Does worry really cause dandruff? Well, worry is another form of stress, and it is easier for me to describe worry as opposed to the highly subjective state of stress. In fact, stress is really worry or fear in disguise: when you feel stressed, the underlying thought process is that you are worried about your ability to cope or manage the situation at hand.

You may not consciously think, "Gosh, I'm worried," but the next time you feel stressed, experiment by telling yourself something positive and strong. For example, stand up straight with good posture and stick your nose in the air as if you are posh, then shout (or think to yourself in an assertive manner): "Of course I'm strong enough to get through this problem! I'm clever and capable; I will survive this!" And mean every word of it. I guarantee that for a split second or two you won't feel any stress or anxiety.

4. Consume fewer sugar, dairy, and alcohol products

The sad fact is that fungus loves sugar and milk sugars. Fungus literally can't live without them. If you have a fungus problem, whether it is dandruff or *Candida albicans*, you will most likely crave sugar and/or carbohydrates, such as breads and pastries. And this craving or addiction is often so strong that when you have one sugar-free day, you wind up feeling crabby and tired, and you may even want to lash out at others. But this addiction is a fungus-triggered craving, because the fungi are dying and they need a sugar hit to live. Processed carbohydrates, such as white bread, white rice, and white flour products, all supply your body with a big dose of sweet glucose so your yeast freeloaders stay well fed. Fungi also love dairy and thrive off the milk sugar.

Did You Know?

Sugar Cravings

If you have sugar cravings, add cinnamon to your meals and take a chromium supplement. Chromium and cinnamon help to keep your blood sugar levels normal. There is less sugar floating around in the bloodstream so your fungi starve quickly. For more information about chromium, see Guideline #3 (page 82).

Q. How much sugar is too much?

A. Some experts say you have to avoid all sugar, even fruit sugars, to kill off out-of-control fungi, but it is quite possible to get the little buggers under control without having to avoid all forms of sugar (which is very good news). You see, if you are a relaxed person who is great at managing stress, gets plenty of sleep, and eats garlic regularly, you can still have small amounts of sugar and fruit, as well as drink alcohol moderately, without your immune system being affected. On the other hand, if you are a stress-head, a worrywart, an insomniac, or you have immune suppression, you will probably have to strictly avoid sugar, fruit, and alcohol for at least 3 months. Trust me: learning how to relax is a much easier option.

5. Counteract the negative effects of medications

Certain medications, such as corticosteroids, birth-control pills, and antibiotics, suppress the immune system, allowing fungi to multiply rapidly. Antibiotics are administered to kill a bacterial infection, but they also kill your good bacteria, annihilating a vital part of your defence system. Most antibiotics don't kill fungi, so they soon have free rein of your skin and bowels. If you have taken a course of antibiotics in the last 6 months, it is important to take a probiotic supplement to replace the good gut flora and win the war against dandruff.

Did You Know?

Probiotic Support

What has taking probiotics got to do with fixing the dandruff on your head? Everything. Probiotics take the load off an overworked immune system by offering a helping hand — it is like having a million tiny 'bouncers' making sure fungus and bacteria don't shack up in too many areas of your body. For more information on the right probiotic for you, refer to Guideline #1 (page 51).

How to eliminate yeast infections

If you are a relaxed type (or a new fan of relaxation), this is how you can eliminate yeast infestations:

- Eat no more than one piece of fruit daily (no fruit leather or fruit juices other than fresh lemon juice).
- Avoid or only drink alcohol once a week (no binge drinking).
- Eat whole-grain bread and whole-grain products.
- Reward yourself with a sweet treat occasionally (but not every day). To do this successfully, give yourself strict guidelines, such as "Sunday is sweets day."
- Substitute sugar with the natural herb stevia to sweeten your food and drinks. Honey is also a better choice than sugar because it contains minerals.
- Eat protein with every meal (fish, eggs, skinless chicken, legumes, beans, and lean red meat); eat lots of fresh vegetables and drink plenty of water (or just follow the Healthy Skin Diet).
- Liquid chlorophyll and apple cider vinegar, which are used in the Healthy Skin Diet, also work to prevent microbe overgrowth.

Step 3: Exercise to Improve Scalp Circulation

Being a couch potato can be so much fun, especially on a rainy day when you can sit in front of the TV watching your favorite action movie and munching on popcorn. But couch potatoes are more likely to have dandruff, and dandruff is not a bucket of fun, so when it stops raining you need to move out the door and into a park or gym for some of your own blood-pumping action.

Busy people may not be couch potatoes, but they suffer from the same type of dandruff because they can either have poor circulation from lack of exercise or a poor immune system from overworking. Yes, the people who suffer from the "busy flu" (an insidious disease that prevents them from looking after their own body) can end up with busy fungi on their scalp.

Exercise junkies should be praised for their motivation — they put their body first all the way and everything else comes a poor second. Four hours of exercise is not a problem for the gym bandit, but for some reason their immune system eventually shuts down in protest. No, overexercising is not the answer to good health either (if you're a professional athlete, you're exempt, of course, as you're probably getting super health advice from experts to minimize the risk of burnout). Moderate exercise is good for your immune system. Moderate exercise basically means to exercise but not overdo it. Overdoing it would be exercising for more than 2 hours without specialized coaching, or running a marathon. Fifteen to 30 minutes of high-impact exercise can be beneficial, or 1 hour of walking or a similar low- to medium-impact workout would be good for your immune system. Your aim is to improve circulation to your scalp without depleting your immunity. You can also improve circulation to your scalp by doing headstands. Go to a yoga class to learn how to do it correctly.

> Yes, the people who suffer from the "busy flu" (an insidious disease that prevents them from looking after their own body) can end up with busy fungi on their scalp.

> You can also improve circulation to your scalp by doing headstands.

Activity

Grab your diary or planner right now and book in 15 minutes of exercise for today or tomorrow. Find out more about moderate exercise routines in Guideline #5 (page 101). Also schedule in some time to learn the breathing exercises from the Beauty Breathing chapter because they reduce stress (page 281).

Step 4: Eat Moisturizing Foods

The Healthy Skin Diet can help you eliminate dandruff, but you don't have to go overboard with dietary changes; you can simply add some fabulous foods to your existing diet, especially foods that moisturize from the inside.

Moisturizing Foods for Managing Dandruff

1. Salmon, trout, sardines, mackerel. Oily fish are a great source of omega-3 fatty acids, which are vital for healthy, flake-free skin.
2. Ground flax seeds and flaxseed oil. They are also a good source of omega-3. Have them on the days you don't eat fish. Make the Flaxseed Lemon Drink in the recipe section at least 3 days a week because it is specific for immune system health.
3. Garlic, onions, avocado, basil, and radishes have anti-fungal properties. There are plenty of snack and lunch recipes containing avocado.
4. Anti-Aging Broth and Therapeutic Chicken Soup naturally boost the immune system.
5. Horseradish and ginger. These foods have antiseptic properties and they are also good for the immune system.
6. Raw, salt-free sauerkraut. Sauerkraut is a natural probiotic.

Supplements for Preventing Dandruff

Good anti-dandruff foods may need to be supplemented in some cases with these vitamins, probiotics, biotin, and chicken.

- Omega-3 fish oils, which are high in DHA and EPA (see Guideline #2 for more information).
- B vitamins, especially vitamin B_6 and biotin. There is a Biotin Deficiency Questionnaire on page 224.
- As mentioned earlier, take a suitable probiotic supplement. Not all probiotics treat low immunity, so look up the correct one for your needs in Guideline #1.

Recipes for Managing Dandruff

To get more omega-3 in your diet: Add flax seeds, flaxseed oil, fish, and omega-3-fortified eggs to your diet. Suitable recipes include Flaxseed Lemon Drink (have it three times a week); Designer Muesli; Gluten-Free Muesli; Vitamin E Muesli; Mango and Buckwheat Crêpes; Smoked Salmon and Eggs; Tuna and Avocado Wrap; Salmon Steaks with Peas and Mash; Marinated Whole Steamed Trout; Rainbow Trout with Honey-Roasted Vegetables.

To increase the zinc in your diet: Eat fresh oysters at your next social function.

To increase biotin in your diet: Eat egg yolk and make the Creamy Mayonnaise recipe.

To boost your immune system: Make the Anti-Aging Broth or Therapeutic Chicken Soup every week until your dandruff clears up.

Quick Review of the Dandruff Management Program

Step 1: Check your hair-care products

- Wash your hair regularly with a natural shampoo and conditioner and avoid using hairspray or gel products. Avoid using a hair dryer if your scalp is overly dry and flaking. See Guideline #8 (page 126) for more information on hair-care products.

Step 2: Look after your immune system

- Learn how to relax. See Guideline #7 (page 115) and the chapter on beauty breathing (page 281).
- Drink Green Water and the Flaxseed Lemon Drink three times a week.
- Eat anti-fungal foods, such as garlic, sauerkraut (salt-free), and onion
- Prepare the Anti-Aging Broth and Therapeutic Chicken Soup.

Step 3: Exercise to improve scalp circulation

- Improve circulation to the scalp with moderate exercise and hair brushing. See Guideline #5 (page 101) for more detailed information.

Step 4: Eat moisturizing foods

- Eat a healthy diet (follow the Healthy Skin Diet)
- Increase omega-3 EFAs in your diet. See Guideline #2 (page 55) for more information.

Eczema Care

Eczema is also known as atopic dermatitis. Its distinguishing feature is a maddening itch — an itch that begs for scratching if only for a moment's relief. Other symptoms include dry red patches and cracked skin. In severe cases, weeping, bleeding, and crusts may form in the elbow creases and behind the ears and knees, and bacterial infections can occur. Having a family history of eczema, hay fever, or asthma increases your chances of inheriting eczema. A mighty flare-up can be triggered by stress, anxiety, chemicals, food intolerances, and allergens, such as dust mites.

The eczema management program shows you how to eliminate atopic dermatitis from the inside out. It describes effective supplements and lifestyle changes. This unique and exciting program can allow you to have a normal life, free of eczema. This program also strengthens your body to the point where you may stop getting minor allergies and intolerances so you can eventually eat a wider variety of foods if you wish.

Did You Know?

Prevalence and Incidence

Approximately 15 million Americans suffer from eczema at any given time. In developed countries, atopic eczema affects more than one in 10 children.

Foods to Limit, Avoid, and Increase with Eczema

- Limit saturated fats, nuts, vegetable oils, seeds, salicylates
- Avoid dairy, margarine, fried foods, white bread, and other high-GI foods
- Eat foods with fewer leukotrienes and more beneficial prostaglandins for healthy, rash-free skin.
- Increase moisturizing foods: omega-3, salmon, trout, sardines, flaxseed oil/ground flax seeds; dark green leafy vegetables.

Eczema Management Program

• •

This section shows you how to identify triggers and irritants that may be contributing to your condition. It also gives you information on allergy testing and how to soothe your skin with topical treatments. Most conventional eczema treatments prescribed by specialists end here, but this anti-eczema program details the other vital steps that can actually prevent eczema from occurring. *Note:* There is a lot of information listed in the eczema management plan, but you don't have to follow every bit of advice. Decide what's relevant to your condition and keep it simple and as doable as possible. The anti-eczema steps (steps 4, 5 and 6) are the most important ones to follow.

Q. When my eczema flares up, I get unbearably itchy. What can I do to stop the itch?

A. If you're having an itch attack, there are several remedies you can try.

- Fill a plastic bag with ice cubes and hold it next to the skin.
- Add $\frac{1}{4}$ cup (60 mL) of baking soda to a lukewarm bath and soak in it.
- Immediately after bathing, pat skin semi-dry and then apply moisturizer to your entire body, plus a thick ointment over the itchy areas.

Step 1: Identify Triggers and Irritants

Your genetics play a major role in whether you will end up with an inflammatory condition or two. If you have a family history of hay fever, asthma, sinusitis, or arthritis and both parents have had eczema at some point in their life, you have an 80% chance of developing eczema.

Common Triggers of Eczema and Other Inflammatory Conditions

- High chemical exposure
- Illness
- Food intolerances and allergies
- Drugs such as aspirin
- Dietary deficiencies
- Eating excess saturated fats
- Eating too many processed vegetable oils
- Aging
- Carbohydrates with a high GI rating
- Chronic stress

Avoiding Triggers and Irritants

High chemical exposure

Pest-control sprays, household cleaning products, perfumes, hairdressing chemicals, and crop sprays can cause toxic buildup in the body. When you breathe in or ingest too many chemicals, they can block enzyme reactions and lead to eczema. A chemical trigger could be caused by something as simple as cleaning the oven with a heavy-duty chemical cleaner or not ventilating your house for a few weeks during winter. Furnishings and carpets give off mild gases that can build up in your home over the weeks, so open the windows daily to keep your chemical exposure low.

Illness

Bacterial and viral infections, such as glandular fever, or fungal infections, such as *Candida albicans*, can deplete the body of nutrients and weaken the immune system. This can trigger hypersensitivity to harmless substances, causing an increased incidence of allergies and intolerances.

Food intolerances and allergies

Allergies, intolerances, and sensitivities can cause an inflammatory response in the body. Food intolerances generally occur when you have a weakened immune system (from illness or poor diet) or digestive disturbances. These factors must be addressed.

Aspirin

Aspirin is a type of salicylate that can block an enzyme reaction called cyclooxygenase in the body. This causes an excess of leukotrienes, the pathway in the body that makes eczema.

Dietary deficiencies

Omega-3, vitamin C, vitamin B complex (including biotin), zinc, and magnesium are all needed for eczema-free skin. These nutrients work as little helpers to assist enzyme reactions in series 1 and series 3 prostaglandins. See Guideline #2 for more information on prostaglandins and skin health.

Symptoms or Conditions Associated with Salicylate Sensitivity

- Eczema and other skin rashes
- Irritability
- Hyperactivity disorders (ADD, ADHD)
- Behavioral problems
- Migraines, frequent headaches
- Irritable bowel syndrome
- Rheumatoid arthritis
- Asthma
- Anxiety
- Depression
- Insomnia, poor sleep
- Fatigue

Q. I have eczema and I was told to avoid salicylates. What are they?

A. Your diet may contain up to 200 mg of salicylates, or the equivalent of one aspirin tablet, per day without irritating your eczema. If you have aspirin sensitivity, you can bet you have salicylate sensitivity. Salicylates are found in many fruits and vegetables, as well as sauces and gravies. Salicylates occur naturally in plant foods and they function as a pesticide and preservative, offering the plant some protection from insects and spoilage. So salicylates are beneficial for plant survival and help to keep fruits and vegetables fresher for longer.

Salicylates don't usually pose a problem to our health; in fact, many wonderful cancer- and heart-protective foods, such as blueberries and spinach, contain salicylates. However, salicylates can cause problems if your liver doesn't process these chemicals quickly enough. If your liver already has a high chemical load to deal with (from high chemical exposure) or if your liver has low phase 2 detoxification, then salicylates and other chemicals are able to build up in your system.

Eating excess saturated fats

Saturated fats from meat and dairy products supply arachidonic acid, the building block for inflammation (series 2 prostaglandins).

Aging

As you get older, your body produces fewer enzymes, especially digestive enzymes, and this can lead to poor digestion and nutritional deficiencies, causing drier skin and increased risk of inflammatory conditions.

Did You Know?
....
Too Many Trans Fats and Processed Vegetable Oils
Trans fatty acids, heated or burnt vegetable oils, and foods that are fried or deep-fried in oil contain damaged fats. Trans fats are found in some margarines, shortenings, and partially hydrogenated cooking oils. These damaged fats can make damaged prostaglandins. They cannot promote healthy cell function. One study found that children who consumed margarine had an increased risk of eczema or allergic sensitization (such as hay fever).

Carbohydrates with a high GI rating

High-GI foods, such as white bread, jasmine rice, cookies, pastries, and alcoholic beverages, rapidly break down into glucose. This influx causes losses in vitamin C and prevents utilization of essential fatty acids, so high-GI foods can indirectly cause skin inflammation. See Guideline #3 for more information on the glycemic index (GI).

Chronic stress

Chronic stress can be caused by many things, including grief, emotional breakdown, and a busy life, coupled with not enough relaxation or a negative disposition (focusing on the bad in your life more often than appreciating the good). Chronic stress is incredibly harmful to your health. It blocks valuable enzyme reactions in the body (such as series 1 prostaglandins), so you are more likely to suffer from skin inflammation, dry skin, irritability, poor sleep, and anxiety. You will have a heightened sense of pain when you are stressed.

Chronic stress is incredibly harmful to your health. It blocks valuable enzyme reactions in the body (such as series 1 prostaglandins), so you are more likely to suffer from skin inflammation, dry skin, irritability, poor sleep, and anxiety.

Activity

Think back to when your eczema first appeared — what was going on in your life at the time? For example, were you exposed to a new chemical or food? Did you move? Did you renovate or put in new carpets in your home? Was your home or office sprayed for pests or were the carpets chemically cleaned? Were you under great financial or personal pressure? Were you feeling rundown from a virus? Or if you have a child with eczema: Did your baby start drinking formula or milk just before the rash appeared? Did your baby start on solids or did your child go to a birthday party and eat brightly colored party foods, flavored chips, or sweets? Sometimes it's just not possible to work out the exact trigger for your condition. If this is the case, don't worry, because the anti-eczema program is designed to address all the triggers of eczema.

Eczema Aggravation

Now that you have looked at the triggers of eczema, you need to work out what may be aggravating your current condition. Not all of these aggravating factors will apply to you, so you may want to check off only the ones relevant to your experience. Avoid these aggravating factors whenever possible.

External factors that may aggravate eczema:

- Air conditioning
- Chlorinated water/pools
- Dust mites
- Nickel (if allergy present)
- Overheating
- Pet allergy (cat/dog/bird)
- Sand
- Soaps, shampoos, laundry detergents
- Some cosmetics and toiletries
- Some synthetic and woollen materials
- Some grasses, molds, and pollens
- Stress
- Tobacco smoke
- Weather conditions (hot/humid/cold/dry/season changes)

Internal factors that may aggravate eczema:

- Alcoholic drinks
- Chemical food additives
- Citrus fruits
- Dairy products
- Eggs (if allergy present)
- Food colorings (especially red and yellow)
- Food preservatives
- Nut allergy or rancid nuts
- Salicylates and MSG
- Seafood (if allergy present)
- Stress
- Wheat products
- Nitrates (in ham/bacon)

Foods that can cause or contribute to eczema flare-ups:

According to my own research and client feedback. MSG is the abbreviation for the form of monosodium glutamate that occurs naturally in the plant, not the chemical additive.

Food Item	Irritant
Avocado	Very high in salicylates
Chocolate	Caffeine, dairy, amines
Oranges/citrus fruit	Salicylates
Dairy	Acid-producing, lactose
Dried fruit	Preservatives
Grapes	Very high in salicylates, MSG
Sultanas/raisins	Salicylates, MSG
Kiwifruit	Very high in salicylates
Stone fruit — plum, apricot, peach	Very high in salicylates, MSG

continued...

Food Item	Irritant
Tomato	Very high in salicylates, MSG
Soy sauce/tamari	MSG
Honey/jam	Very high in salicylates
Wine, especially red	Very high in salicylates, MSG, preservatives
Broccoli, spinach	Very high in salicylates, MSG
Mushrooms	Very high in salicylates, MSG
Prune juice	Very high in salicylates, MSG

Short-Term Relief

If you are suffering with severe eczema, there are many short-term activities you can do to help minimize your discomfort. See a doctor if your rash becomes infected.

- Wear 100% cotton clothing
- Avoid wearing synthetic or woollen fabrics
- Avoid using soap and foaming cleansers
- Avoid bubble baths and normal shampoos
- Avoid fragranced toiletries and perfume
- Use lukewarm water for showering and bathing
- Use gentle, non-chemical bath oils
- Avoid stress and overtiredness
- Find a gentle, non-irritating skin cream
- Avoid stuffed toys (they harbor dust mites)
- Use rubber gloves with cotton lining
- Take off tags from clothing
- Use 100% cotton bedding
- Avoid using duvets (overheating)
- Use cotton sheets and woollen, breathable blankets in winter
- Change bedsheets weekly
- Avoid feather-filled pillows
- Vacuum carpets regularly
- Avoid cigarette smoke
- Use detergents for sensitive skin
- Use natural cosmetics if necessary

> Reducing the chemical load in your body, as a step on its own, may clear up your skin condition.

- Keep away from freshly cut grass
- Keep the house well ventilated
- Avoid using electric heating (dries skin)
- Apply moisturizer up to five times a day
- Avoid artificial chemicals and additives

An important part of the management plan is to reduce your chemical load and avoid problematic food additives. This is necessary because additives and chemicals not only trigger the onset of eczema but can also aggravate eczema on a daily basis. If your eczema is only mild or occasional, reducing the chemical load in your body, as a step on its own, may clear up your skin condition. See the list of Additives to Avoid (page 459).

Did You Know?

Climate Factor

You may notice your skin clears up when you go on holidays to sunnier, more tropical climates. This can also occur when you simply get out of the big city and go somewhere quieter and slower. Eczema can improve in certain climates, but the reason is more likely to be exposure to cleaner air, away from pollution and industrial zones. There is also evidence that salt water baths and swimming in the ocean can reduce eczema symptoms, especially if your rash is oozing or infected. This may be because sea water is a weak antiseptic and promotes healing. Swimming in salt water and exposure to sunshine (ultraviolet light) can also have a therapeutic effect, but your eczema may also clear up simply because when you are on holidays, you stop stressing and actually relax!

Step 2: Identify Allergies

You may already know if you are allergic or sensitive to something, especially if it causes physical reactions, such as swelling or redness of the skin. However, if you are unsure, you can speak to your general practitioner about allergy testing.

Skin Prick Test

Your doctor can refer you for a skin prick test. This test involves an allergy specialist putting onto your forearm about a dozen little dots of liquid samples containing potential allergens. Then the specialist pricks your skin where each dot of liquid sits. This test can help to identify if you are allergic to cats, dogs, dust mites, dust, certain nuts, dairy, soy, and so on. The skin prick test, or "scratch" test, is useful, but it only tests a small number of potential allergens and it only measures immediate IgE (immunoglobulin E) reactions or histamine reactions (involving skin swelling and redness), not sensitivity reactions (which can take hours to show up). The skin prick is not 100% reliable, so you need to trust your instincts. For example, if you feel unwell after eating a food (a couple of times in a row) or if you get a flare-up when you eat a food, listen to your body and stop consuming it for a couple of months.

Step 3: Soothe Your Skin with Topical Treatments

Topical creams and ointments are used to temporarily soothe flaky, irritated skin and reduce the itch. Oil-based moisturizers are especially useful because the lipids and fatty acids supply nutrients and trap moisture. This helps to keep out unwanted bacteria, irritants, and allergens, and can restore the skin's barrier function, which allows healing to occur. Your topical treatment options include ointments, creams and lotions, bath treatments, medicated creams, and wet bandaging.

Ointments

Ointments are thick and greasy. They are useful for scaly skin and extremely dry patches and may temporarily soothe itchy skin. Ointments can also protect your skin from stinging when you go for a swim in the ocean or chlorinated pool if a thick coat is applied beforehand. However, ointments can also stain your clothes if not used sparingly.

Creams and Lotions

> Creams, ointments, and oil-based moisturizers help to keep out unwanted bacteria, irritants, and allergens, and can restore the skin's barrier function, which allows healing to occur.

These are much thinner in consistency and soak into the skin better than an ointment. On the down side, creams and lotions wash off faster so they need to be reapplied more often (two to four times per day, or more if necessary). Lotions are even thinner than creams in consistency, so they may not offer enough moisture for severely dry and itchy skin. Although there are many eczema creams on the market, there are only two basic types to choose from. First, there are conventional creams containing synthetic and natural ingredients designed to coat the skin and trap moisture with as little irritation as possible. Second, the more natural oil- and herb-based products provide nourishment and anti-inflammatory ingredients to help heal the skin.

Positive Reports on Creams and Lotions:
- Calendula-based creams
- Zinc-based creams
- Papaya-based ointments
- Ointments containing grape seed oil; sorbolene cream; almond oil and creams containing evening primrose oil and licorice root

Negative Reports:
- Sorbolene creams
- Oatmeal-based creams
- Creams containing alcohol or too many herbs

Through talking with my clients who have had eczema, I have found that they all have differing opinions about what types of creams soothed their eczema and what creams irritated their

Bath Treatments

Bath oils coat the skin and lock in moisture; however, keep the bath lukewarm and brief so you don't dry your skin out further. After bathing, pat skin semi-dry with a soft towel and then apply a suitable moisturizer over your irritated skin. Apply your moisturizer when your skin is still a bit wet.

When choosing a bath oil, look for these ingredients:

- Sweet almond/almond oil
- Olive oil
- Coconut oil
- Apricot kernel oil
- Jojoba oil
- Vitamin E
- Borage oil
- Evening primrose oil

condition. If you find a cream that soothes the inflammation and offers relief, then stick with it. I have a list of reviewed eczema products on my website (www.healthbeforebeauty.com).

Q. The bubble bath and soap products I buy claim to be gentle on a baby's skin, so why does my child's skin break out in a rash after I bathe her with these products?

A. There are many reasons why a cleansing or beauty product can cause skin rashes. Some products alter the skin's pH level; others contain synthetic chemicals that irritate the skin. Some products can also have substances that trigger allergic responses in sensitive people. Studies show that soap can break down the skin's valuable barrier function. In fact, normal skin should have a pH of 5.5, but after soap use the skin's pH increases to more than 7.5, which can leave you vulnerable to irritants and allergens. Soap-free washes are not a good substitute to soaps, as they can also mess with the body's pH balance and leave your skin vulnerable to microbes. Also be wary if your cleansing product bubbles and foams with ease. It probably contains a synthetic ingredient called sodium lauryl sulfate (SLS) or one of its close cousins, such as sodium laureth sulfate (which is milder but still problematic in sensitive individuals). Studies have shown that SLS damages the skin barrier function for up to a month after use. So avoid cleansers, soap-free washes, shampoos, and bubble bath containing sodium lauryl sulfate. After SLS damage has occurred, you can use a moisturizer containing natural oils to speed up the healing process.

Bath Tips

1. If you want to have a bath, limit your soaking time to less than 15 minutes because bathing can strip the natural oils from your skin (which is already far too dry). To replace lost oil, add a teaspoon or two (5 to 10 mL) of your oil of choice to bath water.

2. Mix a teaspoon (5 mL) of oil (olive, coconut, or almond) with a teaspoon (5 mL) of your favorite moisturizer and then disperse it into the bath — this helps the oil to diffuse easier.

Healing Bath Recipe

1. Add ½ cup (125 mL) of apple cider vinegar and 6 to 8 drops of rose oil to warm bath water. Vinegar, especially apple cider vinegar, promotes healing of inflammation and helps to restore the skin's acidic pH.
2. Soak in this bath water.
3. Pat your skin semi-dry and moisturize your skin immediately afterwards.
4. Apple cider vinegar may increase itchiness in some individuals; if this occurs, use ¼ cup (60 mL) of baking soda in new bath water to relieve the itch.

Q. My daughter has severe eczema and my doctor prescribed cortisone cream for her. However, I've heard steroids are bad so I feel guilty using it on her. Is it bad for her?

A. I know how awful it is to see your child itching madly and crying from the pain of eczema, but don't feel guilty when using medicated creams. You need to help minimize your child's discomfort and topical steroids are an acceptable short-term treatment.

Medicated Creams

Topical steroids and cortisone creams are commonly used to treat eczema, but the results are split. There are good and bad points to using medications.

Topical steroids
Positive reviews

On the up side, topical steroids temporarily suppress surface inflammation and can offer relief for children and adults who have severe eczema. Short-term use of topical steroids shouldn't cause any long-term side effects. Use topical steroids only in severe cases where temporary relief is necessary, apply sparingly, and follow your medical practitioner's instructions.

Negative reviews

However, long-term use of topical steroids can damage collagen protein, which reduces skin elasticity and thins the skin. Steroids can also cause increased susceptibility to skin and blood vessel damage (similar symptoms to premature aging). I learned this the hard way after years of using cortisone on my face during my teenage years: now my skin has thinned and the underlying blood vessels are more visible. My skin is also extra sensitive to sunlight and prone to sun damage, so I have to take extra special care of it.

Corticosteroids

These steroids increase urinary losses of chromium. Steroids reduce the beneficial effects of vitamin C and reduce vitamin D absorption. You may worry about these factors if you continue to rely solely on steroid creams for your management of eczema. However, you can look at it this way: use the medicated creams for a short period of time while the eczema management program takes effect and each week halve the amount of steroids used. By the fourth week, you shouldn't need to use medicated creams at all.

Anti-fungal creams

These creams can be prescribed by your doctor for eczema that is infected with *Candida albicans*, a fungus that can inhabit the skin. However, long-term use is not recommended, as resistance to treatment can eventually occur.

Colloidal silver

When applied topically, this cream has a similar anti-fungal effect. Use colloidal silver externally only. You should only need it for up to 4 weeks.

Wet bandaging

In some serious cases, medical bandages can offer relief from severe itchiness and help heal lesions. Wet bandaging is often used on children with severe eczema who persistently scratch until they bleed. Speak to your doctor or pharmacist for more information.

Use topical steroids only in severe cases where temporary relief is necessary, apply sparingly, and follow your medical practitioner's instructions.

Q. I've tried eczema creams before and they always sting my skin. How do I know if a skin product is right for me?

A. Patch-testing emollients may help. When testing a product, if your skin swells and burns or feels hot and tingly or slightly more irritated on undamaged skin, then the moisturizer is not right for you. If a reaction occurs, wash the product off and apply something soothing, such as a plain ointment. If no reaction occurs, apply a small amount of moisturizer to your eczema. As your skin is damaged, this is likely to sting. Stinging shouldn't last longer than 3 minutes (usually between 1 and 3 minutes), and you should stop reacting to a cream within three applications. For example, if you apply the moisturizer twice a day, by the end of the second day your skin shouldn't sting at all. If your skin continues to hurt after the fourth application, you might be reacting to an additive in the product and you should wash the cream off and discontinue use.

How to apply a topical product

When applying a moisturizer to damaged skin, there is a very specific method, according to Professor Hywel C. Williams from the British Association of Dermatologists. Professor Williams says this can help to prevent your hair follicles from clogging and becoming infected.

1. Apply a moisturizer when your skin is still damp from a shower or bath to trap extra moisture within your skin. If you don't want to have a shower or a bath, you can always gently apply lukewarm water to your skin with a quick splash or by patting it on with a wet cotton cloth before moisturizing.
2. Don't rub it on in a circular motion as you would a normal emollient
3. Apply the moisturizer in one direction only by wiping it onto your skin in the same direction as the hair growth.

Ingredients for Eczema Moisturizers

Moisturizers can be very useful for managing the symptoms of eczema. Studies have shown that the damaged barrier function, as seen in eczema, can be restored or partially healed with oil-based creams and ointments. When choosing a moisturizer or eczema cream, look for the following ingredients:

- Calendula
- Sweet almond oil/almond oil
- Beeswax
- Evening primrose oil
- GLA (gamma-linolenic acid)
- Rosehip oil
- Vitamin E
- Apricot kernel oil
- Extra virgin coconut oil
- Zinc oxide
- Licorice root
- Shea butter
- Cocoa butter

The following can cause irritation or allergic reaction in some individuals:

- Chamomile
- Rosemary
- Aloe vera
- Manuka honey
- Borage oil

Q. I always get rough, dry hands after gardening; they also peel and it takes ages for them to soften. What can I apply to help speed up the healing process?

A. If you have dry and rough hands, there are several great hand scrubs on the market. Look for one that contains natural ingredients, such as sea salts, sodium bicarbonate (baking soda), and oils derived from apricot seed, grape seed, and rosemary. You can also try this hand scrub recipe:

Hand Scrub Recipe

This recipe exfoliates dry skin and moisturizes at the same time. Afterwards you can add extra moisturizer to protect your skin from dehydration. **Caution:** Don't use this remedy on raw and sensitive skin, open sores, or weeping skin (ouch!).

1. Mix a small amount of finely ground sea salt (less than 1/4 teaspoon/ 1 mL) with 2 teaspoons (10 mL) of olive oil. Don't make the scrub with too much salt or it will be too rough. Begin with less salt, and you can apply more if you need to.

2. Apply a teaspoon (5 mL) of the mixture to your hands and rub gently.

3. Rinse and dry your hands.

Did You Know?

No Cure for Eczema

This program eliminates eczema symptoms; however, I cannot claim to permanently cure eczema. It will disappear on the Healthy Skin Diet, but eczema can reappear if you don't look after your well-being in the future. If you have a genetic tendency for eczema, it can be retriggered by poor health, poor diet, high chemical exposure, or a severe bout of stress. Ongoing nutritional supplementation may be required to sustain clear skin.

Step 4: Take Anti-Eczema Supplements

This is a very important step toward ridding yourself of eczema. This step can also prevent food sensitivities from occurring so you can eat a more varied diet after the 8-week Healthy Skin Diet program. Supplement your diet with these products:

- Glycine (taken during weeks 1 to 8 of the Healthy Skin Diet)
- Probiotics (weeks 1 to 8)
- Biotin

Glycine

The most wonderful news I found while doing eczema research was that there is an amino acid called glycine that helps the body to eliminate salicylates safely and effectively. Amino acids are the main components of protein foods, and glycine is classed as a non-essential amino acid because the body is supposed to be able to manufacture its own supply. However, in the case of eczema and salicylate sensitivity, this may not occur.

Caution

Please note that Step 4 is specifically for adults. Don't give adult supplements to children or babies. Speak to a nutritionist or naturopathic doctor before buying a supplement for your child. You will find the Children's Clear Skin Program starting on page 263, which discusses suitable foods and supplements for children with eczema.

Glycine deficiency

The salicylates stay in your body and can cause skin rashes and even hyperactivity in some people, especially kids. Too many salicylates can also trigger an asthma attack. However, salicylates aren't the bad guys — it is a deficiency in glycine and other liver detoxification helpers that is the underlying problem. If you have good glycination, your body can effectively process and remove salicylates, benzoates (food preservatives), and phenylacetic acid (found in nuts and cigarettes). Glycine supplementation can effectively reduce salicylate sensitivity in eczema sufferers.

The recommended dosage is 2000 mg (2 g) per day, but check with your doctor before taking glycine. See the caution box below. Take glycine for 8 weeks. It may be necessary to supplement with glycine on a long-term basis, at a reduced dosage.

Caution

Do not take glycine if you are on blood-thinning medications, such as aspirin, because glycine will reduce the effects of aspirin. If you have any condition and are taking medications, seek medical advice before taking liver detoxification supplements. Newborn babies may develop cradle cap, which shows up as thick yellow crusts on the scalp. See the cradle cap discussion (page 183) and the children's program (page 263).

Did You Know?

Aspirin Overdose

Aspirin is an infamous salicylate. Medical studies have shown that glycine is effective at treating aspirin overdose. In hospitals, glycine is also used in combination with activated charcoal to treat aspirin overdose. The liver should store a supply of glycine and use it for chemical detoxification as necessary. For example, when you eat salicylate-rich fruit, such as oranges, strawberries, or kiwifruit, your liver uses glycine to detoxify and remove the salicylate portion through a process called glycination (a liver detoxifying pathway).

Other nutrients that help the liver process salicylates:

Vitamin B$_6$, also known as pyridoxine, is another nutrient that is useful in reducing salicylate and monosodium glutamate (MGS) sensitivity.

Magnesium is a mineral known as "the great relaxer" because it relieves muscle tension. Magnesium helps to prevent inflammation, so it is a valuable mineral for the treatment of eczema. This mineral is also a vital component of your bones; in fact, calcium can't make strong bones without magnesium's presence. Magnesium is another component needed for glycination in the liver. You will get enough magnesium in your diet if you drink Green Water daily because chlorophyll is a rich source of magnesium.

Calcium carbonate can also counteract a salicylate reaction. Since the Healthy Skin Diet is a dairy-free program, look for a soy milk alternative that is fortified with calcium carbonate.

Liver Detoxification Product

If you have chemical sensitivity (such as an aversion to perfumes, chemical household cleaning products, amines, MSG, or food additives) and/or a salicylate sensitivity, I highly recommend taking a specific liver detoxification supplement. Two weeks of taking a liver detox product can assist your liver with clearing out excess chemicals so you can handle them better in future. This works wonders, but the detox supplement must include magnesium, vitamin B$_6$, and a therapeutic dose of glycine. (Note: a therapeutic dose is the recommended dose for a particular supplement and taking a lower dosage may not have the desired effect.) If your liver detox supplement does not have a therapeutic amount of glycine, you can take an extra dose of glycine separately. A liver detox/cleansing supplement should only be necessary for 2 weeks.

Q. I'm so sensitive to chemicals! I can't even use furniture polish without feeling dizzy and ill, and perfumes make me sneeze. I'm also sensitive to salicylate, so I can't eat tomato, citrus, soy sauce, or strawberries without getting a flare-up. Is there anything I can do to feel well and have a more normal life?

A. Yes, you can take a liver-cleansing supplement that contains a therapeutic dose of glycine. Glycine deficiency can be caused by inadequate digestion of protein, poor diet, genetics, and/or high chemical exposure. Without adequate reserves of glycine (plus vitamin B_6 and magnesium), glycination cannot occur. You then get a flare-up.

Detox ingredients

If you have chemical or salicylate sensitivity, look for a good detoxification or cleansing supplement that includes:

- Amino acids, such as glycine, cysteine, glutamine, and taurine
- Vitamins, such as vitamin B_6, B_2, B_{12}, folic acid, biotin, and vitamin C
- Minerals, such as magnesium, calcium saccharate (glucarate), zinc, and selenium
- Herbs, such as St Mary's thistle (milk thistle, *Silybum marianum*). Milk thistle is a useful liver detoxification herb, but it contains salicylates, so it must be used with 1 to 2 grams of glycine to help process the salicylates.

Two weeks of taking a liver detox product can assist your liver with clearing out excess chemicals so you can handle them better in future.

Probiotics

Microscopic bacteria that are beneficial to health are found in the gastrointestinal tract of healthy people. These friendly flora work by adhering to your gut wall and policing the bad microbes so they can't multiply and thrive. However, studies have found that this is not always the case. People who have eczema are more likely to have an uneven balance of friendly bacteria and harmful microbes, with an increase in bad bugs and a near absence of good bacteria. Probiotic supplements supply a dose of friendly bacteria needed for healthy bowels. Common types of probiotics that you've probably seen on television commercials include acidophilus and bifidus. See Guideline #1 (page 51) for the full details about how probiotics work.

Q. I've heard probiotics are good for eczema but I tried one and it didn't work. Did I choose the wrong supplement?

A. You may have chosen the incorrect supplement, because not all probiotics are specific for treating eczema. In the *Journal of the Australian Traditional Medicine Society*, naturopathic doctor Jason Hawrelak compared the scientific research on probiotic supplements. He found the benefits you get from probiotics are strain-specific: this means they don't all treat the same conditions. Probiotics can be used therapeutically for treating eczema, but you need to know the specific strain that has been scientifically proven to suit your needs.

Probiotics proven to reduce the severity of eczema

- *Bifidobacterium lactis* Bb12 (it's now called *Bifidobacterium animalis*)
- *L. fermentum* PCC
- *L. rhamnosus* GG or *Lactobacillus* GG (it must be the GG variety)
- *L. paracasei* shirota.

Well, now the answer for eczema is as clear as mud! To remove confusion, Hawrelak also listed where to find the specific strains of good bacteria. However, product companies can change their supplement formulas, so I have listed the specific brands on my website so this information can be updated if necessary (www.healthbeforebeauty.com). If your local pharmacy or health food shop tries to convince you to buy another brand or strain of probiotic, politely say, "No, thanks," and keep looking for the "key" probiotics.

Dosage

Take one capsule three times a day on an empty stomach. For example, have your capsule 15 minutes before breakfast, lunch, and dinner. Probiotics should be ingested with room-temperature water or lukewarm rice milk/soy milk. Avoid having probiotics with excessively cold or hot drinks as extreme temperatures may damage the beneficial bacteria. It is essential to take a probiotic supplement for the duration of the Healthy Skin Diet.

Liquid Chlorophyll

As mentioned in Guideline #1, green vegetables are about the only foods that contain chlorophyll, a substance that appears as a green pigment. Chlorophyll is plant energy, converted from sunshine in a process called photosynthesis. This plant pigment is available in a liquid supplement that has an alkalizing effect when you consume it. It is this alkalizing effect that is especially important, because people with eczema tend to have an incorrect acid and alkaline balance. An acid–alkaline imbalance in the body can also result in inflammatory conditions.

> **It is this alkalizing effect that is especially important, because people with eczema tend to have an incorrect acid and alkaline balance.**

Causes of Acid–Alkaline Imbalance

- Inflammation (eczema)
- Genetics
- Eating too many acid-producing foods and not enough alkalizing vegetables
- Not coping well with stress or not looking after your well-being
- Not getting enough sleep and rest
- Medical drugs
- Chemicals
- Overexercising as well as a lack of exercise

Chlorophyll and apple cider vinegar remedies for eczema

1. Drink Green Water to help restore your acid and alkaline balance. I recommend making up a 6-cup (1.5 L) bottle of water, adding liquid chlorophyll (start with the lowest dose) and a therapeutic amount of glycine, and sip it throughout the day.

2. Since liquid chlorophyll and apple cider vinegar are high in salicylates, only use them after the glycine and probiotic supplementation has taken effect. This should happen by week 8 of the Healthy Skin Diet. However, avoid them if you are sensitive to salicylates or sulfates, because they could worsen your eczema. See Guideline #1 for dosages and cautions. Apple cider vinegar (ACV) also has an alkalizing effect in the body, so it can be useful for treating eczema. Add ACV to salad dressings. See suitable salad recipes on page 229.

3. Keep on drinking chlorophyll and ACV after you have completed the 8-week program because they will help you to keep the correct acid and alkaline balance and stay free from eczema.

Causes of Biotin Deficiency

- Excessive alcohol intake
- Frequent use of antibiotics
- Smoking
- Low-calorie diets
- Excessive junk-food intake
- Lack of friendly bacteria in the gut
- Egg white injury

Q. I've had dermatitis and dry skin for a while, but recently my skin has started looking grayish and I'm tired all the time. What is wrong with me?

A. It sounds like you may have biotin deficiency. Biotin is a B vitamin that is essential for rash-free skin. The first signs of biotin deficiency include scaly dermatitis and dry skin. Biotin can be manufactured by friendly bacteria in healthy intestines (as with many of the B vitamins); however, this bacteria can easily be destroyed by antibiotics, including the second-hand antibiotics you get from eating chicken and other non-organic meats that are fed antibiotics. Friendly bacteria can also be wiped out if you have a bout of diarrhea or illness, or if you have a poor diet.

Did You Know?

Egg White Injury

Regularly eating raw egg whites can cause egg white injury, which is a biotin deficiency. Raw egg whites contain a protein called avidin that latches onto biotin, making it too large for absorption in the body. The more raw egg white you consume, the more biotin you need to avoid deficiency symptoms. Raw egg white is found in certain food products, but you won't always know you are eating your way to a deficiency. For example, if you order a sandwich or fish burger made with mayonnaise, you could be eating raw egg white because it is often used in whole-egg mayonnaise. If you are eating party dips, such as baba ganoush or tuna dip, you could be eating raw egg white. Hollandaise sauce on eggs Benedict, chocolate mousse, and icing on traditional wedding cakes also contain raw egg white.

Occasionally having raw egg white won't give you a biotin deficiency. However, it is a good idea to avoid raw egg white or limit it to once a month if you have eczema. Once you limit eating raw egg white, your body will absorb biotin better. The good news is that when egg whites are cooked, the avidin is deactivated, so it does not affect biotin, making cooked eggs a healthy option. Egg yolks are also a rich source of biotin, making them generally good for eczema.

Biotin Deficiency Questionnaire

Complete the following questionnaire to see if you have any biotin deficiency signs. Check off any symptoms you have on a regular basis (three or more times per week):

- ☐ Scaly dermatitis/eczema*
- ☐ Dry skin*
- ☐ Grayish skin*
- ☐ Rash around the mouth and nose
- ☐ Redness and hardening around
- ☐ Eyes
- ☐ Dandruff
- ☐ Muscular pain
- ☐ Lack of energy
- ☐ Depression
- ☐ Hair loss (not including hereditary baldness)

If you have more than three symptoms and two of them are marked with an asterisk, then you may have a biotin deficiency.

Biotin Supplements

Adults require approximately 100 to 300 mcg per day, though there is no official RDI (recommended daily intake). A therapeutic dose for adults with biotin deficiency is 1 to 5 mg per day for 4 to 5 days only. Then reduce the dosage to 100 mcg per day for the duration of the Healthy Skin Diet. If you cannot get high-dose biotin, just take 100 mcg per day until your symptoms cease. Speak to your doctor before taking biotin to confirm dosage and if symptoms persist.

Caution

As with all B vitamins, if you are taking biotin for longer than a few weeks it should be taken with all the B vitamins (in a B complex supplement) to avoid causing other B vitamin deficiencies. If you are on medication, speak to your doctor before taking B vitamins.

Step 5: Eat Moisturizing Foods

When eczema occurs, it is partly due to the fact that your cells can't hold fluids properly. They leak — and as a result the skin barrier becomes dry, cracked, and inflamed. Omega-3 EFAs are anti-inflammatory and can reduce pain and inflammation when combined with an anti-inflammatory diet. Omega-3 also draws fluid back into your cells so they remain hydrated. See Guidelines #2 and #4 and the cellulite care section (page 167). You can literally moisturize your body from the inside out with the right types of foods. See the recipe ideas on page 229.

Step 6: Go on an Elimination Diet

If you suffer from eczema, you need to avoid or limit certain foods that can exacerbate your condition. Having eczema means you will be more prone to food chemical sensitivity, and dairy products will contribute to inflammation whether you have an allergy to them or not. In fact, the most dramatic results I see when treating eczema patients are when dairy is eliminated from their diets. This is why I now include this step for everyone with eczema.

Elimination Diet Plan

Follow this very basic elimination diet for 2 months. First avoid or limit specific offending foods, and once your eczema has cleared up, reintroduce these foods to see which ones affect your skin health. Your eczema should clear up within this time, although you should continue to avoid consuming artificial additives, margarine, and preservatives.

Foods and Drinks to Avoid

- Food colorings (especially red and yellow)
- Food preservatives, bread preservatives
- Nitrates (ham, bacon)
- Chemical food additives (see Additives to Avoid, page 459)
- Dairy products
- Chocolate (contains dairy and sugar)
- Citrus (oranges, mandarins, limes)
- Dried fruits (preservatives)
- Kiwifruit
- Strawberries
- Stone fruit — plums, apricots, peaches
- Tomatoes
- Grapes, sultanas, raisins
- Avocados
- Soy sauce/tamari/oyster sauce
- Anything containing raw egg white
- Alcohol, especially red wine
- Margarine
- Some saturated fats (including milk, cream, cheese, fatty meats, pork/ham/bacon, many desserts, doughnuts, fried eggs, and anything deep-fried)

Food and Drinks to Limit

- Mushrooms
- Prunes
- Red meat
- Sauces
- Certain vegetable oils (including safflower, sunflower, corn, canola, soy, and sesame oils because they contain omega-6 EFAs that can convert to arachidonic acid and cause inflammation).

Q. When do I reintroduce these foods back into my diet?

A. Two weeks after your eczema clears up, you can to begin to reintroduce these foods. When reintroducing foods or drinks, do it gradually and only when you are relaxed, because a bout of stress will make you more likely to react negatively to these foods. I find that eczema sufferers, once their eczema has cleared up, can go back to eating the Foods to Avoid list as long as they don't overindulge in them. For example, having a dairy milkshake, cheese, and a creamy dessert all in one day may cause itchiness; however, one serving of plain yogurt or milk in your coffee should be fine.

Q. My eczema first appeared when I took on a stressful job minding four children. The eczema practically covers my whole body now, and I constantly overheat and feel uncomfortable. I'm also very busy, so I need simple ways to get rid of my eczema. What can I do?

A. If stress is your trigger, you need to implement good relaxation techniques and also look after yourself a bit better. I understand this may not be so simple, especially if you believe it is not possible to slow down and be good to yourself. But remember that chronic stress is harmful to your health. You can't work or look after a family effectively if you become sick and debilitated through lack of self-care.

Relieving Stress

Relaxation: Daily relaxation is vital for your health. All you have to do is spend 15 minutes at the end of your day (or in the middle of the day if that is when you're most stressed) relaxing with one of the recommended techniques. The relaxation techniques for eczema sufferers include breathing exercises and taking lukewarm baths with natural bath oils (if bathing is not too uncomfortable for you). Spend 15 minutes indulging in relaxation each day and you will be more likely to cope with daily stress, such as screaming children, bad traffic, and lineups. See the discussion of stress in Guideline #7 (page 115) and the breathing exercises in Beauty Breathing (page 281).

Exercise: Another way to decrease the effects of stress is to exercise. You get a double bonus, as moderate exercise decreases blood levels of arachidonic acid (AA), which may help prevent eczema. Exercise also induces sweating, which has a mild anti-bacterial effect on the skin and helps to release toxins from the body. You literally sweat them out. As you can imagine, this can initially make your complexion look worse, but this is only temporary. Your skin will soon improve after the toxin load in your body has decreased. Trust me, it's worth the wait. I recommend you sweat for at least 15 minutes each day for beautiful, clear skin. The key is consistency. You must sweat nearly every day to change your health status. See Guideline #5 for further information.

> You get a double bonus, as moderate exercise decreases blood levels of arachidonic acid (AA), which may help prevent eczema.

Quick Tips for Eczema Management

Increase your glycine intake naturally by eating foods such as fish, eggs, chicken, red meat, and legumes.

1. Increase your glycine intake naturally. Glycine is an amino acid that occurs naturally in protein foods, such as fish, eggs, chicken, red meat, and legumes, although you need to be able to digest your food properly to get a dose of glycine from these foods. If you are on medication (or have poor digestion), you can get a daily dose of glycine simply by drinking the Anti-Aging Broth (see recipe section). This broth is a rich source of glycine, so sip 1 to 2 cups (250 to 500 mL) of it per day during the 8 weeks of the Healthy Skin Diet. Chamomile tea also increases glycine stores in the liver. However, be cautious. Chamomile may initially irritate your eczema because it is high in salicylate (and chamomile allergy is possible).

2. Familiarize yourself with the foods to avoid and the foods to limit (page 226), including additives and preservatives, and anything containing raw egg white. Be aware of which foods you should steer clear of when you are eating out.

3. If you want to drink alcohol during the Healthy Skin Diet, avoid all wines and beer, and favor vodka and lemonade (unpreserved lemonade), whisky and soda or gin and soda/lemonade (a splash of fresh lemon would be okay). Vodka, whisky, and gin (and soda) are all very low in food chemicals, such as salicylates, but they are still alcohol, so they need to be limited during the Healthy Skin Diet.

4. Eczema sufferers need to get adequate amounts of omega-3 from food sources. You don't need to take a fish oil supplement if you eat enough fish (especially salmon, trout, sardines, and tinned tuna are okay). Other food sources rich in omega-3 include flax seeds and omega-3-fortified eggs. I have reversed eczema without using fish oil supplements, but I find it is important for eczema sufferers to consume food sources of omega-3, such as flaxseed oil or ground flax seeds, daily and eat oily, deep sea fish.

Recipes for Managing Eczema

To increase omega-3 EFAs in your diet: Consume Pear Flaxseed Drink for Sensitive Skin; Calcium-rich Smoothie; Smoked Salmon and Eggs; Salmon Steaks with Peas and Mash; Rainbow Trout with Honey-Roasted Vegetables; and Marinated Whole Steamed Trout (avoid the sauce as it contains soy sauce/tamari). Cook with rice bran oil.

To include a variety of omega-3 EFAs: Cook rich fish two to three times a week. On the days you don't eat fish (or if you can't eat fish at all), add 1 to 2 tablespoons (15 to 30 mL) of flax seeds to your food or use flaxseed oil in salad dressings. You can also add flax seeds (ground or whole) to the following recipes: Designer Muesli; Gluten-Free Muesli; Vitamin E Muesli; Pear and Buckwheat Crêpes. To get the most out of your high-omega-3 diet, it's necessary to concurrently reduce your intake of saturated fats. This helps to balance the hormone-like prostaglandins in your body. You can still have up to two servings of meat per week, but it is necessary to avoid all dairy products during the Healthy Skin Diet.

> **To get the most out of your high-omega-3 diet, it's necessary to concurrently reduce your intake of saturated fats.**

To increase the nutrient content of your meals: Eat fresh oysters, which contain lots of zinc vital for healthy skin. Biotin-rich egg yolk can help prevent dermatitis if you have biotin deficiency, so make Creamy Mayonnaise (homemade only as it cannot contain any raw egg white/whole egg).

To get more antioxidants in your diet: Eat Sweet Chicken Stir-Fry; Roasted Sweet Potato Salad and Tasty Spinach Salad; however, use Omega Salad Dressing instead of the ones recommended. Enjoy dairy-free carob, decaffeinated coffee (no more than two cups a day), dandelion tea and chamomile tea.

To remain hydrated: Are you drinking plenty of water? Water is vital for elimination of waste and it hydrates your skin. You will get all the information you need on water in Guideline #1. Other suitable drinks include Skin Juice for Sensitive Skin No. 1 and No. 2; Skin-Firming Drink; Green Water (from week 3); ACV Drink (from week 3); and Anti-Aging Broth.

Quick Review of the Eczema Management Program

Step 1: Identify triggers and irritants

- Limit chemical exposure, use natural cleaning products, and wash fruits and veg.
- Eat fewer processed, chemical-laden products and eat more fresh food.

Step 2: Identify allergies

- Identify allergies and avoid offending foods and environments.

Step 3: Soothe your skin with topical treatments

- Moisturize your skin as often as needed (two to four times a day).
- Have a healing bath once or twice a week.

Step 4: Take anti-eczema supplements

- Have a therapeutic dose of glycine daily (look for a glycine supplement that also contains magnesium and vitamin B_6).
- Take a probiotic supplement that is specific for eczema.
- **Optional:** If you have signs of biotin deficiency, take a supplement for 8 weeks, and if you present with chemical sensitivity, take a liver detoxification supplement for 2 weeks.

Step 5: Eat moisturizing foods

- Drink plenty of water — 8 to 10 glasses a day.
- Consume omega-3 EFAs every day.
- Adults with severe dry skin should also take an omega-3 supplement. See Guideline #2 (page 70) for dosage and cautions.

Step 6: Go on an elimination diet

- Limit saturated fat intake — avoid pork and dairy products and limit red meat intake (have one to two servings of meat a week, each serving smaller than the size and thickness of the palm of your hand).
- Avoid foods that are likely to cause flare-ups. Especially limit the types of fruit you eat. Favor pears, banana, and papaya as they are salicylate-free, and eat small amounts of apples and blueberries. Avoid all other fruits.
- Reduce omega-6 EFAs by avoiding margarine; safflower/sunflower/sesame/corn oil; nuts and seeds. You can use small amounts of ghee, butter, or extra virgin olive oil in cooking.
- Increase non-dairy sources of calcium (see page 66). Use soy milk that is fortified with calcium carbonate. Butter and ghee are the only acceptable dairy products, unless you have a diagnosed dairy allergy.
- Relax.
- Sweat for 15 minutes every day.
- In week 3, introduce Green Water and apple cider vinegar into your routine.

After your eczema has cleared up

- Celebrate!
- Gradually reintroduce dairy products into your diet. Have one serving only per day, such as plain yogurt, and see if it causes a flare-up. This step is necessary to identify whether you should avoid or limit dairy for the long term.
- After you have tried dairy products and have experienced no reaction, add more foods back into your diet, including tomato, grapes, and lemon. Introduce one new food every 3 days. If you get a flare-up, limit or avoid that food for another month, then retest.
- Reduce supplement dosages gradually. Stop taking probiotic, biotin, and liver-cleansing supplements (if you haven't already).
- **Important:** Keep consuming omega-3-rich foods every day (fish, flax seeds etc), and continue having one bottle of Green Water (with added glycine and 2 teaspoons/10 mL of chlorophyll) three to five times a week (or daily if desired).

Psoriasis Care

Silvery scales were meant for fish, not femmes fatales. Psoriasis (pronounced sor-RYa-sis) is an inflammatory skin disorder that can look silvery or red, and it can occur on any part of the body. As mentioned previously, skin cells mature in approximately 4 weeks, but with psoriasis they can mature in as little as 3 to 4 days, resulting in flaky buildup. It's as if the skin is desperate to expel something irritating from within, so it prematurely forces skin cells to the surface. Psoriasis can be itchy and occasionally painful, but it is not contagious. People with psoriasis usually have an underlying genetic tendency that makes them susceptible to getting the condition. However, psoriasis can lie dormant for many years and may never appear unless it's awoken by some sort of trigger.

Did You Know?

Prevalence and Incidence

- Up to 7.5 million Americans have psoriasis, according to the US National Psoriasis Foundation.
- Approximately 2% to 3% of the world's population is affected by psoriasis (at the time this statistic was calculated, it totaled approximately 125 million people!)
- Psoriasis commonly develops between the ages of 15 and 40, but it can occur at any age. Approximately 75% of psoriasis cases occur before the age of 40.
- Psoriasis is more common in fair-skinned people.
- You are less likely to get psoriasis if you live somewhere tropical and sunny. It's a good excuse to move to the Bahamas.

Psoriasis Triggers

Psoriasis can be triggered by the following factors:

- High chemical exposure
- Injury
- Throat infection/poor health
- Drugs/medications
- Physical stress
- Emotional stress

Activity

If your psoriasis appeared during adulthood or in your later childhood years, it is a good idea to try to figure out what may have triggered it. Think back to when your psoriasis first appeared — what was going on in your life at the time? For example, were you exposed to a new chemical or food? Did you move? Did you renovate your house or put in new carpets? Was your home or office sprayed with pesticides or were the carpets chemically cleaned? Were you under great financial or personal pressure? Were you feeling rundown with a virus or throat infection? Were you prescribed a new drug or were you using pain-killers or another kind of medication? Were you self-medicating with alcohol or cigarettes? It's important to work out what may have switched on your psoriasis gene so you can see if you're still being exposed to the problem. For example, if you figure that stress triggered your psoriasis, you can make sure you include relaxation techniques in your healthy skin program. If your trigger was a throat infection, you can support your immune system with relaxation and supplements, such as probiotics and zinc, as well as certain foods, such as garlic and the Anti-Aging Broth (page 392). If you suspect it may have been triggered by a prescribed drug (and you are still taking it), speak to your doctor about possible alternatives (DON'T stop taking the drug without speaking to your doctor first).

Psoriasis Aggravations

Psoriasis symptoms can be aggravated by these behaviors and conditions:

- Alcohol, heavy drinking
- Anxiety and worry
- Chemical exposure
- Chemical cleaning products
- Illness, serious throat infection
- Medications/drugs
- Severe stress, trauma, inability to cope
- Trauma to the skin (scratch/surgery)
- Vitamin and mineral deficiencies
- Cold climates
- Poor digestion, bowel toxemia
- Impaired liver function
- Eating excess meats/saturated fats
- *Candida albicans*
- Cigarette smoke

Psoriasis Management Program

This management program details how psoriasis can be managed, soothed, and calmed. You can use WOL (water, oil, and light) therapy in conjunction with this anti-psoriasis program. This program is like an insurance policy that helps to prevent your psoriasis from returning. Please note that this is an adult program for anyone over the age of 15 years only. For a suitable children's program, see the Children's Clear Skin Program (page 263). Children with psoriasis should also use WOL therapy 4 days a week.

Step 1: Use Water, Oil, and Light Therapy

Q. I have psoriasis, it's extremely uncomfortable and I'm shedding skin everywhere. What can I do to get some relief and reduce flaking?

A. A common therapy for treating psoriasis is sunlight therapy, and when you combine this treatment with water and oiled skin, you can quickly reduce scales and get some relief. Water, oil, and light therapy (I like to call it WOL therapy) is natural, it doesn't have the negative side effects that corticosteroids have, it is practically free (the price of a jar of oil), and it can be highly effective — it may even temporarily eliminate your psoriasis. However, I recommend using WOL therapy in conjunction with the diet and supplement advice in the anti-psoriasis program for long-term results.

Did You Know?

Warm Bath and Vitamin D Research

An 8-week study published in the *International Journal of Hypothermia* found that warm bath treatments were also very effective in healing flaky lesions in psoriasis patients. Seven people were asked to take very warm baths twice a week and three of them showed a rapid improvement in symptoms; the other four were told to increase bathing to every second day and three out of the four had improved symptoms. Only one person's lesions did not improve with bath therapy, and coincidentally he was the only person in the study who was also using doctor-prescribed drug therapy. So WOL therapy may not work in conjunction with conventional psoriasis medications, but please speak to your doctor first before discontinuing your prescribed drugs. Back to the "warm bath" study…

Not only were psoriatic lesions completely healed in six out of seven of the people, swelling (edema) was also markedly reduced and itching was relieved in all patients during the treatments. This relief lasted for up to several months after treatment. An unexpected (and some would say positive) side effect was increased melanin content in the skin, which increased tanning ability in sun-exposed skin.

Another study found that people with severe psoriasis have decreased blood levels of vitamin D, compared with clear-skinned people and people with mild psoriasis. You can obtain a daily dose of vitamin D by simply going out in the sun because UV rays from sunlight trigger vitamin D production in the skin. (Being covered from head to toe with sunscreen can block vitamin D production, so skip the heavy-duty sunscreen during WOL therapy, but use sunscreen if you are spending more than 15 minutes in the sun.) I don't recommend sun-baking for long periods. Keep sunshine therapy to a healthy minimum, which is about 10 minutes a day.

WOL Therapy Step by Step

1. Begin by wetting your skin with warm water — either by having a very warm bath or a shower or by splashing yourself with water. Keep in mind that it is best to allow the water to soak into the skin for a few minutes. Bathing is also a safe and effective way to gently remove some of the excess skin.

2. Pat your skin semi-dry, leaving some moisture on the skin, then rub in tiny (must be tiny!) amounts of olive oil, ointment, or coconut oil. When applying the ointment or oil, remember that the less you use, the better it works. Gently rub in the ointment/oil until it is completely absorbed. According to psoriasis specialist Dr David Cohen, the more you rub it in, the better this treatment should work.

3. Once you have applied a thin, well-rubbed-in layer of ointment or oil onto the affected areas, you may notice that these areas end up feeling dry again. IMMEDIATELY, while the skin is still partially moist, rub another smidgen of ointment over the same spots of scaly skin. Rub in thoroughly once again.

Topical Treatments

There are a number of beneficial topical treatments that can be used for WOL therapy:

Extra virgin olive oil. Extra virgin means it is less processed and has higher vitamin E content (an antioxidant that is good for the skin) than regular olive oil. Apply a capful to bath water for WOL therapy. Use organic oil if possible. It is inexpensive and effective.

Extra virgin coconut oil. Contains capric acid, which is anti-fungal, and also contains anti-microbial lauric acid, which is naturally found in sebum. It is one of the most respected oils found in the British Pharmacopoeia. Protects the skin from microbes and dryness. Suitable for WOL therapy.

Ointments. Ointments and balms are thick and greasy. Look for beneficial ingredients, such as papaya, triglyceride wax, grape seed oil, beeswax, and vitamin E. Useful for scaly skin and extremely dry patches. May temporarily soothe itchy skin. Ointments can protect your skin from stinging when you go for a swim in the ocean or a chlorinated pool if a thick coat is applied beforehand. However, ointments can also stain your clothes if not used sparingly. Natural ointments are available from health food shops. May be suitable for WOL therapy.

Sweet almond oil/almond oil. These are anti-bacterial and contain fatty acids and triglycerides to moisturize the skin. Soothes irritation and dryness. May be suitable for WOL therapy.

4. Follow this procedure at least twice a day for best results. For severe psoriasis, you can repeat this process up to five times a day for maximum relief. When symptoms markedly improve, you can reduce this routine to once a day.

5. For accelerated results, which may also put your psoriasis into remission, use natural sunlight therapy daily after one of your ointment applications: 10 minutes of sunshine daily, after wetting and moisturizing the skin, is enough to encourage healing.

6. After short sun exposure, don't wash off the oil by having a shower. Instead, if it is necessary, you can gently blot any excess oil/ointment with a wet cloth (don't rub harshly).

7. Don't try to remove dry patches of skin unless they are first wetted with water. There is little or no benefit to putting a cream or oil onto the skin unless the skin is moist.

Caution

Avoid psoriasis products that contain coal tar, as this ingredient is a skin and eye irritant that has promoted cancer in animal studies (keeping in mind that this has not been proven in human studies).

Step 2: Improve Your Liver Health

As I have mentioned before, I've had a personal relationship with psoriasis, so I realize how ostracized you can feel when you have this skin condition. My psoriasis was triggered when I flea-bombed the house with a strong chemical concoction bought from the supermarket. I have a family history of eczema, contact dermatitis, arthritis, and heart disease (lots of inflammation in the family tree), so getting psoriasis was no big surprise. Psoriasis can also be triggered in people who have no family history of the condition and no genetic tendency, if they're exposed to a large dose of stress or chemicals. Let's first consider psoriasis that is caused by chemical exposure.

Psoriasis can also be triggered in people who have no family history of the condition and no genetic tendency, if they're exposed to a large dose of stress or chemicals.

Chemical Exposure

We were never meant to inhale or ingest large amounts of toxic substances. In fact, even low but regular exposure to chemicals puts a great burden on the liver (and immune system). Your liver is designed to deactivate chemicals, toxins, hormones, and drugs, safely removing them from your blood. To demonstrate this, picture your liver as a big sponge that filters the blood — chemicals go in and then they exit the other end of the sponge in a different form as they are now deactivated so they can be removed from the body. This is called detoxification.

Detoxification Process

To deactivate chemicals, the liver needs little "helpers" — tiny worker nutrients, such as B vitamins, minerals, omega-3 and amino acids — to assist with the detoxification process. But what happens if you're not getting enough of these helpers in your diet? Your liver cannot work on its own, and if it runs out of helpers — the essential nutrients — the liver will send chemicals back into the bloodstream without deactivating them, so they stay in the body.

Imagine what happens over time … your body has more and more chemicals in the blood, and to prevent damage they have to be stored in your body's tissues. What happens to this excess waste? Your body wants to remove unwanted materials any way it can. Another way to do this is through the skin. Chemicals are expelled through the skin, which may explain

CASE STUDY

After my chemical exposure, I ended up with a small circular patch of flaking skin on my neck and it didn't go away. It quickly spread over my chest, and my torso ended up completely covered within a month of the first patch appearing. I was embarrassed about my patchy red scales, and going for a swim at the local pool became a test in confidence as I exposed my mottled skin. With the help of the anti-psoriasis program and WOL therapy, my psoriasis completely disappeared within 4 weeks. My psoriasis has never reappeared, not even a single patch.

the exceptionally fast skin-turnover process in psoriasis sufferers. The skin may shed quickly to help eliminate excess chemicals.

Nutrient Support of Detoxification

To help your liver recover from chemical exposure, drugs/ medicines, alcohol, illness, or a stressful period in your life, you need in your diet nutrients such as omega-3, selenium, vitamin E, zinc, magnesium, vitamin B_6, glycine, taurine, and vitamin C. If you are not getting these nutrients in your diet, your liver can't do its job properly.

Glutathione: The antioxidant enzyme glutathione peroxidase is abnormally low in many psoriatic patients, and this can result from the excessive loss of skin cells or other factors, such as alcohol misuse and eating too much greasy fast food. Low glutathione is bad news for you because glutathione is vital to keep you looking young and gorgeous. It is an antioxidant that is vital for liver detoxification of pesticides, alcohol, and heavy metals. The antioxidant mineral selenium, when combined with vitamin E, can bring glutathione levels back up to normal levels.

Liver detoxification supplement: This is the first line of defense or the first supplement to use when treating psoriasis. A good liver detox supplement (and one that is suitable for psoriasis) should contain selenium, vitamin E, vitamin A (beta-carotene), zinc, magnesium, vitamin B_6, glycine, taurine, glutamine, and vitamin C. Take a liver detox supplement for 2 to 4 weeks.

Exercise, adequate sleep, and drinking plenty of water also help the liver to function at full speed.

Step 3: Improve Your Digestion and Bowel Health

Poor digestion of protein can contribute to psoriasis. If your digestive system does not break down and absorb protein correctly, high levels of amino acids and polypeptides are left in the bowel. You don't have to remember their names; just know that they are converted by bowel bacteria into toxic substances, such as polyamines.

Hydration

Make sure you're drinking enough water and other hydrating liquids to keep your skin looking gorgeous and clear of psoriasis. Other hydrating liquids include herbal teas, fresh vegetable juices, mineral water, dandelion tea, and any of the drinks listed in the recipe section (page 343).

Q. What are polyamines?

A. Increased polyamine levels have been found in psoriasis sufferers, which may explain why psoriatic skin cells mature too quickly. Psoriasis sufferers have incorrect cell division caused by not enough cyclic AMP and too much cyclic GMP (both are internal control compounds). Polyamines decrease production of cyclic AMP, which contributes to skin cells maturing too quickly (causing scaly, rough skin). Polyamines may sound a bit confusing, but all you have to do is focus on the remedies for inhibiting these toxic substances — the main remedy being to improve your protein digestion, as this is the true source of the problem. This may involve relaxing more often, chewing your food better, and drinking the Papaya Beauty Smoothie to improve digestive juices. You can also protect yourself against toxic polyamines by taking vitamin A and the herb goldenseal (*Hydrastis canadensis*). Check with your doctor before taking this herb. People with psoriasis are often deficient in vitamin A and zinc — both of these nutrients are vital for healthy skin. When buying a liver detoxification/cleansing supplement, make sure it contains vitamin A, or beta-carotene, and zinc.

Bowel Health Questionnaire

Let's see if you have any signs of poor bowel health. Check any signs or symptoms that you experience on a regular basis (weekly):

- ☐ Foul-smelling gas and/or stools
- ☐ Excessive gas
- ☐ Excessive burping
- ☐ Bloating
- ☐ Food allergies, food sensitivities
- ☐ Abdominal discomfort/pain
- ☐ Chronic fatigue
- ☐ Premature aging
- ☐ Constipation and/or diarrhea
- ☐ Nausea
- ☐ Unexplained back/shoulder/abdominal pain

If you have checked off more than three symptoms, you may have poor bowel health that could be caused by poor digestion, poor diet, not enough water/hydration, *Candida albicans* (yeast infection), poor bowel flora, or parasites. If you have any concerns, see your doctor, especially if you have pain. Refer to Guideline #1 to see what you can do to keep your gut in good working order.

Step 4: Consume Omega-3 Fatty Acids

According to an international study, psoriasis sufferers have decreased levels of omega-3 EFAs in their blood. Omega-3 is absolutely essential for gorgeous skin. Your cells need EFAs, such as omega-3 (linoleic acid), to function properly because without adequate EFAs skin cells can become rigid. Skin cells may also leak fluids, which can irritate the surrounding tissues, causing redness and swelling. Omega-3 is anti-inflammatory, so it can reduce the inflammation seen in psoriasis.

Omega-3 needs to convert to EPA and DHA in the body before it can be used to prevent inflammation and dry, flaking skin. If taking an omega-3 fish oil supplement, it is important to get a therapeutic dose of EPA and DHA. Fish oil works better than flaxseed oil when treating psoriasis, but you can also add this omega-3-rich seed oil to your diet. For correct dosages of omega-3 supplements, see page 70.

Step 5: Stress Less and Relax More

As mentioned earlier, psoriasis can be triggered by emotional stress and anxiety, but don't get me wrong, stress isn't always a bad thing: short-term stress can give you a boost of energy and motivate you to excel. But chronic emotional stress and bouts of anxiety can cause all sorts of health problems. Stress and anxiety have the ability to drain your body of essential nutrients.

For example, you are panicking about your high school end-of-year exams and you can't sleep. You worry about failing, and by the time you have completed your tests, your body is so depleted of B vitamins and liver-detoxifying minerals that your liver hasn't got enough "helpers" to keep your blood clean, so you end up with psoriasis. Your skin bears the burden if your liver and immune system are overworked.

Dealing with Your Stress

So you have identified that you are prone to stress, but you can't possibly give up your busy life to go and meditate for a week in Nepal. What else can you do? There are plenty of alternatives to help you temporarily switch off your inner "busyness" and find some inner peace.

1. **Warm bath recipe.** Have a warm bath at the end of your action-packed day. A bath is fantastic for psoriasis, as mentioned in the WOL therapy section, and it also helps your body switch to the rest and digest part of your nervous system. Having a humble bath is truly good for you. Have a relaxing bath three to four times a week. You can combine this with WOL therapy. Fill the bath with warm water and add the following: 1 cup (250 mL) Epsom salts, 1 tablespoon (15 mL) extra virgin olive oil or coconut oil. Bathe for 10 to 20 minutes and do nothing but breathe in and out and look at the water. For a moment, forget your life and your worries — they can wait. Remember, bath time is your precious time out, not time to make a "to do" list.

2. **Relaxing breathing exercises.** They are also fantastic for inducing relaxation. But I'm not talking about any old breathing in and out, I mean true diaphragmatic breathing that tricks your body into thinking it is calm and happy, if only for a few moments. Mastering a few of these techniques can be useful for when you're at work and you have a panic attack or if you're feeling overwhelmed. Just sit at your desk and focus on very specific inhalations and exhalations and you'll soon feel better. These breathing exercises are covered in the chapter on beauty breathing (page 281).

3. **Regular exercise.** Physical activity is one of the best ways to reduce stress. See Guideline #5 (page 101) for suitable exercise regimens.

4. **Good sleep.** Getting adequate sleep is a great way to counter stress. When you sleep, your body heals itself. Your cells are like little doctors and nurses, working though the night, making you all better. However, when your sleep is disturbed by lights or sunlight (if you're a shift or night worker), noise, or insomnia, then your skin won't be able to rejuvenate itself properly. Wounds may not heal effectively and you end up aging prematurely. Make sure you get to bed by 10:30 p.m. and have about 8 hours of quality sleep. If you are having trouble getting to sleep, see Guideline #4 (page 95) for more information.

> Psoriasis can be triggered by emotional stress and anxiety. Your skin bears the burden if your liver and immune system are overworked.

Recipes for Managing Psoriasis

To get more vitamin A and beta-carotene in your diet: I recommend you simply eat more carrots, eggs, and colorful vegetables rather than taking a supplement. After all, one carrot contains approximately 20,253 IUs (international units) of beta-carotene. Try recipes from the Healthy Skin Diet such as Roasted Sweet Potato Salad; C-Rich Apricot Chicken; Sweet Raspberry, Avocado and Watercress Salad; ACE Smoothie; Spot-Free Skin Juice; Mango and Buckwheat Crêpes; and Perfect Poached Eggs.

To get more zinc in your diet: Eat oysters and liver. Snack on a small handful of Brazil nuts twice a week. They also contain selenium.

To increase omega-3 (EPA/DHA) in your diet: Eat deep sea/oily fish at least twice a week. Recipes include Marinated Whole Steamed Trout; Salmon Steaks with Peas and Mash; Rainbow Trout with Honey-Roasted Vegetables; Creamy Salmon Mornay; Smoked Salmon and Eggs; Tuna and Avocado Wrap. Essential: Add 1 to 2 tablespoons (15 to 30 mL) of flax seeds to your food or use flaxseed oil in one of the following skin drinks: Flaxseed Lemon Drink; Pear Flaxseed Drink for Sensitive Skin; Berry Beauty Smoothie; Papaya Beauty Smoothie; Calcium-Rich Smoothie; Apple Omega Drink.

Quick Review of the Psoriasis Management Program

Step 1: Water, oil, and light therapy

- Use WOL therapy approximately four times a week.

Step 2: Improve liver health

- Follow the Healthy Skin Diet (either the standard 8-week program or the structured menu).
- During the first 2 weeks, take a liver detox/cleansing supplement. Look for one that contains selenium, vitamin E, vitamin A/beta-carotene, zinc, magnesium, vitamin B_6 (and other B vitamins), glycine, taurine, glutamine, and vitamin C.

Step 3: Improve your digestion and bowel health

- Improve bowel health with a probiotic supplement (see page 51).
- Drink plenty of water and other hydrating fluids.

Step 4: Consume omega-3 EFAs

- Take an omega-3 fish oil supplement containing EPA and DHA. Make sure you're having a therapeutic dose (page 70).

Step 5: Stress less and relax more

- Have relaxing baths once or twice a week.
- Relax for at least 10 minutes a day
- Do breathing exercises (page 281).
- Sweat daily and exercise three to four times a week (page 101).
- Get adequate sleep (page 95).

Rosacea Care

Rosacea sufferers are not only blushing like a beet, they are also suffering with an uncomfortable skin disorder that may eventually disfigure their face. Rosacea (pronounced rose-AY-sha) first appears as a mild redness of the skin that looks like sunburn, but the redness doesn't disappear. Rosacea is not contagious or infectious. The rosiness is actually caused by enlarged blood vessels under the skin, as these blood vessels fail to function like normal ones. Rosacea sufferers may also develop pimples and have dry, burning and gritty sensations in the eyes. A thickening of the skin, caused by enlarged sebaceous glands, can also lead to the nose becoming larger and disfigured (bulbous). Rosacea is said to be irreversible once it becomes chronic, but I believe any stage of rosacea can be eliminated or at least minimized and controlled with the right health program.

Facial Blood Vessel Function and Structure

Rosacea is primarily a disorder of the facial blood vessels. Facial skin contains hundreds of blood vessels of different shapes and sizes, but with rosacea, where the facial skin becomes easily flushed, the underlying facial blood vessels don't behave as they should. To understand rosacea better, it is important to look at the functional and structural changes that occur in the blood vessels of rosacea sufferers. You don't have to fully understand the structural and functional changes in rosacea to be able to treat your condition; you just need to remember things that make your condition worse so you can limit your exposure to them. This is important because you can help to prevent your blood vessel functional changes from becoming permanent structural changes. Structural changes are bad news, so you want to treat this condition as early as possible.

Normal Function of Facial Blood Vessels

- Facial blood vessels deliver essential nutrients and oxygen to the skin. Just like the postman delivers letters to your home each day, your blood vessels transport and deposit vitamins, minerals, fats, and oxygen to your outer layer throughout the day (and night) so your skin can function properly.
- Facial blood vessels remove waste products that have been produced by facial skin cells. Just as you put out your household garbage each week for collection by the local garbageworkers, your facial skin cells also put out their garbage daily and the bloodstream takes these waste products away for removal from the body.
- Facial blood vessels help to regulate internal body temperature. If your body's internal temperature gets too high, it triggers the blood vessels to dilate. This expansion of the vessels allows an increase in blood flow, which releases large amounts of heat from the skin's surface. This helps the internal body temperature to normalize and, afterwards, healthy blood vessels return to their regular size.

Abnormal Function of Facial Blood Vessels in Rosacea

- Rosacea blood vessels expand (dilate) when exposed to ordinary substances that normal blood vessels do not respond to.
- Rosacea blood vessels can expand wider than normal blood vessels.
- Rosacea blood vessels can continue to dilate for abnormally long periods.

These three changes cause an abnormal increase in blood flow to facial skin, and this results in facial flushing. In rosacea, the functional changes occur first, and if these functional changes are left untreated, then more serious structural changes may eventually occur.

Normal Structure of Facial Blood Vessels

- Blood vessels are hollow tubes that transport blood that is rich in nutrients and oxygen from the heart to the body's outermost organ — the skin.
- Facial blood vessels contain vascular smooth muscle cells and endothelial cells, which work to control blood flow and change the blood vessel diameter.

Abnormal Structure of Facial Blood Vessels in Rosacea

- Rosacea facial blood vessels may become permanently dilated from dysfunctional endothelial cells — like a balloon that has been blown up and let out so many times that it eventually fails to deflate back to its original size.
- Damage may occur to vascular smooth muscle.
- New blood vessels may branch out from existing blood vessels (angiogenesis), and more blood vessels near the surface of your skin will make your skin appear red.

Activity

Imagine that vascular smooth muscle cells and endothelial cells are like nightclub bouncers. A bouncer acts as a regulator, usually increasing the flow of people through the door when the club is empty but restricting the amount of patrons who come through the door when they get instructions from management to do so. In a similar way, normal blood vessels should dilate and constrict on cue, to meet the body's demands and maintain good health.

Rosacea Triggers

Let's identify factors that can aggravate rosacea. This will vary from person to person. See if you can identify some of your facial flushing triggers from this list. Check off behaviors, substances, and other triggers you have experienced recently:

- ☐ Allergies (triggering histamine release)
- ☐ Alcohol
- ☐ Anxiety and worry
- ☐ Dairy products
- ☐ Embarrassment
- ☐ Exposure to sunlight
- ☐ Extreme temperatures
- ☐ Foods containing histamine
- ☐ Hot drinks
- ☐ Illness
- ☐ Laughing, crying
- ☐ Poor diet and lifestyle
- ☐ Saunas or hot baths
- ☐ Sudden temperature changes
- ☐ Sunshine
- ☐ Some medications (such as topical steroids)
- ☐ Spicy and hot foods
- ☐ Skin-care products
- ☐ Stress, inability to cope
- ☐ Vitamin and mineral deficiencies
- ☐ Windy weather
- ☐ Physical activity (physical activity aggravates rosacea, but exercise should not be avoided as it is an important part of recovery)

Rosacea Management Program

In the rosacea management plan, you will find out how to look after your skin condition and minimize discomfort. The management plan details factors that can exacerbate rosacea, as do the what to avoid and topical treatments sections. I have listed heaps of information below, but you don't have to follow every bit of advice; you should decide what is relevant to your condition and keep it as simple and as "doable" as possible. This anti-rosacea program takes a deeper look at why rosacea may appear in the first place. It goes way beyond trying to soothe the hot flush and looks at possible causes so you can eliminate the root of your problem and improve your blood vessel function and structure. This program shows you how to improve your health and clear up your skin condition from the inside out. This program is divided into six steps.

The supplement advice in this program is designed for adults. If you have a child with rosacea, you can read this section, but you should follow the Children's Clear Skin Program (page 163) and implement a daily exercise routine for your child.

> This program shows you how to improve your health and clear up your skin condition from the inside out.

Step 1: Limit Histamine Reactions

Because the redness of rosacea is created by enlarged blood vessels under the skin, we'll look very closely at histamine foods and their ability to enlarge blood vessels. Histamines are able to cause such havoc in your body because they are present in almost all body tissues, waiting for a trigger to release them into the bloodstream. Histamine is stored in the skin, lungs, intestinal lining, mast cells, and basophils. Histamine has the ability to signal to your body to enlarge the blood vessels and allow maximum blood flow, which leads to a facial flush. Headaches can be caused by histamine-containing chocolate because histamine causes the blood vessels in the brain to dilate, which increases pressure in the head.

> Histamines are able to cause such havoc in your body because they are present in almost all body tissues, waiting for a trigger to release them into the bloodstream.

Histamine Triggers

- The release of histamine can be triggered by anything your body deems an allergen, including drugs, chemicals, inhaled particles (such as pollen), insect venom, and some foods.
- Histamine release can also be triggered by stress. If you are an anxious worrywart, you are probably flooding your body with havoc-wreaking histamines.

Histamine/Amine Sensitivity Questionnaire

Read and fill in the following questionnaire to identify whether you have a histamine or amine sensitivity.

QUESTION	Always	Sometimes	Never
If you eat too much chocolate, do you get a headache or migraine? OR do you suffer from frequent headaches or migraines but don't know the trigger?	10	5	0
Does alcohol, especially red wine and beer, cause increased flushing of the face, excess body heat, swelling of the tongue/throat/face, or is there any other sensitivity reaction?	10	5	0
Do you notice a reaction when you eat cheese, raw egg, or citrus?	10	5	0
Do you notice a reaction when you eat fish, deli meats, or sausages?	10	5	0
Do you notice a reaction when you eat preservatives (in breads, etc.)?	10	5	0
Do you react to perfumes, household cleaners, or pesticides?	10	5	0
TOTAL SCORE:			

Score Card

If you scored 20 or above, you may have an amine sensitivity. If you scored over 30, then you are highly likely to have amine sensitivity. However, even if you scored lower, I believe all people with rosacea should limit their intake of histamine-containing foods to prevent the progression of rosacea.

Histamine Release

When you have an allergic response, the substance you have come into contact with stimulates the release of antibodies, which then attach to your mast cells and cause histamine to be released. For example, you might be allergic to the yellow food coloring found in the packaged dessert you just ate, so your body goes into panic mode and releases the antibodies that attach to mast cells. Then histamine is freed into your bloodstream, which causes your skin to itch and flush with redness.

Histamine/Allergic Symptoms

- Itchy nose
- Sneezing and increased mucus production
- Watery or burning sensation in eyes
- Skin rashes or hives
- Congested sinuses
- Headache or migraine
- Wheeze in lungs or spasms
- Stomach cramps
- Diarrhea
- Skin itchiness
- Skin flushing/redness

Did You Know?

Histamine Exposure

Histamine can trigger facial flushing in rosacea sufferers. There are two ways you can be exposed to histamine. First, histamine is released within the body when exposed to stress or an allergen (an allergen causes an allergic histamine reaction, such as redness or swelling). Second, histamine is naturally found in many delicious foods and drinks, such as wine, cheese, and chocolate.

Histamines in Foods and Drinks

As mentioned earlier, histamine is naturally found in many foods and drinks, in varying amounts. Large amounts can be found in chocolate, cheese, wine, spicy food, and beer, which is why they are more likely to cause a reaction than other histamine-containing foods. It is not necessary to avoid all of these foods, but you must limit them. Also take note of any negative reactions that occur after eating any of these foods. If hot flushes or heart palpitations happen after eating a particular food, avoid that substance for the duration of the Healthy Skin Diet.

Histamine-Rich Foods and Drinks

- Anchovies, sardines, tuna
- Avocado
- Beer, brandy, liqueur, port, rum, sherry
- Canned foods
- Cheese
- Chocolate, cocoa powder/drinks
- Ciders, cider vinegar, vinegar
- Cola soft drinks
- Eggplant
- Fermented drinks
- Fermented foods/yogurt/soy sauce
- Fish (colored, not white-fleshed)
- Gherkins
- Jams and preserves
- Meats, cooked or processed
- Mushrooms
- Olives
- Oranges, orange juice
- Sour cream
- Spinach
- Tomatoes, tomato juice and sauce
- Wines, especially red wine
- Yeast extract

Histamine-Releasing Foods, Which Cause a Histamine Reaction

- Alcohol
- Bananas
- Certain nuts
- Chocolate
- Eggs
- Fish
- Milk/dairy products
- Papaya
- Pineapple
- Shellfish
- Strawberries
- Tomatoes

Amine-Free Foods — ENJOY!

Legumes
- Lentils, beans , peas
- Soy milk, tofu
- Carob

Seeds and nuts
- Sunflower oil
- Cashews

Most vegetables and fruits
- Garlic
- Shallots
- Apples
- Custard apples (cherimoya, sweetsops)
- Mangos
- Apricots
- Peaches
- Rhubarb
- Berries
- Cherries
- Currants
- Guava
- Lychees
- Nectarines
- Pomegranate
- Watermelon
- Pears

Meat
- Freshly cooked beef
- Skinless chicken
- Lamb, veal
- Rabbit
- Fresh white fish

continued...

Beverages
- Lemonade
- Decaffeinated coffee
- Coffee, tea
- Peppermint tea

Grains
- Arrowroot
- Barley
- Buckwheat
- Cornmeal, polenta

- Malt
- Rice, rice flour
- Rolled oats
- Rye
- Wheat

Herbs and flavorings
- Vanilla
- Honey
- Maple syrup

Note: Amine levels increase during storage of cooked meats, so avoid eating cooked leftovers that have been stored/refrigerated overnight.

Q. What is sulfation?

A. Histamines may not be the initial cause of your rosacea, but they usually play a role in exacerbating the problem. In a properly functioning body, the liver helps to safely remove histamines by a process called sulfation, and people with rosacea may have poor sulfation ability. When sulfation and other liver detoxification reactions are overburdened, histamine is not removed from the body fast enough and problems, such as vasodilation, may be the result.

Sulfation in the liver sounds a bit confusing, but whenever I explain liver detoxification, I liken it to a horse race around a race track. Histamine is the race horse that is traveling along the blood vessels, and it needs to be sternly guided to the finish line for safe removal from the body. Now, histamine "race horses" can't find the finish line all by themselves — horses just aren't that disciplined on their own — they need jockeys to steer them in the right direction. In your body, sulfur is the jockey that can ride histamine horses safely to the finish line. When sulfur is available in the body, histamine is quickly removed from the bloodstream so only the appropriate amount of blood vessel dilation can occur.

Did You Know?

Celebrations
If you want to drink alcohol for a special occasion, your best choices would be gin, vodka, or whisky because they don't contain amines (although they can still cause a histamine reaction). You can drink them with soda or mineral water (but not tonic water or any other mixer). However, you really should avoid alcohol until your condition improves.

Improving Sulfation

Poor sulfation (not enough jockeys) in the liver detoxification (race track) can make you more susceptible to environmental illness, rheumatoid arthritis, and nervous system problems, such as Parkinson's disease and motor neuron disease. You can improve sulfation (and histamine removal from the bloodstream) by including sulfur-rich foods, such as garlic, onion, and cabbage, in your diet. Sulfur-containing amino acids (methionine, cysteine, and taurine) are found in protein-rich foods, such as chicken. All of the other detoxification pathways need support to take the burden off the sulfation pathway in the liver, so also take the other liver jockeys — omega-3 EFAs, glycine, magnesium, B vitamins, selenium, and vitamin C.

Step 2: Soothe Your Skin

You may need to soothe your skin with anti-inflammatory and moisturizing topical treatments to minimize discomfort. When choosing a moisturizing and cleansing product, look for the following key ingredients:

- Omega-3 (linolenic acid)
- Chamomile
- Calendula
- Vitamin E
- Blackcurrant seed oil
- Sweet almond oil
- Evening primrose oil
- Rosehip oil
- Sea buckthorn berry oil
- Hemp seed oil
- Gamma-linolenic acid (GLA)
- Grape seed extract/citrus seed
- Vitamin C
- Licorice

See Guideline #8 (page 126) for further descriptions and information on what product ingredients to avoid.

Q. I get awful facial flushing, especially in summer. What can I do to quickly relieve the flush?

A. People with severe rosacea produce a lot of body heat, so they feel hot and uncomfortable much of the time. If you are having a facial flush or experiencing excessive heat, try the following:

- Suck on an ice cube.
- Wet your skin with cold water or fill a plastic bag with ice cubes and hold next to the skin.
- During a flush, if you have no ice cubes or access to cold water, visualize bathing in a swimming pool filled with ice cubes. This works because studies have shown that the brain can't tell the difference between what is real and what is vividly imagined. Picture bathing with ice cubes floating around you, even pretend to shiver, and you will cool down in no time.

Q. I have rosacea and my skin gets itchy all the time. Is there anything I can do to get some relief?

A. If you're feeling itchy, try the following:

- Fill a plastic bag with ice cubes and hold next to the skin.
- Add 1/4 cup (60 mL) of baking soda to a lukewarm bath and soak in it. See bath recipe on page 212.
- Immediately after bathing, before the skin is totally dry, gently dab sensitive-skin moisturizer or ointment on the affected areas.
- Take a supplement containing quercetin and vitamin C (see Step 5, page 259).

Step 3: Exercise!

CASE STUDY

Exercise is essential for eliminating rosacea. I found this out the hard way... My own personal experience is with mild rosacea. It wasn't so bad because luckily I found a way to get rid of it before it had a chance to get worse. The first signs of rosacea began to appear 8 years ago; my chin was always red and I had to camouflage it with makeup. But my skin color suddenly improved after I took dairy products out of my diet.

I had a skin prick test and blood test for allergies and intolerances and modified my diet slightly, so I enjoyed having a clear complexion for a while. However, a few years later, even without having dairy in my diet, I started getting facial flushing. If the gas heater was on in winter, I would flush. I was also overly sensitive to the summer heat, and I couldn't splash my face with warm water in the morning without my face being pink for the rest of the day.

I also got patchy, red flushing during and after exercise. This was embarrassing, so I used to apply makeup before going to the gym, just so I wouldn't look like a blushing beet. Not that I ever exercised much! As I've mentioned before, I just never liked exercise; it always fatigued me and sometimes brought on cold and flu symptoms so I'd feel rotten for a whole week. However, whenever I did stick to an exercise routine, my rosacea would magically disappear. Then I would find another excuse to ditch the regimen and my rosacea would soon return.

Exercise Tips

- When you start to exercise, you will flush and feel uncomfortable, but this reaction will eventually disappear.
- If possible, exercise in air-conditioned space or go swimming to avoid negative symptoms.
- Exercise and sweat for at least 15 minutes a day. However, keep your routines moderate and under 1 hour until your rosacea has cleared up. See Guideline #5 (page 101) for more information.

Did You Know?

Rosacea Exercise Research

The Rosacea Support Group website states that "many rosaceans have noted that moderate (not strenuous) exercise seems to help alleviate their rosacea symptoms." Other specialists have reported that many patients with rosacea have experienced the same results from exercise, which could be due to increased sympathetic constrictor tone to the facial blood vessels.

- Moderate exercise burns up the body's lipid stores, which potentially leaves less fat available for the inflammatory response. However, excessive exercise, such as running a marathon, does the opposite and promotes inflammation in the body. Moderate exercise decreases blood levels of arachidonic acid (AA) from meat and dairy, which can promote inflammation in the body. It is important to reduce AA levels by exercising and avoiding dairy if you suffer from rosacea.
- Exercise enhances the amount of anti-inflammatory endorphins in the bloodstream.
- Exercise reduces blood glucose levels; high levels can damage blood vessels.
- Regular exercise also improves blood circulation, and good circulation is vital for healthy skin. An efficiently pumping circulatory system is necessary to carry nutrients and oxygen to your skin. If you have poor circulation, your skin literally becomes starved of nutrients because you are giving it an inadequate supply of essential fatty acids, antioxidants, and oxygen.

Q. How does skin that is starved of nutrients survive?

A. Think about it... skin that lacks oxygen and nutrients will rot and die (as is the case with gangrene). So when your blood supply is sluggish or hampered in some way, the skin needs extra blood vessels to supply more nutrient-rich blood and it needs wider blood vessels to allow more flow with less effort. Poor circulation also means there is an inefficient removal of bodily wastes, such as industrial toxins, pollution, dead cells, and chemicals. Increased waste and skin cell turnover can cause the facial oil glands to become blocked and enlarged. This can eventually lead to nose and skin disfigurement seen in chronic rosacea.

Step 4: Promote Good Intestinal Health

Rosacea may also be exacerbated by poor gastrointestinal tract health and intestinal permeability. Ideally, your intestines should only allow tiny particles (that have been extracted from properly digested foods) to enter the bloodstream. These microscopic amino acids, glucose, vitamins, minerals, and fatty acids are small enough to pass through a healthy gut wall, while the larger particles stay in the intestines and pass through to the colon for removal in the feces. When the intestinal wall is unhealthy, it can develop larger than normal holes that allow the wrong-sized particles into your blood vessels. All rosacea sufferers should make sure they have good digestion and intestinal health. A probiotic supplement and chewing your food properly may help. See Guideline #1 (page 29) for more information.

Activity

To get a clear idea of what I mean, picture that you are in a kitchen, you have cooked some rice, and you are now using a strainer to drain the water from the rice. The rice ends up in the strainer and the liquid passes through. Imagine what would happen if the colander holes were too large: when you strained the rice, some of the grains would pass through. This is not ideal. When your gut lining is permeable, foreign particles pass though, enter your bloodstream, and cause an immune system response. Your body panics at the invasion and a cascade of histamines is released from your cells. And as you know, histamines cause blood vessel dilation that affects skin health.

Step 5: Take Supplements That Promote Healthy Blood Flow

These supplements include natural antihistamine, omega-3 fish oil, and chlorophyll.

Natural Antihistamine Supplements

There are many nutrients that have an antihistamine effect. Here are the top two: quercetin and vitamin C.

Quercetin

Quercetin is anti-inflammatory and a natural antihistamine, making it ideal for rosacea sufferers. Quercetin is the most studied flavonoid because it is abundant in nature. Quercetin is found in high doses in red onions, and it is an antioxidant that is more potent than vitamin E. Flavonoids — sometimes referred to in the media as "bioflavonoids" — are fruit pigments; they give berries and other fruit and vegetables their color. Flavonoids have antioxidant properties, so they help to protect your cells from oxidation and cancer. Apart from red onions, quercetin is found in apples, leafy vegetables such as spinach, green cabbage, cranberries, kale, grapes, pears, garlic, and grapefruit.

> **Quercetin is anti-inflammatory and a natural antihistamine, making it ideal for rosacea sufferers.**

Dosage

Take 500 mg of quercetin twice a day with foods to reduce histamine buildup in the body, and eat quercetin-rich foods. If you have a histamine reaction, such as hay fever or facial flushing after eating an amine-rich food or beverage, you can have one extra dose of quercetin and vitamin C.

Vitamin C

Vitamin C also has an antihistamine effect and is a well-known antioxidant. The human body can't manufacture its own supply of vitamin C, so we must consume it every day. Vitamin C is abundant in vegetables and fruit, fruit being the original sweet treat before candies and cake were invented. Without vitamin C, your skin would come "unglued" and you'd bleed (this is a deficiency disease called scurvy). So your desire for sweets may be an ancient life-preserving craving for fruits that contain vitamin C (and no, cake doesn't have vitamin C in it).

If you want to see vitamin C work its magic, just give 1000 mg to an adult who is acutely suffering from hay fever and see how quickly the symptoms disappear (see caution box)!

Dosage

Take 1000 mg of vitamin C three times a day during an acute rosacea attack. Reduce dosage to 500 mg per day once rosacea begins to improve.

It's more convenient to buy one supplement that contains both quercetin and vitamin C.

Caution

Vitamin C is an acid, so don't buy chewable vitamin C tablets, as they will wear away tooth enamel and leave your teeth feeling sensitive (this is painful!). Vitamin C thins the blood, so don't take a vitamin C supplement if you are on blood-thinning medications (heart medications, aspirin, etc.), are a hemophiliac, or are undergoing surgery. If you have any medical condition requiring drugs, speak to your doctor before taking vitamin C. Also do not rely on natural antihistamine treatments if you have a life-threatening histamine reaction (swelling of the lips, tongue, or throat). Please continue to strictly avoid anything that causes swelling and get advice from your doctor or allergy specialist.

Omega-3 essential fatty acids

Omega-3 fish oil supplements can increase peripheral circulation because they thin the blood. Omega-3 also decreases skin inflammation because it alters inflammation-making hormone-like substances (prostaglandins), so it is very specific for rosacea. Omega-3 can also be obtained from non-fish sources, such as flax seeds, flaxseed oil, and freshly shelled walnuts. Tiny amounts are found in dark leafy vegetables.

Dosage

See Guideline #2 (page 70) for dosage and cautions.

Chlorophyll

Chlorophyll is the green pigment in plants. Liquid chlorophyll supplements are useful for improving red blood cell health. See Guideline #1 (page 50) for more information, as chlorophyll is an essential treatment for rosacea.

Step 6: Eat a Healthy Diet

Don't forget to follow the 8-Week Healthy Skin Diet. There are histamine-containing foods in the Healthy Skin Diet, but not as many as the average Western diet, so you shouldn't have any problems enjoying the delicious recipes. I am not giving you an amine-free diet, as you want to be able to eat amine-containing foods and be rosacea-free. Exercising on a daily basis and taking the essential supplements will help you to achieve this.

Recipes for Managing Rosacea

- **If you need more omega-3 EFAs in your diet:** You can get a fantastic dose of omega-3 (EPA and DHA) from oily fish, such as salmon, trout, herring, sardines, and mackerel. Eat fish twice a week, but remember that fish contains histamines, so don't overindulge and don't eat fish if you have a fish allergy. Omega-3 is also found in flax seeds, flaxseed oil, and walnuts, and in tiny amounts in dark green leafy vegetables. Eat one serving of these daily — one serving would be 1 to 2 tablespoons (15 to 30 mL) of flaxseed oil, 1 to 2 tablespoons (15 to 30 mL) of ground or whole flax seeds — and one small handful of freshly shelled walnuts a couple of times a week. Eat two handfuls of dark green vegetables every day. Recipes high in omega-3 EPA and DHA include: Salmon Steaks with Peas and Mash; Rainbow Trout with Honey-Roasted Vegetables; Creamy Salmon Mornay. Add 1 to 2 tablespoons (15 to 30 mL) of flax seeds to your food or use flaxseed oil in one of the following skin drinks: Flaxseed Lemon Drink; Pear Flaxseed Drink for Sensitive Skin; Berry Beauty Smoothie; Calcium-Rich Smoothie; Apple Omega Drink. Also drink plenty of filtered water.

- **To help your liver detoxify amines/histamines:** Drink Green Water twice a day and eat sulfur-rich foods, such as garlic, onion, and cabbage. Recipes include Anti-Aging Broth; Therapeutic Veggie Soup; Herb and Garlic Chicken Casserole; and Therapeutic Chicken Soup.

- **Add quercetin-rich produce,** such as red onions, apples, grapefruit, and cabbage, to the shopping list.

> Eat fish twice a week, but remember that fish contains histamines, so don't overindulge and don't eat fish if you have a fish allergy. Omega-3 is also found in flax seeds, flaxseed oil, walnuts, and in tiny amounts in dark green leafy vegetables.

- **Snack on amine-free foods,** such as Amine-Free Fruit Salad, lychees, watermelon, apples, pears, peas, mangos, berries, rockmelon, carob, rice and rolled oats (review the list of amine-free foods on page 252).

Quick Review of Rosacea Management Program

Step 1: Limit histamine reactions

- Avoid alcohol, chocolate, cheese, oranges, spicy food, and allergy foods.
- Stress and anxiety also trigger histamine release. See the Beauty Breathing section (page 281) for effective relaxation techniques.

Step 2: Soothe your skin

- Use a cleanser and moisturizer that contain anti-inflammatory ingredients.

Step 3: Exercise!

- Improve your circulation. Exercise for at least 15 minutes every day. Sweat and breathe deeply.
- Exercise is the most essential step to improving your rosacea; without it, all other steps will only offer minor benefit.

Step 4: Promote good intestinal health

- Take a probiotic supplement if necessary; chew your food properly; drink water.

Step 5: Take supplements that promote healthy blood flow

- Take a quercetin and vitamin C supplement; drink Green Water; and take an omega-3 supplement.

Step 6: Eat a healthy diet

- Follow the Healthy Skin Diet for 8 weeks.
- Improve liver function with garlic, onion, cabbage, and omega-3-rich fish.
- Include flaxseed oil in your diet.
- Eat dark green leafy vegetables every day.

Children's Clear Skin Program

This program is suitable for children with eczema, psoriasis, hives, rosacea, and allergies. If a treatment is for a specific condition, it will be mentioned by name. If your child has an undesirable skin condition, you can begin by following the relevant advice in the eczema management program for adults — Steps 1 to 3 (pages 202–215). Here is a brief recap of information from that chapter.

Step 1: Identify Triggers and Irritants

- Limit chemical exposure. You can do this by using natural cleaning products and washing fruit and vegetables in a bowl of water with a splash of vinegar (the vinegar helps with pesticide removal). You can also wash your child's clothes with sensitive-skin laundry detergent and avoid all bath products containing chemicals and artificial foaming agents.

> **Feed your child fresh foods that don't contain artificial additives.**

- Feed your child fresh foods that don't contain artificial additives. Avoid food colorings, preservatives, and flavor enhancers. See the Additives to Avoid (page 459).

Step 2: Identify Allergies

- Have your child allergy tested if age-appropriate. Talk to your doctor.

Step 3: Soothe Your Child's Skin with Topical Treatments

- Moisturize your child's skin as often as needed (two to four times a day).
- Apply creams in the same direction as the hair growth on your child's skin.
- Give your child healing baths at least three times a week. If you bathe your child in a baby-sized bath, see the Baby Bath Recipes (below), or if your child is old enough to bathe in an adult-sized bath, then follow the Big Bath recipes opposite.

Baby Bath Recipes

1. For bacterial infections and healing of lesions: Add 1 tablespoon (15 mL) of sea salt to a lukewarm baby-sized bath. Bathe your baby for approximately 5 minutes. Pat skin semi-dry (allowing some moisture to remain). Then apply moisturizer or a thick barrier cream to affected areas. Do not use vinegar, because it can increase itchiness. Do not use oils, because they can make bath surfaces slippery.

2. For severely itchy skin: Add 2 tablespoons (30 mL) of baking soda to a lukewarm bath. Bathe for 10 minutes. Afterwards, pat skin semi-dry and apply moisturizer or a thick barrier cream.

3. For dry, flaky, itchy skin: Add 1 capful (1 teaspoon/ 5 mL) of oil or oil blend to a lukewarm bath. Suitable oils include jojoba oil and evening primrose oil. Bathe for 10 minutes. Pat skin semi-dry afterwards and apply a moisturizer or barrier cream to affected areas.

Big Bath Recipes

When children are older, they can bathe in an adult-sized bath, although keep the bath fairly shallow so less measured ingredients are needed.

1. For bacterial infections and healing of lesions: Add ½ cup (125 mL) of sea salt to a lukewarm bath. Bathe for 5 to 15 minutes. You may need to rinse the skin afterwards if your child suffers from itchiness. Pat skin semi-dry with a towel, and then apply moisturizer or a thick barrier cream to affected skin.

2. For severely itchy skin: Add ¼ cup (60 mL) of baking soda to a lukewarm bath. Bathe for 5 to 15 minutes. Afterwards, pat semi-dry and apply moisturizer or a thick barrier cream.

3. For dry, flaky, itchy skin: Add 1–2 capfuls (teaspoons/5–10 mL) of natural oil or oil blend to a lukewarm bath. Suitable oils include jojoba oil and evening primrose oil. Bathe for 5 to 15 minutes. Pat skin semi-dry afterwards and apply a barrier cream.

Never use bubble bath, antiseptics, or soap because they will irritate the condition further. They also exacerbate vulvovaginitis (vagina inflammation, common in young girls). A vinegar bath is most suitable for this condition.

Apply Topical Evening Primrose Oil

For babies and children with eczema, follow this procedure for applying evening primrose oil as a moisturizer:

1. Pierce one capsule of evening primrose oil and mix it in with your child's usual skin cream and then apply the mixture to unbroken skin (to test for reactions).

2. If there is no swelling or redness, apply the emollient directly to the eczema-affected areas so your baby can absorb the beneficial oils through the skin.

3. Look out for good moisturizers that include evening primrose oil, blackcurrant seed oil, or borage oil because these oils contain gamma-linolenic acid (GLA), which is beneficial for your child's skin.

Step 4: Give Your Child Suitable Supplements

All children can benefit from taking a probiotic supplement.

After you have reviewed the first three steps, move on to Step 4. Supplements are necessary for children with inflammation for three main reasons:

1. Skin inflammation causes a high amount of nutrient loss in children — the body burns up vitamins and minerals in its bid to repair the damaged skin. The stress caused by having itchy or uncomfortable skin also depletes nutrients in the body.

2. A deficiency in B vitamins, glycine, magnesium, and/or essential fatty acids can cause skin conditions because the liver needs these nutrients to safely remove chemicals, hormones, and carcinogens (cancer-causing substances) from the body.

3. A deficiency of healthy bacteria in your child's gastro-intestinal tract can cause a proliferation of unhealthy microbes, and this can hamper your child's digestion and absorption of foods. Poor digestion can prevent essential fatty acids, such as omega-3, from being absorbed properly, and B vitamins cannot be manufactured by your child's body if friendly bacteria are not present.

Suitable Supplements for Children

Please note that some supplements are essential only for certain skin conditions:

- Glycine (essential for eczema, salicylate, and chemical sensitivity, psoriasis, hives, and may be beneficial for nut sensitivity).
- Probiotic supplement (essential for all skin conditions, lowered immunity, allergies and sensitivities). If an adverse reaction occurs, discontinue use.
- Liquid chlorophyll (essential for all skin conditions, allergies and sensitivities).
- Children's omega-3 fish oil supplement (essential for psoriasis, rosacea, and hyperactivity).

Glycine

As I mentioned in the Eczema Care chapter, glycine helps the liver to safely process salicylates and other chemicals. Glycine can help your child tolerate a wider variety of foods without getting an adverse skin reaction, so it can help them to have a more normal diet! Glycine is available from most health food shops. Glycine is sweet and pleasant-tasting. You can add it to Green Water in week 4 of the Healthy Skin Diet. Be sure to discuss with your doctor the dosage and safety of glycine for children.

Dosage

For babies under 1 year: 100–200 mg of glycine, added to formula or water.

For children over the age of 1 year: 600–800 mg per day, added to liquid.

Older children: 1000 mg per day; begin with a glycine dosage of 600–700 mg per day in divided doses. After the skin has cleared up, give your child one to two maintenance doses a week to ensure there is always enough glycine stored in the liver for salicylate removal.

Probiotic supplement

There is excellent scientific research showing that certain strains of probiotic bacteria can successfully reduce inflammation in many (but not all) people suffering from atopic and allergic conditions. All children can benefit from taking a probiotic supplement. Probiotic strains that have solid evidence of usefulness in infantile eczema and food allergies include:

- *L. fermentum* PCC (VRI-002)
- *B. lactis* Bb12 (now called Bifidobacterium animalis)
- *L. rhamnosus* GG, Lactobacillus GG (it must be the GG variety)
- *L. paracasei* shirota

Again, this information is confusing when presented on its own, but when combined with brand information it becomes easy to find the right supplement for your child. As products and formulas can change at any time, you can find up-to-date information at my website (www.healthbeforebeauty.com).

Did You Know?

Breastfeeding

Salicylates end up in breast milk, so babies with eczema and salicylate sensitivity may benefit if their breastfeeding mother takes a glycine supplement. If you are breastfeeding, you can take glycine on its own or with magnesium and vitamin B_6 (see the adult dosage in the Eczema Care chapter). You can also drink the Anti-Aging Broth twice a day because it is naturally rich in glycine.

Q. Are probiotics suitable for babies with eczema?

A. Yes. Plain probiotic supplements are safe for babies. There are a couple of ways to administer probiotics if your baby is under the age of 1. If you are still breastfeeding, you can take the probiotic yourself (as it may alter the flora in your breast milk) and you can also put a few grains of probiotic on your nipple before your baby breastfeeds (do this twice a day). If your baby is bottle-fed, you can add a measured dose of probiotic to his or her bottle, twice a day.

All babies should naturally develop healthy gut bacteria in their gastrointestinal tracts soon after birth. This helps them to have a healthy immune system and good digestion. However, this flora proliferation doesn't always occur, especially if the baby was born by cesarean or prematurely, or if the mother had a yeast infection in the vaginal tract at the time of giving birth. If babies don't have enough of the right gut bacteria, then *Candida albicans* (fungus/yeast) and other undesirable microbes attach to the gut lining. This increases your baby's chance of illness, allergies, and skin conditions, such as eczema (not forgetting that genetics also play a role). A suitable probiotic can help to improve a baby's gut health, reduce some allergic responses, and promote good digestion and proper immunity.

Dosage

From birth to 7 months: 1 pinch ($\frac{1}{8}$ capsule) of probiotic grains sprinkled onto nipple or bottle nipple before suckling.

Eight months to 1 year: $\frac{1}{4}$ capsule ($\frac{1}{8}$ teaspoon/0.5 mL) added to a lukewarm bottle or room-temperature water. You can also sprinkle probiotic grains onto cooled baby rice cereal (never add probiotic to overly warm foods).

Two to 7 years old: $\frac{1}{2}$ capsule (or less than $\frac{1}{4}$ teaspoon/1 mL) added to liquid.

Over the age of 8 years: 1 full capsule opened (or $\frac{1}{2}$ teaspoon/2 mL) added to liquid.

If you're unsure of the dosage, refer to the manufacturer's instructions for the appropriate measure for your child's age. Give your child a suitable probiotic supplement twice a day, before breakfast and in the afternoon, preferably on an empty stomach (or about 15 minutes before food). Add a measured dose of probiotic to rice/soy milk, water, or diluted apple/pear juice, twice a day. If you're using apple or pear juice, make sure it is preservative-free and diluted with water. Juices and rice milk generally aren't good for children's teeth, so you should brush their teeth afterwards or before sleep.

A 1-year-old boy had severe eczema on the back of his legs, on his back, chest, and ears, and his arms and face were extremely dry. His dermatologist previously said the eczema wasn't food-related and prescribed a medicated cream and the avoidance of dust mites. The child was later brought to our clinic by his mother because his eczema still wasn't getting any better. Dietary changes were prescribed — no dairy/tomato/high-salicylate fruits such as grapes/sultanas — and he was to take a probiotic and a children's supplement containing glycine. His eczema completely cleared up within 2 months of taking the supplements and making dietary changes. His mother happily reported that she threw away the medicated cream. After his eczema cleared up, his mother reintroduced foods one by one so she could identify trigger foods that caused flare-ups (these were orange juice, tomato, and dairy). His diet was expanded to include healthy alternatives so he could continue to be eczema-free.

Caution

Chlorophyll is not suitable for babies under the age of 6 months. Liquid chlorophyll may initially cause a flare-up because it contains salicylates. To reduce the chance of this happening, do not serve Green Water until your child is 4 weeks into the program. Flare-ups should not occur if glycine is used concurrently.

Children's omega-3 fish oil supplement

Chewable omega-3 fish oil supplements are good for children over the age of 1 year who have psoriasis, rosacea, or hyperactivity. Omega-3 from fish oil supplements and food sources can also enhance brain development, according to recent scientific studies. Omega-3 also helps to hydrate skin cells, as omega-3 can literally draw fluids back into cells (where it should be).

> Omega-3 also helps to hydrate skin cells, as omega-3 can literally draw fluids back into cells (where it should be).

Dosage

One year or above: 50–150 mg of omega-3 marine triglycerides per day. Please refer to the packaging for the appropriate dosage for your child's age.

For other skin conditions: if your child eats deep sea fish at least twice a week, an omega-3 supplement may not be needed. If your child has a fish allergy or if you are a vegetarian family, she can have flaxseed oil or ground flax seeds (see Step 5).

Caution

Always supervise young children while they're taking chewable vitamins. If your child has allergies, speak to your doctor before giving your child an omega-3 fish oil supplement.

Step 5: Feed Your Child Moisturizing Foods

When you have eczema, your skin lacks the ability to hold adequate moisture. Even though this can occur genetically from enzyme insufficiency, specific foods can literally moisturize your child's skin from the inside out.

Omega-3

All children with dry, irritated skin should have flaxseed oil or ground flax seeds daily (unless they have an allergy to flax).

Omega-3 from food sources and supplements has a beneficial effect when consumed in high enough doses to exert a therapeutic effect. Omega-3 helps to produce the good prostaglandins and it also suppresses the bad ones. However, omega-3 will not work effectively if your child is consuming lots of saturated fats, fried foods (containing trans fats), and omega-6-rich vegetable oils, nuts, and margarine. As I mentioned in the last chapter, a study found that margarine users were more likely to suffer with eczema than butter users, making butter a slightly better choice.

All children with dry, irritated skin should have flaxseed oil or ground flax seeds daily (unless they have an allergy to flax). On page 271 is a formula that shows you how to use omega-3-rich products to decrease skin inflammation.

Dosage

For children over the age of 1 year: Give your child omega-3-rich fish three times a week (tinned sardines or salmon, or fresh, boneless salmon/trout) and flaxseed oil or a children's fish oil supplement on the days when fresh fish is not consumed.

Flaxseed oil dosage: 1 teaspoon (5 mL) mixed into calcium-fortified rice milk, cooled breakfast cereal or vegetables (flaxseed is a pleasant-tasting oil). See caution box, below.

Tip: Flaxseed oil goes rancid very easily. Only buy refrigerated flaxseed oil and choose one that's packaged in dark glass (not plastic). To keep it fresh, always refrigerate the oil and use within 5 weeks. Flaxseed oil can be stored in the freezer to keep it fresh for longer. Heat damages flaxseed oil, so never heat it or add to hot food.

Caution

If your child has multiple allergies, especially seed allergies, then speak to an allergy specialist before giving your child flaxseed oil. Allergy is rare but possible. Fish oil and flaxseed oil naturally thin the blood, so avoid supplemental omega-3 if your child has hemorrhaging problems or is undergoing surgery. If diarrhea occurs from flaxseed oil, reduce the dosage and improve your child's digestion with a suitable probiotic.

Tips for Breastfeeding Mothers

- Improve the omega-3 content in your breast milk by regularly eating omega-3-rich foods including salmon, trout, sardines, herring, mackerel, and freshly ground flax seeds or flaxseed oil. Eat a variety of omega-3-rich foods, one serving daily.
- Avoid nuts, caffeine, chocolate, tomato, dried fruits, oranges, and spicy foods.
- Avoid foods you are allergic to.

Choosing Baby Formulas

If your baby is drinking formula, make sure it contains the amino acids taurine and glycine. Like glycine, taurine helps the liver detoxify chemicals, and taurine is also essential for brain development. When choosing a goat's milk or cow's milk formula, make sure it contains added vitamins, minerals, and omega-3, taurine, and glycine. NEVER give standard milk to a baby under the age of 1 year, because regular milks, on their own, are not nutritious enough to sustain a baby's health.

Calcium Supplement

During this time, make sure your child is having 500 to 800 mg of calcium daily to ensure proper bone and teeth development. Calcium sources include rice or soy milk that has added calcium. Other sources suitable for children over the age of 1 year include the Anti-Aging Broth and Calcium-Rich Smoothie (give them one to two small cups per day, plus additional calcium-rich foods and drinks). Calcium can be found in many non-dairy sources. See page 66 for a list of non-dairy sources of calcium.

Dosage

One to 4 years: 500 mg of calcium per day
Over the age of 4: 800 mg of calcium per day

Step 6: Put Your Child on an Elimination Diet

This step can work on its own, but it is enhanced when combined with the other steps. Your child's skin condition should completely disappear within 8 weeks using dietary changes alone and much sooner if all six steps from this chapter are implemented. This is great news — your child won't have to suffer with eczema anymore.

Foods for Babies with Skin Conditions

Every 3 days, introduce a new food separately, which will help to identify any allergies as you go.

When your child is 5 or 6 months old, you can introduce solid food (baby food that resembles mush). Begin with plain rice cereals mixed with cooled boiled water (it is necessary to pre-boil water to kill microbes). Baby rice cereal can be mixed with cooled boiled water, breast milk, or formula. Every 3 days, introduce a new food separately, which will help to identify any allergies as you go. If a vegetable contains salicylates, look for a reaction within 48 hours of consumption and discontinue if there is a reaction.

First Solid Foods

5 to 6 months

Serve puréed, 1 to 3 teaspoons (5 to 15 mL). Begin with one and gradually increase.

- Rice cereal. Serve once a day for the first week, then twice a day in the second week.
- Stewed peeled pear. Serve third week, cooked, then puréed or mashed.
- Very ripe banana. Serve third week, mashed with a fork.
- Mashed potato. Serve fourth week, cooked, then puréed or mashed.
- Carrot. Serve fourth week, cooked, then puréed or mashed (contains salicylates).

Continue to breastfeed or formula-feed your baby.

6 to 9 months

At 6 to 9 months old, solid meals should be given to babies before milk feeding so they have a better appetite for their solid foods. Start with three mushy meals and three to four milk feeds (breast milk and/or formula) per day. If a vegetable contains salicylates, look for a reaction within 48 hours of consumption. Your baby needs to have at least one serving of iron-rich foods daily, such as lamb, chicken, or lentils to prevent anemia. Make sure you remove the skin and fatty sections before puréeing or chopping finely (food can be a little bit lumpy as your child needs to get used to textured foods).

- Dried peas, cooked and mashed
- Kidney beans, cooked and mashed

- Steamed fish without bones
- Steamed free-range/organic chicken
- Cooked lamb
- Plain full-fat yogurt mixed with stewed fruit
- Lentils, pre-soaked overnight, then cooked
- Pumpkin, mashed (contains salicylates)
- Sweet potato, mashed (contains salicylates)
- Papaya, mashed

Caution

Avoid larger fish that contain high levels of mercury. See Guideline #2 (page 69) for a list of suitable fish. Fish allergy is possible in sensitive individuals.

9 to 12 Months

By this age, each mealtime should include carbohydrates (cereal/bread/rice), fruit or vegetables, and protein (fish/meat/lentils/tofu/beans/egg) to make it a balanced meal. Make sure breads are preservative-free and whole-grain (get them used to eating brown bread). NEVER leave children alone with any food. They may choke and need your help. At 9 to 12 months old, you can also give your baby three solid meals, including finger foods, and three milk feeds a day (approximately $2^{1}/_{2}$ cups/600 mL in total).

- Mashed green peas (contains salicylates)
- Stewed peeled apple (contains salicylates)
- Brown rice (well cooked so it is very soft)
- Tofu
- Egg yolk (make Egg Soldiers and dip toast)
- Crusts of bread, fingers of toast
- Steamed vegetables cut into slices
- Pieces of banana
- Macaroni pasta (no cheese or sauce)
- Casseroles with meat/beans/veggies (see recipe section)
- Sweet Banana Porridge (see recipe section), omit honey

After the Age of 1 Year

If your child has skin inflammation after the age of 1, it is essential to stop giving formula and switch to non-dairy milks for 2 months only. You can continue to breastfeed if you wish, but you may have to modify your own diet slightly (follow the adult guidelines in Step 6 of the Eczema Care chapter).

Preventing Skin Inflammation

To help prevent skin inflammation (and for optimal health in all children), it is important to avoid giving your child artificial additives, such as bread preservative, food colors, and flavor enhancers, found in certain products, such as seasoning mixes, flavored chips, and crackers. These additives offer no benefits to your child and, according to the scientific research, they can promote bad behavior, poor concentration and learning skills, and skin inflammation.

Also avoid giving your child too many salicylate and MSG-rich foods ("flare-up foods") such as tomato, stone fruit, citrus, grapes, dried fruits, kiwifruit, avocado, soy sauce/tamari,

CASE STUDY

A 4-year-old girl with a history of eczema and dust mite allergy had a severe flare-up when she ate colored candies and chocolate at her birthday party. Previously, her eczema had been controlled by having a low-salicylate diet and by avoiding dairy, colored sweets, and preservatives. This diet ceased to work after the party and her eczema continued to get worse for the following 2 months. Glycine, chlorophyll, and probiotics were prescribed, and ground flax seeds were added to her breakfast cereal. Her eczema cleared up within 5 weeks, and she could eat a more varied diet, which included salicylate fruits, such as mango, watermelon, and lemon, and other foods that previously caused flare-ups. She could eat small amounts of dairy, tomato, and party food without her eczema returning. Another positive result was that after taking the supplements she no longer had reactions to dust mites and she could sleep with her fluffy toys for the first time in years.

Did You Know?

Growth and Development

After the age of 1, your child needs a wider variety of solid foods. Growth can be hampered if a child has too many bottles of milk (four or more per day) and not enough solid foods, such as meats, fish, vegetables, and carbohydrates. Give your child two bottles of calcium-fortified non-dairy milk per day. Your child also needs protein with every meal, such as beans with whole-grain toast or tuna, egg, or chicken sandwiches.

To help prevent skin inflammation (and for optimal health in all children), it is important to avoid giving your child artificial additives.

Q. My child loves sweets, but she has eczema and rosacea and they seem to make her skin worse. Are there any treats that won't aggravate her condition?

A. Colored candies are notorious for causing skin rashes because they contain artificial additives. Yellow food colorings are particularly bad for the skin: FD&C Yellow #5 can cause allergic reactions, skin rashes, hyperactivity, and headaches, and FD&C Yellow #6 can cause skin rashes, sunlight allergy, and upset stomach. Red, green, and blue food colorings can also cause adverse reactions in children. Flavored chips, instant noodles, and seasoning mixes often contain flavor enhancers, such as monosodium glutamate. These additives are not suitable for infants and small children because they can induce hyperactivity, skin rashes, stomach upsets, irritability, insomnia, and asthma attacks in sensitive individuals.

Luckily, there are suitable alternatives. If your child is going to a party or if you want to give your child a treat, favor products that are free from food colorings and artificial flavors. The best choices include:

- Plain lemonade popsicles
- White marshmallows
- White jellybeans
- Plain potato chips
- Plain corn chips
- Plain rice crackers
- Oat or plain cookies
- Homemade cakes with no food coloring

gravies, and nut or chocolate spreads. For a full list of these problematic food products, see the Foods and Drinks to Avoid and Foods and Drinks to Limit in adults in on page 226. Always check the ingredient panel for suspect additives.

Recipes for Children's Meals and Therapeutic Drinks

For children from age 1 to adolescence

Essential drinks: Pear Flaxseed Drink for Sensitive Skin; Anti-Aging Broth; filtered water; calcium-fortified rice or soy milk twice a day in drinks, such as Calcium-Rich Smoothie.

Breakfasts: Gluten-Free Muesli (no nuts); Pear and Buckwheat Crêpes; Egg Soldiers; Sweet Banana Porridge; Kids' Creamy Beans on Toast; Sardines and Lemon on Grainy Toast; Kids' Scrambled Eggs; Delicious French Toast (modified).

Lunches and dinners rich in omega-3: Creamy Salmon Mornay; Salmon and Salad Sandwich; Salmon Steaks with Peas and Mash; Rainbow Trout with Honey-Roasted Vegetables; Marinated Whole Steamed Trout (avoid the marinade/sauce); Fish and Steamed Vegetables; Roasted Sweet Potato Salad; Kids' Creamy Beans on Toast.

Other meals and snacks: Fruit Salad with Flax Seeds; Perfect Poached Eggs; Sweet Chicken Stir-Fry; Therapeutic Veggie Soup; Salad Sandwich with Creamy Mayo; Lean Meat and Three Veg; Colorful Non-Fried Rice (without the sauce: alternatively, flavor it with natural sea salt); Tasty Vegetable Casserole; Therapeutic Chicken Soup; Tuna and Salad Wrap (no avocado). And for special occasions: Banana Cake; Carrot Cake; Rhubarb Crumble (modified: use pear and juice instead of rhubarb and lemon); Stewed Pears with Vanilla Soy Custard; Sweet Banana and Carob Spread (makes delicious popsicles, cake filling/icing, or a light pudding).

Baby Massage

Your child's skin will profit from regular body massages. Massaging your baby promotes relaxation: it calms an itchy, irritated child and increases bonding.

- Gently massage your baby's or child's shoulders and scalp with natural oil, such as calendula and coconut oil.
- Don't massage directly over the affected skin.
- Massage for at least 5 minutes a day.
- Give extra hugs!

Did You Know?

Hug Therapy

Give your child lots of hugs. Kids with skin inflammation need more cuddles and encouragement than usual because they are very sensitive. A really warm and loving hug is basically touch therapy, which has been proven to trigger the release of endorphins. Endorphins help to reduce inflammation in the body, so give hug therapy a try. This will help you and your child to remain calm. Skin inflammation sufferers are particularly sensitive to stress, so try not to shout at your child or argue in front of him, because stress promotes the enzyme blockage that increases arachidonic acid and inflammation. Of course, you can calmly discipline children if they are being naughty. Clearly set boundaries are also vital for a child's development.

Quick Review of the Children's Clear Skin Program

Step 1: Identify triggers and irritants

- Limit chemical exposure: use natural cleaning products and wash fruits and vegetables.

Step 2: Identify allergies

- Get allergy testing if age-appropriate.

Step 3: Soothe your child's skin with topical treatments

- Moisturize your child's skin as often as needed (two to four times a day).
- Bathe your child three to four times a week and use therapeutic ingredients.

Step 4: Give your child suitable supplements

- Glycine (for eczema, psoriasis, salicylate, and chemical sensitivity, and hives).
- Probiotic supplement (for all skin conditions and lowered immunity and digestive complaints).
- Liquid chlorophyll (for all skin conditions and for allergy sufferers and reflux).
- Children's omega-3 supplement (for psoriasis, rosacea, and hyperactivity).

Step 5: Give your child moisturizing foods

- Ensure your child has plenty of water to drink throughout the day.
- Give your child a daily omega-3 intake: fish two to three times a week (salmon, trout, sardines) and flaxseed oil or ground flax seeds at least four times a week.

Step 6: Put your child on an elimination diet

- Limit saturated fat intake: Avoid pork and dairy products for 2 months.
- Avoid foods that are likely to cause flare-ups, such as sauces containing dairy, tomato, or soy sauce/tamari/oyster sauce. Also familiarize yourself — and your

children, if they are old enough — with the foods to avoid and the foods to limit as specified for adults (page 226), including the list of Additives to Avoid (page 459).

- Reduce omega-6 EFAs: Avoid giving your child margarine, safflower oil, sunflower oil, peanut oil, sesame oil, or corn oil. Limit intake of nuts and seeds until eczema has disappeared. You can use small amounts of butter, ghee, and extra virgin olive oil in your cooking.

After your child's skin condition has cleared up

- Celebrate!
- Wait a couple of weeks and then reintroduce dairy into your child's diet. Do this gradually to avoid flare-ups. This step is necessary to identify whether dairy should be avoided for the long term. If a flare-up occurs or if your child gets itchy skin (inflammation under the surface), avoid dairy and wait for your child's skin to clear up before testing the next food item.
- After you have tested dairy (and your child's skin is clear of rashes), test all of the other foods you have taken out of your child's diet (such as tomato, grapes, and honey). Introduce one new food every 3 days. DO NOT test your child with allergy foods to which you know your child will have an anaphylactic reaction. This allergy may be permanent (and dangerous), so see an allergy specialist for guidance.
- Continue to avoid margarine, poor-quality cooking oils, white bread, preservatives, and artificial additives.
- Reduce supplement dosages gradually. Supplement with glycine and probiotics twice a week, on an ongoing basis if necessary.
- Serve your child alkalizing vegetables daily. For children who suffer from eczema, serve iceberg lettuce, celery, green beans, red cabbage, white potato, carrots, sweet potato, and cos lettuce (and avoid problematic vegetables such as broccoli, mushrooms, and spinach, which are rich in natural "itchy" chemicals, including MSG and salicylates).
- Avoid most fruits. The best fruits for children who have eczema or hyperactivity are banana, peeled pear, peeled Red Delicious apple, and papaya. Avoid all other fruits and dried fruits until the eczema improves.
- Keep giving your child omega-3-rich foods daily (fish or flaxseed).
- Use a moisturizer if necessary.

Part 5

Being Beautiful and Healthy

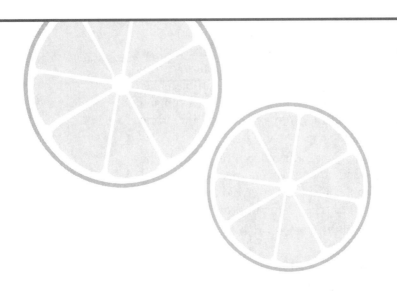

Beauty Breathing

The person with strong lungs has soft, lustrous skin and glossy hair. Skin that is dry, dull or rough is a sign of lung imbalance.

— *Paul Pitchford, author of* Healing with Whole Foods

Feeling stressed? Stress triggers your fight or flight nervous system to kick in. This is the hyped-up part of your nervous system, but you don't want it to be switched on for too long. If you are chronically stressed or always shallow breathing, the stress hormone cortisol will be released. High or continual cortisol levels accelerate aging and decrease the body's ability to fight bacteria and viruses. Fight or flight stress responses can also prevent your body from making beauty-boosting prostaglandins (remember, prostaglandins were covered in Guideline #2). No wonder stress makes you look and feel older. However, if you know a couple of simple breathing techniques, you can make yourself feel relaxed in an instant. In fact, good-quality breathing can enhance your health in many ways, which is why breathing exercises are an important part of the Healthy Skin Diet. Invest at least 5 minutes each morning in practicing breathing exercises. Schedule it into your diary or planner now.

Health Benefits of Correct Breathing

- Reduces stress and anxiety, which decreases the likelihood of skin rashes caused by stress-induced inflammation.
- Increases circulation of the lymph and blood flow to the skin, giving you a fresher-looking complexion. The lymphatic system is also responsible for immunity and resistance to disease.
- Enhances oxygen and nutrient flow to the skin, which facilitates wound healing and cell renewal.
- Teaches you to breathe correctly during exercise, making it easier to do strenuous activities for longer and work up a sweat for gorgeous skin.
- Improves digestion and absorption of nutrients so that more essential fatty acids and antioxidants can get to your outermost organ — the skin. The skin is the last organ to receive nutrients supplied by your meals.

Many doctors and psychiatrists are now prescribing breathing exercises to their patients as a part of their wellness programs.

Deep and Shallow Breathing

Breathing exercises are a useful tool if you suffer from anxiety or depression. According to the principles of traditional Chinese medicine (and mounting evidence), clouded emotions and thoughts can be cleansed by long, deep breathing. Many doctors and psychiatrists are now prescribing breathing exercises to their patients as a part of their wellness programs.

Q. My doctor said I am a shallow breather. What does this mean and what can I do about it?

A. Weak, or shallow, breathing, where you predominantly breathe into your upper chest and only partially inflate the lungs, is becoming a common problem for many in our community. According to renowned breathing teacher Sophie Gabriel, author of *Breathe for Life*, poor breathing habits can be triggered by a variety of factors, such as an inability to cope with stress and anxiety, tense muscles, a sedentary lifestyle, illness, injury, and smoking. Even poor posture, where you slouch for long hours toward your computer (or this book) can decrease your breath quality and lead to chronic upper chest breathing.

To change your pattern of shallow breathing, you need to first become aware of it. You can check your posture and learn some simple breathing techniques (later in this chapter). Practice your breathing exercises daily to help retrain your lungs. However, it must be said that simply breathing in deeply cannot make a lasting change to your health: it is the breathing technique or breath quality that makes all the difference.

Throat Breathing

I feel strongly about sharing with you the breathing techniques that Sophie Gabriel has taught me. I have experienced amazing benefits from incorporating them into my life. When I first learned the technique of "throat breathing," I was amazed at how it helped with my yoga practice. If I felt fatigued while doing leg work, I would just consciously start throat breathing, and this increased my stamina so I could keep going during the class.

I also used to be one of the worst students in my yoga class because I could not keep my balance (and there's a lot of balancing poses in yoga). Even the 60-year-olds in my class could stand on one leg with the other leg pointing skyward like elegant statues. But not me. In the class, I was always the one who wobbled and kept my (supposedly skyward) leg hovering so low it would occasionally touch the ground and save me from an embarrassing fall. When I started to use throat breathing, my balance instantly improved — it's a godsend!

Dr. Gabriel says that your balance improves because throat breathing engages the diaphragm, which is one of the body's strongest muscles. The diaphragm system works hard to stabilize balance and enhance core strength (strength around your torso, back, and stomach). Throat breathing also allows you to take in more breath (and with less effort), so it quickly enhances your energy and stamina.

> Throat breathing also allows you to take in more breath (and with less effort), so it quickly enhances your energy and stamina.

CASE HISTORY

Before I read *Breathe for Life*, it was a different story. For years I had heard that breathing exercises were good for you and breathing exercises helped you to relax, and so on. I would try to breathe in deeply a few times and think, "Big deal!" I got nothing from them — or worse. Sometimes breathing exercises would make me feel light-headed, so I thought feeling bad after breathing deeply was normal. Maybe you've tried basic deep breathing exercises in the past and you have not had any positive results, so you've given up too. If so, I want you to know that when breathing exercises are done correctly, they can help you to feel fantastic. I'd be lying if I said that this didn't take practice, but once you grasp the principles of breathing, you really don't have to have much willpower. All you need to do is be more conscious of your breath quality as you walk to the bus stop or sit at your desk. Then, if you notice you feel tense or tired, correct your posture and do a couple of breathing exercises for 30 seconds or more. These exercises are such simple tools for gaining both energy and relaxation. I hope you enjoy the benefits as much as I have.

Throat Breathing Exercises

The sensation of throat breathing automatically happens when good-quality deep breathing occurs.

Throat breathing is a non-technical term used by Gabriel to describe the next breathing exercise. The throat doesn't actually do the breathing, but when breathing deeply, it is where the sensations are felt. It is important to understand throat breathing before learning any other type of breathing exercise, especially the ones that utilize the diaphragm, because it helps you to understand which throat muscles to engage when doing breathing exercises.

Throat breathing is also a fantastic tool to use during meditation and exercise.

During exercise it allows more air to quickly enter the lungs, with less strain, so you have more energy available to you. Meditating with poor breathing habits can leave you feeling tense and frustrated, but using throat breathing (and good posture) during meditation helps to create a sense of relaxation in your body and this can make meditation more enjoyable. The sensation of throat breathing automatically happens when good-quality deep breathing occurs.

Throat Breathing Exercise 1: Prepare for Throat Breathing

Initially it is best to learn this exercise in a quiet environment, breathing in and out of your mouth. This breathing exercise will eventually be done with the mouth closed, breathing in and out of the nose but still achieving the same sound and sensation in the throat area.

Mouth open version

1. Sit in a chair or lie down flat on your back and relax your shoulders.

2. Take three slow, deep breaths and tell yourself to relax on each exhalation.

3. Keep your chest lifted. Relax! Relax! Relax! Now you are ready for the exhalation stage.

Exhalation stage

1. Try not to strain or create tension in your body, and as you exhale, don't let your chest drop at all.

2. Breathe in a nice, slow, deep breath.

3. Then open your mouth wide, and as you breathe out, make a long HHH sound: HHHHHHHHHH.

4. Notice how your throat muscles respond — there should be a feeling of the throat passageway relaxing so the air passes with ease.

Did You Know?

Practice Makes Perfect

Sophie Gabriel claims that learning how to take a good-quality throat breath is the most important part of breathing training. In fact, she does not continue training unless a person has grasped this properly. It is better to spend more time mastering throat breathing before moving on to the next breathing exercise. Remember, this is for your own benefit. Wouldn't you like to have a great tool for boosting your energy when you feel tired and stressed? And having better balance may also be useful, especially if you play sports. Keeping this in mind, go over your throat breathing exercises for as long as necessary until you feel you have mastered it.

5. Try this a few times and take note of how your throat feels (so you can eventually do this with your mouth closed, and so that the air is moving in and out of the nose only).

6. Practice this throat breathing exhalation exercise until you understand how it works.

Inhalation stage

According to Gabriel, everyone finds that the inhalation is harder to grasp than the exhalation, so you'll need a bit more patience with it. The easiest way to approach it is to simply remember what you did with the exhalation, but in reverse. You are still after the same sensation in the throat and the same sound. Voice coach James Hagan uses this inhalation exercise to teach people how to improve voice quality:

1. Look in the mirror.

2. Open your mouth wide and breathe in until the soft pallet (the uvula, or dangly bit at the back of your throat) retracts upwards. This will sound a bit like Darth Vadar's breathing on a good day.

3. See how this looks in the mirror — the throat is opened in a similar manner to the throat exhalation exercise and the tongue feels like it is being pulled down (out of the way) by the throat muscles. If you cannot move your uvula upwards, it doesn't matter as long as you are opening the throat and allowing air to pass in with ease. You'll know you are doing it correctly when you feel the sensation of air passing the roof of your mouth and you will feel your throat relaxing.

4. Practice this in front of the mirror until you have memorized the feeling of what is happening in the throat. When you eventually do this exercise with your mouth closed and you are only breathing through your nose, there will be a more subtle relaxing of the throat. Initially, exaggerating the movement helps you get a clear idea of what you are trying to achieve.

5. Test yourself. Now that you understand and can feel how throat breathing works, do both the inhalation and exhalation exercises without looking in a mirror and see if you can get the same relaxed-throat feeling. Can you feel the air on the back of the throat and sense the throat muscles working?

6. Remember to be careful not to strain your throat. Relax your throat and take your time.

Mouth closed version

The next step is to practice throat breathing without opening your mouth.

1. Close your mouth and breathe in through your nose (remembering to avoid "sniffing" in air).

2. Remember to relax your whole throat area so that the breath passes easily on the way down to your lungs.

3. Breathe out through the nose, remembering to keep the throat relaxed so the breath passes out with ease.

4. Practice this for as long as necessary. Once you understand how the closed-mouth version of throat breathing should feel, you can use it anytime — while you are walking down the street, when you are sitting in front of your computer, or when relaxing by the pool.

There are a
number of
exercises
you can use
to tone your
diaphragm,
enhance your
breathing, and
improve your
skin.

Diaphragm Breathing

There are many ways to improve your breathing quality, including abdominal breathing from the diaphragm. The diaphragm is a thin muscle that sits horizontally between the lungs and the abdomen, like an upside-down dinner plate. It is an important skeletal muscle because it is used to power lung expansion during breathing. However, it can lose some of its flexibility. A more rigid diaphragm makes it harder to take in a good-quality breath, making exercising, singing, and even relaxing more of a challenge. Athletes and trained singers all have strong, toned diaphragms.

There are a number of exercises you can use to tone your diaphragm, enhance your breathing, and improve your skin.

Diaphragm Exercise 1: Observe Yourself

Stand in front of a mirror and relax your shoulders. Now take a long, deep inhale followed by a long, deep exhale. Do this a few times and observe the way your body moves when you breathe in and out.

- Do your shoulders rise up when you inhale? If so, a little, or a lot?
- Is your upper chest expanding upwards when you inhale? If so, a little, or a lot?
- Do your neck and shoulders look strained?
- Are you holding in your stomach and not allowing movement in the abdominal area?
- How does your posture look? (Go on, have another look in the mirror.)
- Take a really deep breath in through your nose: does it sound like you are sniffing in air?
- Take another deep breath in as you look in the mirror: do your nostrils close up slightly?

If you answered yes to any of these questions, this could indicate that you are struggling to take a good-quality deep breath and that your breathing may possibly be shallow. According to Sophie Gabriel, your shoulders should remain relaxed and not move upwards when you breathe in.

Diaphragm Exercise 2: Listen to Your Nose

Throat breathing is the opposite of "sniffing" in air. An exercise in "what not to do," as described by Dr. Gabriel, is to exaggerate the sound of sniffing in air. Pretend you are smelling a bunch of flowers. Sniff in the aroma as you take a deep breath in. Try to sniff your out breath as well. Observe how this feels. Does your nasal passage feel contracted?

When breathing in consists of subtly (or not so subtly) sniffing air into the upper chest, you create tension in the upper body. Less air is mobilized and less energy is created (so you may feel lethargic for no apparent reason). Sniffing in air is what you want to avoid doing at all times. "There is never a need for it," Dr. Gabriel explains, "unless you want to smell brewed coffee, a baked cake, or flowers."

Abdominal Breathing

According to Sophie Gabriel, abdominal breathing is one of the best ways to relax the mind and body because it triggers the rest and digest part of your nervous system. Once you have mastered it, you can use it anytime, so you can call upon this tool to "de-stress" after a big day at work. You can even do abdominal breathing at work if you suddenly feel uptight or anxious. During abdominal breathing, you relax your abdomen and expand your belly as you inhale. It is a little like a small balloon being inflated behind your belly button. Don't worry, your workmates won't even notice you using this relaxation technique, especially if you are sitting behind your desk. This exercise may be called abdominal breathing, but your breath doesn't really end up in your abdomen; it is your diaphragm pushing downward that creates the expansion. However, when you imagine breathing into the abdominal area, it helps you to grasp the exercise.

> Abdominal breathing is one of the best ways to relax the mind and body because it triggers the rest and digest part of your nervous system.

Abdominal Exercises

Gabriel suggests that you initially practice this exercise lying down on your back, and you can bring your knees up, with your feet flat on the floor, if it is more comfortable to do so.

1. Place a small flat pillow or towel behind your head so your neck is comfortably lengthened and your chin moves slightly toward your chest.

2. Place your hands on your belly with fingers resting toward your belly button.

3. Remembering to throat breathe, take a deep and very slowly breath in through the nose, and imagine this breath traveling to the abdomen as it expands.

4. Be aware of the movement in your hands as you breathe. Are they moving outward or skyward as you inhale (they should be)?

5. Keep breathing in and out gently and expand your abdomen slowly. Your upper chest should not be moving. If it is and your belly is stationary, then you need to make sure you are throat breathing because this helps you to use the diaphragm correctly.

6. Continue to visualize the breath inflating your belly and tell yourself to relax as you exhale.

7. Now try the same exercise sitting up or standing in front of a mirror.

Did You Know?

Slow Down

To slow your breathing down during the exercises, imagine that you are slowly breathing in and out through a straw. This is for when you are practicing, not during high-impact exercise. Practice this over and over again so you can master the exercise before you try it standing up or sitting down. And don't be alarmed if you experience difficulty in moving your belly on cue. If you are used to breathing in a shallow manner into your upper chest, your diaphragm may not have good tone and flexibility. But you can still do this exercise with some persistence and patience. Any small improvement is really a breakthrough, so give yourself a bit of praise as you go. Also, you should not force your breathing, and have a break if you begin to feel light-headed.

8. As you inhale and exhale, keep your hands placed on your belly and mentally visualize this area expanding and contracting like a balloon slowly filling up and slowly deflating.

9. If you want to advance to the next stage, try expanding the front of your lower rib cage. Then you may want to try to expand the side and back ribs. (This is a whole new exercise, so you may want to read Sophie's book for more information)

Breathing Technique

When exercising, Gabriel recommends special attention to technique:

- Maintain correct form and posture at all times, even if you're feeling fatigued.
- Breathe through your mouth using good-quality throat breathing for both the inhalation and exhalation.
- Focus on breathing into the diaphragm and allow plenty of movement in the rib cage area (expand your rib cage, especially the lower part). This tip is very useful.
- Breathe appropriately according to the level of exertion and movement; for example, if you're walking your breathing will be slower and if sprinting you will need to breathe in and out faster and more deeply.
- Don't hold on to your breath (unless instructed by a qualified trainer).
- When aiming for endurance, don't exhale or inhale with too much force during exercise if not required because this can upset your body's oxygen and carbon dioxide levels, which can tire you easily and affect stamina. You know you are breathing in or out too forcefully and upsetting your oxygen and carbon dioxide balance if you experience numbness in the feet and/or hands and light-headedness or feeling faint (however, these may also be caused by other factors).

Did You Know?

Athletic Breathing

Gabriel has observed that athletes use specific methods of breathing during their performance. She also compared athletes to unfit people during exercise and noticed the relevant differences, which included the following:

- Athletes maintain good posture when they exercise. They keep their chest and rib cage lifted and open as much as possible, without letting it drop when exhaling. This allows them to breathe with ease.
- Athletes regulate their breathing. They breathe appropriately according to what their sport demands; for example, they breathe deeper if they're doing high-impact exercise, such as sprinting. Athletes do not take in an unnecessarily large amount of air. This means they keep their oxygen and carbon dioxide levels in a constant healthy balance as they exercise.
- Athletes learn the correct way to do an exercise or sport — they consult with experts.
- Unfit people typically have erratic, inappropriate breathing when exercising. They may also have poor posture.

Quick Review of Breathing Exercises

During breathing exercises, you are aiming to achieve:

- Relaxation
- Smooth air flow so breathing is regular
- Ability to breathe more slowly, gently, longer, and deeply, as well as being able to breathe powerfully
- Relaxed throat while breathing
- Inhalation and exhalation similar in length and strength
- Relaxed abdomen and freer movement in your lower rib cage as you breathe in and out. (If this is difficult, then remember the tip "Keep imagining a balloon slowly expanding and contracting in your abdominal area.")

How to Be Beautiful

You can conform, rebel, pine for it, or make judgments about who is (or isn't), but you can't define beauty for the masses.

The definition of beauty is perfect skin, strong jaw line, symmetrical face, white teeth, blonde hair (or at least glossy and fashionable hair), olive skin, blue eyes, and abs to die for. We should all look like Angelina Jolie, Brad Pitt, or Halle Berry (take your pick) and feel bad about ourselves if we don't fit the beauty mold…

Please argue with me: it is ridiculous to think that beauty has a set formula. You can conform, rebel, pine for it, or make judgments about who is (or isn't), but you can't define beauty for the masses. This chapter is broken down into four beauty insights so you can get the edge without surgery, starvation, or orange-stained sheets from a fake tan.

Q. What is beauty?

A. In fact, beauty is a highly debatable topic. Have you ever said, "She is so beautiful," only to have a friend look at you as if you are crazy and retort with, "No she's not." Some people think Kate Moss is gorgeous, while others wonder what all the fuss is about. Geishas are considered the epitome of Japanese beauty. In certain parts of Thailand, hill-tribe women coil massive lengths of brass wire around their necks to make their necks appear giraffe-like. The coils are a decoration of beauty and wealth so that the women can attract a good husband. However, a Western woman would only draw bewildered glances if her neck was elongated with brass coils or her face painted white. So what is beauty? Beauty is subjective. This is probably not what you want to hear, because it creates a new problem: how do you make yourself appear more attractive if everyone has a different opinion of what beauty is? Do you go blonde or red? Do you get a spray tan or bleach your freckles? And are wrinkles finally in this season? What can you aspire to look like if beauty is so damn indefinable?

Insight No. 1: Inner Beauty Is Beautiful to Everyone

External beauty is subjective. It can be difficult to obtain and too easy to lose, because if you live long enough, you will get wrinkly no matter how much nipping and tucking you have. However, on the up side, inner beauty never grows old; in fact, it gets firmer and stronger as time goes by, and it is certainly easier to obtain than abs because no gym membership is required. And best of all, inner beauty is beyond subjectivity because it is adored by everyone.

CASE STUDY

I saw an example of inner beauty recently when I was standing in the checkout line at my local department store. The woman working behind the counter caught my eye; I had seen her many times before and remembered her to be chatty and friendly (which often slowed down her line). On this day, she was undoing a lollipop wrapper for a little boy and chatting with his mom. As I watched her, I became curious. She looked a little disheveled, with frazzled red hair and scabby sores on her arms, and I admit I was wondering if someone loved her. The mother and son left and the frazzled lady began scanning my items. She was chirpy and welcoming as usual. When the photo album I was buying wouldn't scan, she happily said she would scan the refill pages that I was also purchasing and give the album to me for the same price, saving me time and money. She had an ease about her that made me feel relaxed, and as she handed me my receipt, it suddenly struck me: she had loads of inner beauty and, of course, she was loved. I told a close friend about the lovely lady from the department store, and my friend said, "I know exactly who you're talking about; she's amazing! She even remembers my son's name."

As you check your reflection in the mirror each day, you may analyze your skin, fuss with your hair, and curse your bone structure, but does your beautiful personality ever rate a mention? Other people probably appreciate your good qualities more than you do. Shame on you! When you fail to appreciate yourself, you miss out on feeling beautiful.

Beautiful Attributes

There are many ways to be beautiful. Here are some questions to help you identify your beautiful attributes:

- Are you kind to your mother?
- Do you help her around the house and keep your room clean?
- Are you a great home entertainer?
- Do you cook for others?
- Are you a good friend?
- Do you make others laugh?
- Do you remember birthdays?
- Do you do your best to conserve water and recycle?
- Do you pick up your litter? Maybe you also pick up other people's litter because you care about the environment?
- Are you patient?
- Are you grateful?
- Have you ever performed a random act of kindness?
- Do you respect other people's property?
- Do you have kind thoughts toward others?

Activity

Write down 10 positive attributes you have. If you can't think of 10, you are probably not trying hard enough. Then add to your repertoire by doing something kind and thoughtful today. Write this in your diary or planner right now.

Insight No. 2: People Detect Inner Beauty on an Energetic Level

You could spend all your time meticulously choosing the right foods to eat and exercising fanatically to get your external appearance looking good, but you could still be unattractive. If you neglect your inner goodness, you may find yourself exuding the wrong type of energy, one that repels people despite your exterior good looks.

CASE STUDY

After I finished my shopping at that department store and said goodbye to the frazzle-haired lady with inner beauty, I continued my shopping at a material and haberdashery shop. Once I was in the store, I found some material and asked an assistant how much I'd need for the pillowcase I was going to make for my daughter (well, I was buying the material and my mom would do the sewing). She advised me to look at the pillowcases in the linen section. I found a pillowcase and took it out of its plastic packaging to measure it. When I had finished, I folded it and realized the pillowcase would not fit back into the packaging, so I put it back on the shelf unpacked. I admit this was due to a mixture of laziness and lack of coordination when it comes to folding and packing.

I sensed someone watching me. I looked up and thought I saw a well-groomed woman on the other side of the shop glare at me, but she was so far away I thought I was just being paranoid. However, the next thing I knew she was beside me with the unpacked pillowcase in hand (she must have run from the other side of the shop). She immediately launched into a lecture on how to put the pillowcase back into its packaging and she gave me an efficient demonstration. I apologized profusely and said I would be more thoughtful next time. However, she continued to lecture me until I said, "Excuse me, I have already apologized and you don't need to lecture me as if I'm stupid."

She calmed down and said sorry, but I left the shop a bit shaken up at being attacked for such a minor offense. The funny thing was, I felt her aggressive, rather unattractive energy before she had even said a word.

Q. How is it that we can feel other people's energy?

A. This can be difficult to describe scientifically, but there is evidence that different thoughts create varying frequencies in our brain, which can be demonstrated by electroencephalograph (EEG) testing.

- Delta waves are the lowest frequencies (vibrations) emitted from thoughts, recording only 0.1 to 3 Hz on an EEG. Delta waves occur when you are unmotivated, lethargic, and inattentive or when you have attention deficit disorder (ADD) and try to focus. Delta waves are also recorded during sleep.
- Alpha waves create a little more energy, reading between 7.5 and 13 Hz. You can initiate alpha waves by sitting still and shutting your eyes or with deep breathing exercises and meditation. Alpha waves are associated with relaxation, inner awareness, and healing. Alpha waves stop being produced when you engage in thinking, calculating, and physical action.
- Mid-range beta waves increase with alert mental activity (as long as you are not agitated). Mid-range frequencies range from 15 to 18 Hz. If you were thinking agitated thoughts, your brain's energy frequencies would alter accordingly.

Of course in everyday life you can't see the energy you emit with each passing mood, but that doesn't mean such energy doesn't exist. Just like electricity: you can't see it, you can't explain it, but it still has an effect. Flick on a switch and you create energy in the form of light.

Charisma

In humans, we instinctively sense strong and harmonious energy fields in people and we label it charisma. These people have the ability to hold your attention without them having to say a word; they feel "power-full" and we sense it when they walk into a room. On the other hand, the people who feel "power-less" have not learned to harness their energy or they limit it with self-degradation, also known as negative self-talk. As a result, they may feel sad for no reason , and they can feel overlooked or invisible when in other people's company.

> These people have the ability to hold your attention without them having to say a word.

The good news is, everyone has the ability to raise their energy field so they feel more powerful, loved, and appreciated. You just need to know how. "Seeing is believing," so at the end of this chapter I have included three activities that can alter your energy field and increase your inner beauty. Do these activities for 2 weeks and see if people start responding differently to you.

Activity

Assess what type of energy you are emitting on a daily basis. You can tell this about yourself by the way people interact with you in everyday situations.

- Do people generally like you?
- Do you have good friends?
- Do you consider yourself lucky?
- Do you quickly recover from bad situations?

If you answered yes to these questions, you may be giving off positive energy.

OR
- Do you attract arguments?
- Are you unlucky in love or struggling financially?
- Are you accident-prone?
- Do you feel misunderstood?
- Do you feel anxious or depressed?

If you answered yes to these questions you may be giving off inharmonious energy.

There are also shades of gray in between: you may be lucky sometimes, for example, and have great misfortune at other times. Your energy emissions can change as your thoughts and feelings shift. However, if you always seem to be misunderstood or mistreated, you may want to alter your energy emissions and see what happens.

Insight No. 3: As You See and Appreciate Beauty, You Become More Beautiful

Yes, inner beauty is important, but you are allowed to improve your appearance while you work your inner beauty "muscle" (after all, the Healthy Skin Diet is designed to help you achieve beautiful skin). So this insight goes beyond inner beauty and helps you to program yourself to naturally gravitate toward good habits that promote health and beauty, such as nutritious food and exercise. If you have ever sabotaged your health routine or lamented about your poor willpower, this is the secret that you have been waiting for!

CASE STUDY

When I was 4 years old, I was attacked by a dingo, but I can only remember what happened before and after the attack. I was terrified before it occurred, but I told myself to stop running, as the puppy just wanted to play. The next thing I remember is thinking that my mother was hurt because she had blood all over her white T-shirt. However, after that event, if a dog came near me, my heart would race and I'd feel uncontrollable panic, and if the dog growled at me, I would experience physical pain and cry even though I couldn't ever remember the attack itself.

Five years ago, I made an effort to change my experiences with dogs. I did this by taking a friend's dog for a walk on a regular basis. It was fun and I assured myself over and over again, "Most dogs are friendly." In essence, I reprogrammed my responses to dogs. My automatic reactions to dogs eventually changed and I stopped freaking out around them.

Did You Know?

Subconsciousness

Your subconscious mind helps you achieve insights by storing data for you, including the actions you have performed over and over again. For example, practice driving a car every day and pretty soon it becomes automatic. If you do something without thinking, you know your subconscious mind is at work. The subconscious also stores repressed memories and painful things we don't want to deal with. The subconscious mind records the events you have attached strong emotions to (both good and bad). You may reason you are being silly when you react inappropriately to a situation (like me and dogs), but your subconscious beliefs can override your logical, conscious mind. If this occurs, you need to give your subconscious mind new data to draw from, just as I did when I created lots of positive experiences with dogs. Your subconscious mind generally will not record events to which you are indifferent. If you meet a person who interests you, you are likely to remember their face, but when introduced to a person who does not grab your attention in any way, you are likely to forget the meeting ever occurred.

But you'd be surprised how many people program into their subconscious mind the instructions "Beauty is bad and must be avoided!"

Beauty Is Good

Your subconscious mind also affects how beautiful you allow yourself to be. When you appreciate beauty, your subconscious mind records that beauty is a positive attribute. You may think, "Of course beauty is a positive attribute!" But you'd be surprised how many people program into their subconscious mind the instruction "Beauty is bad and must be avoided!" If you acknowledge a beautiful sunset with a few emotionally charged wows, then your subconscious records, "Beauty is good!" If you appreciate a beautiful face: "Beauty is good!" If you genuinely compliment a woman with beautiful skin and feel happiness for her, then, "Beauty is good!" Pretty soon your subconscious mind has formed a new belief: "Beauty is good … I've got to have it!"

Appreciation of beauty, in all its forms, helps you to have more beauty of your own. You can quite literally become more attractive. (Okay, don't take this out of context: your jaw line won't physically change, but you will gravitate toward healthy living, which can promote good skin health and a better waistline.) This is because appreciation of beauty reduces the likelihood of self-sabotage.

Self-Sabotage

Have you ever sabotaged your good looks with binge eating or laziness? Do you often have a conscious goal to enhance your skin health or lose some weight, but then you always fail to stick with your fab new diet? This is called self-sabotage and it is awfully confusing when you're trying to make positive changes to your life.

Let's say you look in a glossy magazine and see a couple of female models with perfect skin. You may think (with lots of gusto), "These models are only skinny because they don't eat, and they're 15 years old, so of course they have perfect skin!' This deduction makes you feel bad (because you have unfairly compared yourself to them). Or you may go to a bar and see a beautiful person enter the room and you subsequently feel bad about yourself. Or you visit the beach and look at someone slimmer than you and you then feel bad. You go to a café and spot someone with better skin than you and you feel bad. And you do this over and over again until your subconscious mind registers that beauty makes you feel awful, so therefore beauty is a negative attribute and one that must be avoided in order to avoid pain.

Restricting Beauty

What's worse is now your subconscious mind has registered that beauty is only available to young people who starve themselves. Of course, your subconscious mind doesn't want you to go hungry or feel bad, so it reasons it must protect you from this detestable thing called beauty. Your subconscious mind subsequently employs self-sabotage or poor willpower to keep you from falling prey to beauty. Same too with other beliefs, such as "Beautiful people are dumb," "Beautiful people get hassled and ogled," and "Beautiful people are fake." And you wonder why you go on a diet, with good intentions to lose weight or clear up your skin, and then sabotage yourself with binge eating, or you could join a gym and never go.

> And you wonder why you go on a diet, with good intentions to lose weight or clear up your skin, and then sabotage yourself with binge eating, or you could join a gym and never go.

Programming Beauty

You think it is your lack of willpower when in fact you have programmed yourself to fail because you've created a subconscious belief that beauty is a negative thing. What are your beliefs about beautiful people? Do you bitch or praise? Are you happy for other people who are beautiful or are you more than a teensy bit jealous? Your subconscious mind helps you achieve your goals, such as getting fit and healthy; it enhances your willpower and prevents you from overeating. Willpower is your subconscious mind following through with your instructions about beauty. Positive observations about beauty = strong willpower when dieting and exercising. It promotes the satiety response so your body will tell you it is full sooner rather than later so you stay slim. You need willpower to change your diet and achieve your beauty goals, but how do you program "Beauty is positive" into your subconscious mind so you get the drive you need, minus self-sabotage?

> Positive observations about beauty = strong willpower when dieting and exercising.

Beauty Is Positive

To program "Beauty is positive" into your subconscious mind, you need to attach strong positive emotions to beauty, and you need to do this over and over again until you have formed a strong belief. As you appreciate beauty and program "Beauty is positive," your subconscious mind helps you become more beautiful: it ensures you stick to the Healthy Skin Diet and it urges you to put on those running shoes!

Insight No. 4: People Detect Inner Beauty by Your Actions and Habits

Now let's get back to the gorgeous topic of inner beauty… your actions and habits have a strong effect on the people around you, even more so than your words. Actions and habits can contradict a spoken lie and reveal the truth for everyone to see. Unfortunately, your habits are largely driven by your subconscious mind, so they are hard to consciously control. This means you cannot fake inner beauty because your subconsciously driven actions will eventually give you away. Your subconscious mind reveals the most when you are relaxed. Alcohol also has a reputation of bringing hidden or suppressed beliefs out in the open and you can ruin your reputation with one drunken rant.

> This means you cannot fake inner beauty because your subconsciously driven actions will eventually give you away.

Poor Interpretations

Where do these subconscious truths come from and how do we get rid of them? Your words and actions don't necessarily come from your daily life experiences; they come from how you interpret them. Say you had a bad experience with a kid from an ethnic minority at school. He teased you and took your lunch money. You could interpret this to mean "All ethnic minority kids are bad," or alternatively you may decide that "Jerry was mean to me, thank goodness not all people are like him," and you could go on to have healthy friendships with others.

Poor interpretations can shape your future and they can also ruin your life. Poor interpretations form unreasonable subconscious truths (true in your subconscious mind but not reality) and they affect your actions in daily life so you can come across as defensive, angry, or unlikeable without you even realizing it. For example, if you've decided that all men are bastards because you have had your heart broken a few times, then you are likely to appear defensive when in the company of men. So on your next date, you may end up sounding arrogant or angry without meaning to. Your subconscious mind has worked against you (another case of self-sabotage) and you are unlikely to be asked out a second time because of your angry-about-men habits. Guess what? This bad outcome once again backs up your

> Poor interpretations can shape your future and they can also ruin your life.

belief that all men are bastards (when in reality most men just don't like defensive behavior). Poor interpretations of your past relationships can lead you to sabotage your future relationships.

Did You Know?

Good Things

A remedy for negative interpretations is to focus on beauty rather than faults. For example, don't spend longer than a few moments thinking about a negative situation; instead, turn your attention to the good things in your life, such as your strengths and positive attributes. If intimate relationships are a problem, focus on your positive experiences with the opposite sex. If you don't have any good memories to draw from, it is time to form some platonic friendships. Have good clean fun and expect nothing from them in return, and you will create positive experiences that will condition your mind for healthy relationships in the future. If you have had negative experiences with beautiful people, forge new friendships with people you consider attractive (who seem kind) so you can create new positive experiences with beauty.

Beautiful Words

People also experience your beauty via your words. When you genuinely care about other people, you make them feel good. Who wouldn't want to be around someone who makes their life more enjoyable? When you say thank you (and mean it), when you show genuine gratitude, and when you offer help and then follow through on your offer, you form strong bonds with people. These bonds cannot be broken easily: not by small arguments, not by distance, and certainly not by you having a bad skin day. The recipients of your kindness will always remember your beauty, and if they don't, then they probably aren't worthy of your friendship.

> These bonds cannot be broken easily: not by small arguments, not by distance, and certainly not by you having a bad skin day.

Transforming Jealousy

What do you think your energy field is like when you're jealous or bitching about another? Do you think it gives you an attractive energy that others are drawn to? Unfortunately it doesn't, as jealousy can temporarily block your inner beauty. Jealousy also makes you feel "power-less" because it is a proclamation of inferiority. It is like holding up a sign

How to bump up your inner beauty in a flash

- Smile.
- Have integrity — be honest and authentic.
- Meditate or do breathing exercises — calm your mind.
- Value the present moment — observe your family, your children, and the world around you and enjoy it now.
- Enjoy being you — like yourself unconditionally.
- Treat yourself with respect — speak kindly of yourself and respect your body. This shows other people how you expect them to treat you.
- Find a charity and support it within your means. If you have time, give time; if you have a special skill, help out; if you have money, give donations.
- Be kind and generous, whether it is an anonymous random act of kindness or saying hello to an old person. Your kindness makes the world a better place.
- Appreciate beauty — expand your definition of beauty and choose to see it more often.
- Wish other people happiness.
- Be happy for other people's good fortune.
- When you glance at yourself in the mirror, look for beauty, not faults.

saying, "I am not as good as the person over there." Jealousy undermines your self-worth, but it is a common feeling that can be hard to ignore. So what can you do when the green-eyed monster suddenly appears?

Be prepared! Start to associate jealousy with weakness and all things bad. You can do this by considering the problems with jealousy:

Say to yourself (with great passion):
"Jealousy makes me weaker."
"Jealousy is a sign I'm feeling inferior or inadequate."
"Jealousy will not bring good fortune into my life."

Your subconscious mind will stop you from striving for something you have perceived as bad. Jealousy is bad! It is a self-sabotaging emotion, so limit it for your own good. The famous Swiss psychoanalyst Carl Jung said that anything about which you feel strong emotions is a part of your shadow self, the suppressed or unacknowledged part of yourself.

For example, when you feel strong positive emotions about another person's charisma, you should realize this quality can be yours too if you stop suppressing it (with negative self-talk) and then consciously cultivate it (with research and practice, practice, practice).

It also works the other way around: when you feel strong negative emotions about a person (such as jealousy of their beauty), your jealousy has nothing to do with the other person, but everything to do with your own negative feelings about yourself. It's fuelled by a suppressed part of yourself. If you are jealous of another person's good looks, you are really envious because you have either suppressed your own beauty or have not acknowledged your own good features. Shame on you! Your beauty is being wasted by your own ignorance.

Do you despise fitness freaks? You may have sabotaged your own health and fitness for years, so you don't like to see it in other people. This belief may come out in the form of jealousy or hate. However, when you allow yourself to be your best, you don't mind if others are also being their best. I find that most people are hard on themselves and don't appreciate their good features, so if this sounds like you, then you're not alone. Instead, when you become jealous, tell yourself: "My jealousy is coming from a suppressed part of myself."

If you see someone whom you consider beautiful, remember your shadow self and say to yourself: "As I see the beauty in you, I allow the beauty in myself." And remember you don't need to compete to be a contender. You will shine when you value your own worth — this simply means you should be happy to be you rather than wishing you were more like someone else.

> When you feel strong negative emotions about a person (such as jealousy of their beauty), your jealousy has nothing to do with the other person, but everything to do with your own negative feelings about yourself.

Sisterhood

About 100 years ago, women were not allowed to vote. We have come a long way, but today there are women who are still being treated like second-class citizens. And I'm sad to say that quite often it is other women who are the main offenders in treating them this way. We should not be putting other women down, as many of them still feel powerless and they need a boost, not a kick.

I believe women should look after each other more and compete less. We are not in competition unless we are behind the starting line at the Olympic Games waiting for the starter gun to go off. We do not need to battle at bars, we are not contenders at clubs, and we are not at war with good-looking women, single or not.

> We should not be putting other women down, as many of them still feel powerless and they need a boost, not a kick.

We should also be looking out for one another. For example, there have been an alarming number of women who have been out socializing and had their drinks spiked with date-rape drugs. When this occurs, they appear drunk and disorderly. If they have been separated from their friends, they often have no one to care for them: instead, onlookers may laugh at their behavior and leave these women vulnerable to predators. It is up to us to make sure that this does not occur, first by making sure our own drinks are not left unattended and second by helping a woman find her friends if she appears drunk and disoriented, or consider calling an ambulance. Don't snigger at someone else's poor judgment and don't compete on a beauty level. Inner beauty is created when you bond, help, and care for another human being.

Inner Beauty Exercises

Here are three exercises to boost your inner beauty and enhance your energetic field or charisma.

Inner Beauty Exercise, Level 1

This walking appreciation exercise is a fantastic tool for expanding your definition of beauty so you can experience more beauty in your life.

1. Go for a brisk walk in a public place, preferably a popular nature walk, beach walk, or park (anywhere will do, just as long as you are walking past other people).

2. Instead of focusing on yourself, focus your attention on the people you pass. Your task is to look for the beauty in others. Look for conventional and unconventional beauty: is there unconventional beauty in their eyes, their appearance, or their smile? Look for inner beauty: strength, happiness, kindness, feminine/masculine power, wisdom, free-spiritedness, loveliness.

3. See the beauty in people of all shapes and sizes (including the overly skinny or overweight). It is your duty to break the size barrier that may exist in your mind — you cannot accuse the media of favoring the slim and beautiful if you yourself cannot see or appreciate beauty in all forms. The key is to look for beauty, not faults.

4. If this activity brings up uneasiness in you, then a more subtle approach may be necessary. Try thinking, "Wouldn't it be nice if I could see the beauty in her (or him)?" If resistance occurs, this is a sign you are suppressing your

own beauty. If this is the case, when you see someone attractive, say over and over again to yourself (with great passion/feeling): "As I see the beauty in you, I see the beauty in myself."

5. As you walk and look for the beauty in others, don't be afraid of eye contact — just smile if a person catches you looking at them.

6. Do this walking appreciation exercise for at least 10 minutes each day. After doing this for several days, you may notice that people seem friendlier and smile at you more often.

Seeing beauty in others is a great way to expand your definition of beauty, and you also bond with your local community without having to utter a word!

Seeing beauty in others is a great way to expand your definition of beauty, and you also bond with your local community without having to utter a word!

Inner Beauty Exercise, Level 2

Insight No. 2 taught us that people detect inner beauty on an energetic level. This activity helps to alter your inner energy so you seem more attractive. You can do this activity as soon as you wake up or when you go for a walk.

1. For 3 to 5 minutes, list everything you are grateful for. You can either do this in your head or out loud, but you must do this exercise with enthusiasm and passion (remember you need to use strong positive emotions to store new information in your subconscious mind). When your subconscious mind records how grateful you are, you will feel happier and emit a more powerful energy. This is the energy that attracts other people and makes you seem more alluring.

2. Now list your positive attributes and strengths. For example, I'm so grateful I have two legs to walk with; I'm so thankful I'm good at table tennis; I really appreciate my green eyes and my perfect eyesight; I'm so grateful I can look after myself; I'm so grateful I'm fit and healthy (even if it's only wishful thinking).

3. Then list what you appreciate about the people closest to you: I'm so grateful for my daughter, she is smart and kind and laughs at all my jokes; I'm so grateful for my partner, he pays the bills and loves me dearly; I'm so thankful for my mom, she is so generous and caring; I'm grateful for my dad, he loves me and supports all my decisions; I'm so lucky I have my sister, she is inspirational as she has overcome so many hurdles and this shows me that anything is possible and I am so thankful that she calls me all the time to let me know she is okay (and so on).

4. List the surroundings that you are grateful for: I'm so grateful for this beautiful beach; I'm so grateful for the warm sunshine; I'm so thankful for this lovely house; I'm so happy to be here today; I'm so lucky to be alive. You will find plenty of things to be grateful for if you start with the small stuff, such as your hands, the food in your fridge, or a pet.

Inner Beauty Exercise, Level 3

This exercise is brilliant for changing your energy frequencies to be more like what you want. You can do this exercise while lying down or anywhere you can close your eyes and concentrate. The idea is to imagine what you would like to achieve as if you've already done it, and then say thanks. Do it with enthusiasm and you will feel great — you will feel the same happiness as if it were real because the brain cannot tell the difference between what is actual and what is vividly imagined. So you may not already have a great life, but you are able to emit the same energy frequencies as someone who is charismatic and rich, with beautiful skin, a great job and is happy. All you have to do is imagine having a good life and feel the associated good feelings.

> So you may not already have a great life, but you are able to emit the same energy frequencies as someone who is charismatic and rich, with beautiful skin, a great job and is happy.

1. Begin by closing your eyes and taking three deep breaths.

2. Spend 5 minutes daydreaming about what you would love to achieve. Since you are reading this book, I assume you want better-looking skin. If so, then imagine you already have beautiful skin.

3. See people complimenting your gorgeous complexion and say thanks and smile because you're so grateful. Imagine looking at your reflection in a mirror and seeing your skin as smooth and fresh-looking. Imagine you have beautiful skin every day during the 8-week program.

4. It is the positive feelings you attach to these daydreams that will raise your energetic pull. So imagine you have beautiful skin and then get very excited about it. You can even cry happy tears and jump for joy in your daydreams (yes, look as silly as possible) so your subconscious mind will record that you love having beautiful skin. This is also a great confidence booster, which is another attractive quality to have.

Reality Checks

Now, you may be able to imagine having perfect skin, but what about reality? What can you do when you catch a glimpse of yourself in the mirror and see all your skin's faults, creases, canyons, and moguls? It is easy to be beautiful. All you have to do is expand your definition of what beauty is, appreciate beauty, and emulate it. Cultivate a good-looking aura with daily inner beauty exercises and remember, as you glimpse yourself in the mirror, to look for beauty, not faults.

> You need to love the skin you're in because it is a vital part of you.

Accentuate the Positive

1. For starters, you should avoid looking at your problem spots as much as possible, so limit using mirrors during the Healthy Skin Diet 8-week program. This is a little tricky at first, but fogging up the mirrors after a shower will definitely help.

2. Don't worry, you can briefly use a mirror to apply makeup or check that you have nothing hanging out of your nose. Do not judge yourself. Keep it brief and functional, and make sure you are dressed properly and well groomed. Once you look good, you can compliment yourself, but you DO NOT want to comment on any imperfections. You can't feel good about yourself if you are constantly putting yourself down. And you can't hate yourself into having better skin!

   Alternatively, each day look at a good patch of skin that is smooth and clear, such as the inside of your arms, and affirm, "I'm having a great skin day!" or "I have gorgeous skin!" You need to love the skin you're in because it is a vital part of you. Loving all parts of you, no matter how imperfect they seem to be, is imperative for your inner beauty and it is the key to true self-confidence, which is one of the most attractive qualities you can possess.

3. Do all three inner beauty exercises, levels 1 to 3, daily and try to keep the happy feelings they create with you throughout the day. If at any time you begin to feel stressed, counteract that negative feeling by listing the things you are grateful for. Within a few weeks, you just may see a shift in the way people respond to you.

   - Inner beauty is beautiful to everyone.
   - People detect inner beauty on an energetic level.
   - As you see and appreciate beauty, you become more beautiful.

> If at any time you begin to feel stressed, counteract that negative feeling by listing the things you are grateful for. Within a few weeks, you just may see a shift in the way people respond to you.

- People detect inner beauty by your actions and habits.
- Jealousy makes you feel powerless as it's a proclamation of inferiority.
- Smile and laugh more.
- Be kind and thoughtful, and look after each other.
- Inner beauty exercise level 1: As you walk past people, look for beauty, not faults.
- Inner beauty exercise level 2: For 3 to 5 minutes each day, list everything you are grateful for.
- Inner beauty exercise level 3: Spend 5 minutes daydreaming about having beautiful skin. Imagine you already have it and say thanks.
- Avoid critiquing yourself in the mirror. Don't affirm what you hate about yourself, because it will ruin your self-confidence. You can't hate yourself into having better skin.
- Look at a good patch of skin and compliment yourself on having a gorgeous complexion. This will raise your energy field to an attractive level.

Part 6

The Healthy Skin Diet Program

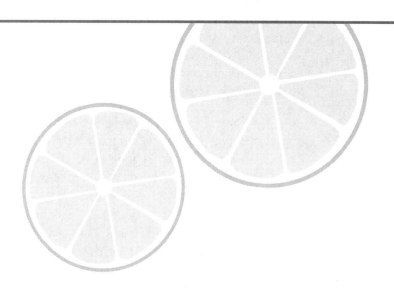

Planning for the Healthy Skin Diet Program

· ·

Now it is time to get practical and do some planning. The Healthy Skin Diet Program runs through four stages during 8 weeks. The first is a planning stage for establishing a set of rules for new eating habits. This is followed by a 3-day alkalizing cleanse that restores healthy pH and probiotic levels in the blood and digestive tract. The third stage involves stocking your kitchen with the best ingredients for the recipes featured in this diet – and taking stock of the physical, breathing, and inner beauty exercises that will carry you through this program. This is followed by a 14-day menu and activity plan, which leads into the recipe section. That's when the fun begins as you prepare a list of delicious recipes that will help your skin become radiant. Here you will find a wide variety of meals you can prepare quite easily, not just for 14 days but for each day of the 8-week program and beyond.

Step 1: Plan Your Diet

You may not be accustomed to planning your diet. There are many reasons why the Healthy Skin Diet works so well to improve skin health and overall vitality. One reason is good planning. A new diet takes planning, so if you don't have a personal assistant to tell you, "Now it's time to eat/relax/go for a walk," or a chef to prepare your meals, then you'll need to write things down in a diary or planner. A bit of organization will help you achieve fabulous-looking skin.

- Browse the best ingredient list and the 14-day menu and activity plan now and make a list of any new foods you may need to stock in your kitchen. Choose the recipes you are going to have for the first week and shop for ingredients.
- Write down your new daily activities, your physical and breathing exercises, as well as your inner beauty exercises. Schedule these activities in your day planner on your desk or in the computer so you keep on track.

- Choose when to start. You will need to work out what day you are going to begin your Healthy Skin Diet routine. Will it be Saturday, so you can relax on the weekend and quietly cleanse? Or will Monday be the first day you start the Healthy Skin Diet — a day when you will be in work mode and far from the influences of your party pals? Once you have picked "Diet Day," you can calculate the finishing date, exactly 8 weeks after starting.

Step 2: Get Rid of Bad Habits

- Gradually cut down on cigarettes, coffee, tea, and cola (caffeine), and reduce your alcohol intake. If you are a big coffee/caffeine drinker or a pack-a-day smoker, you may get withdrawal symptoms if you suddenly stop having them, so it is best to begin cutting down at least 1 week before starting the Healthy Skin Diet.
- List any other habits, including your current eating habits, that may impede your new diet.
- Use deep breathing and inner beauty strategies to help make positive changes to your lifestyle.

Q. What utensils do I need to prepare these foods?

A. When cooking for the Healthy Skin Diet, you will need the following:

- Large nonstick frypan. A small pan would also be good for making crêpes.
- Large steamer. This could be a large pot with a strainer on top, plus a lid. Make sure the pot/steamer is big enough to steam a small rainbow trout. If you are vegetarian, a medium-sized steamer would be suitable for steaming vegetables.
- Storage containers. Empty jars for seed mix and small containers for frozen mango or other fruit.
- Strainer. For straining rice and other foods.
- Juicing machine. This is optional, as you can also buy fresh vegetable juices or simply eat plenty of fruit and vegetables.
- Tea strainer. An enclosed, ball-shaped one for making dandelion or herbal tea.
- Coffee/seed grinder. This is essential for grinding up fresh flax seeds and it is also handy for making bread crumbs. Remember, don't buy pre-ground flax seeds or FSA; they must be fresh.

Step 3: Establish New Eating Habits

There are eight basic eating habits or rules that will guarantee the success of your new diet. You may notice that some of these rules are similar to the eight guidelines for healthy skin in Part 1.

Rule 1: Begin and end each day with an alkalizing drink.

I can't stress enough the need to restore pH balance in your blood for the success of the Healthy Skin Diet. Take the time now to review Guideline #1 and stock your cupboards and refrigerator with alkalizing foods listed there (page 52).

Rule 2: Eat breakfast every day

Don't skip breakfast, which most dietitians and physicians call the most important meal of the day. If you don't eat breakfast every day, you may find you overeat later in the day. If you have no appetite in the morning, drink one of the recommended healthy drinks. If you have a good appetite, you can also have one of the drinks plus a moderate-sized breakfast, approximately one plateful, minus the 30% required by the Healthy Skin Diet Program. Make sure you get some protein with each meal, and choose whole-grain foods instead of processed white flour products. If you are on a specific diet from the Specialized Programs section

> Don't skip breakfast, which most dietitians and physicians call the most important meal of the day.

Take-Away or Café Options for Breakfast

If you don't have the time or the ingredients to eat breakfast at home, try these café or take-away options:

- Freshly squeezed juice (containing more vegetable than fruit) plus a handful of fresh raw almonds or Brazil nuts
- Fresh fruit (as long as it has not been treated with preservatives)
- Muesli with soy milk and fresh fruit, no added sugar
- Poached or boiled eggs (one to two) on whole-grain toast or sourdough, with a side of spinach.
- Salmon and avocado on sourdough or whole-grain toast.

(page 146) or have nutritional deficiencies, you may need to take a supplement or two during breakfast. Take probiotics 15 to 30 minutes before breakfast.

Rule 3: Eat lunch every day

Likewise, don't skip lunch. Have lunch between 12:00 p.m. and 2:00 p.m. (approximately 5 hours after breakfast). Finish before 2:00 p.m., unless you do shift work. If you do shift work, have your first meal after you wake up and eat your lunch 5 or 6 hours later.

Serving size: Depending on your appetite at lunchtime, either go for something light and colorful, such as an antioxidant-rich salad with a serving of protein, or pick something hearty and satisfying, but as always, the meat serving should be no bigger than the size of your palm — yes, a big palm means you can have a bit more.

Take-Away or Café Options for Lunch

- Tuna, avocado, and salad wrap
- Turkey, cranberry, and salad wrap or whole-grain sandwich (sourdough is also okay)
- Chicken and tabbouleh wrap (free-range or organic chicken only)
- Sushi rolls, spinach, edamame, miso soup, and green tea; falafel in a Lebanese wrap/kebab with tabbouleh, onion, tomato, and hummus (don't even think about getting the meat variety!)
- Tuna and salad sandwich with avocado instead of butter (on whole-grain or sourdough bread). Turkey meat, tofu ,or vegetarian patties are alternatives if you don't eat fish.

Rule 4: Eat a mid-afternoon snack

Many people feel tired at around 3:00 p.m., so this is a good time to have a snack that contains some protein or slow-release carbs to energize you. If you don't feel tired around 3:00 p.m., you can skip this snack, but this snack also helps to combat overeating at dinner time.

Rule 5: Eat dinner every evening

To aid digestion, take a probiotic supplement 15 minutes before dinner. Eat dinner at least 2 hours before bedtime so you have time to digest your food. You can also have one of the healthy desserts if you choose. If you tend to overeat, eat 12 fresh raw almonds or one of the drinks containing flaxseed oil about 20 minutes before dinner. The beneficial fats switch on the satiety response (this takes approximately 30 minutes to kick in) so you are less likely to overeat when your main meal arrives.

Restaurant Options

When eating out, avoid sauces because you don't know how much sugar, fat, additives, or dairy is in them. Choose from the following:

- Any salad (except Caesar salad). Ask for the dressing on the side, and if it is dairy-free and homemade, you can use a small amount of it (olive oil and lemon is ideal).
- Steamed or grilled fish (preferably salmon or trout, not high-mercury fish. See page 69.
- Stir-fried vegetables with fish, tofu, beans, or skinless chicken
- Steamed vegetables with fish, tofu, beans, or skinless chicken
- Fresh oysters (snack)
- Uncooked spring rolls (snack)
- Skinless chicken and vegetables
- Any vegetarian dish that's not deep-fried or overly processed, no sauces
- Side serving of vegetables with a protein food (fish, chicken, tofu, or beans)
- Vegetable soups, as long as they are dairy-free
- Lean meat (no bigger than the palm of your hand) and vegetables

Rule 6: Moderate desserts

If you crave something sweet, you can choose from a range of dessert recipes in this book. However, please follow these rules:

- Have no more than three desserts per week.

- If you have a heavy meal, such as Creamy Tuna and Mushroom Mornay, choose a light fruit dessert, such as Mango Ice.
- If you have a light meal, such as a salad, then you can have a heavier dessert, such as Rhubarb Crumble or Carrot Cake.

3-Day Alkalizing Cleanse

● ●

This cleanse is a distinguishing stage in the Healthy Skin Diet program. The cleanse prepares your body for your new diet. Unlike many cleansing or detoxification programs, this one does not involve excessive food restrictions or purging the bowels; rather, you are encouraged to eat healthy but very basic meals, three times a day, with a wake-up beverage and small snacks. Instructions for preparing the recipes involved in the 3-day cleanse can be found in the recipe section. There are two related cleanses, a salad-based and green drink cleanse for warmer weather and a root vegetable and broth cleanse for colder weather. A salad-based cleanse is ideal in warmer weather because it is cooling in nature, but in cold weather you need warm, soupy broths and casseroles to cleanse effectively. Please note that children under the age of 15 years should not follow any detoxification program, including this one.

> Unlike many cleansing or detoxification programs, this one does not involve excessive food restrictions or purging the bowels; rather, you are encouraged to eat healthy but very basic meals, three times a day, with a wake-up beverage and small snacks.

Did You Know?

● ●

Liver Detoxification

If you suffer from chemical sensitivity, acne, or psoriasis, I highly recommend you take a liver detoxification supplement for the first 2 weeks of the program. Liver detoxification supplements help to decrease the chemical load in your body. Good liver detox supplements include the following nutrients: glycine, magnesium, vitamin B_6, selenium, cysteine, glutamine, taurine, vitamin B_2, vitamin B_{12}, folic acid, vitamin C, zinc, and the herb St Mary's thistle (otherwise known as milk thistle or *Silybum marianum*). However, if your skin is in reasonably good condition, you can simply drink dandelion tea every day because it stimulates digestion and promotes healthy liver function.

Preparing for a Cleanse

1. Determine if the warm or the cold version of the 3-Day Alkalizing Cleanse is most appropriate for your circumstances and the season, and then plan which day you would like to begin.
2. If you don't work on the weekends, you might want to start the program on a Saturday so you have time to rest during the cleanse. However, if you want to socialize on the weekend and you work during the week, I'd recommend beginning the program on a Monday, after the weekend, so you have no temptations during your cleanse program.
3. During the first 3 days, do not exercise vigorously. This is a time to eat alkalizing foods, master the beauty breathing exercises, and take relaxing baths.
4. Get plenty of rest because your body is restoring your health during this time.
5. Avoid caffeine and alcohol because they are highly acidic and may negate some of the healing effects of the cleanse. Gradually cut down on both of these substances before you begin the program so you don't suffer withdrawal symptoms.
6. Freeze some fresh fruit (such as a 1 cup/250 mL of diced mango or peeled whole banana) to use in the Skin-Firming Drink and desserts recipe.
7. Make the Anti-Aging Broth ahead of your starting time.
8. Grind up 1 cup (250 mL) of fresh whole flax seeds, place in a jar, and store in the refrigerator ready to add to meals to increase your omega-3 essential fatty acid intake.

Warm Weather Version

> Remaining well hydrated is essential to the success of the cleanse.

Remaining well hydrated is essential to the success of the cleanse. Drink two bottles of Green Water throughout the day, ideally before breakfast and in between meals.

Essential beverages

Fresh water: 8 cups (2 L) of water, sipped throughout the day
Flaxseed Lemon Drink: 3 glasses made fresh daily — this drink is fabulous for your immune system and it is completely alkaline
Green Water: Before breakfast and during the day (if you have eczema or salicylate sensitivity, also add glycine to this drink to prevent salicylate reaction).

Optional beverages

Pau d'arco tea; dandelion tea (may stimulate your digestion, which can make you feel hungry); vegetable juices containing cabbage, celery, parsley, carrot, and ginger.

Days 1 to 3
Before breakfast

As soon as you wake up, drink 1 small glass of Green Water, initially making it up with a low dosage of 1 teaspoon (5 mL) of chlorophyll. Also make a bottle of Green Water (1 teaspoon of chlorophyll to 6 cups/1.5 L of water) and sip throughout the day. If you have eczema, also add glycine. See the Eczema Care chapter for dosage (page 217). Take your first dosage of probiotics 15 to 30 minutes before breakfast.

Breakfast

Fresh raw almonds: 1 small handful
Flaxseed Lemon Drink: 1 glass

If you have any signs of parasites, also eat ¼ cup (60 mL) of green pumpkin seeds. This can be a combination of white pumpkin seeds and pepitas. However, the white ones are usually highly salted. You can wash off most of the salt or just have the green pumpkin seeds on their own. Eating pumpkin seeds during the 3-day program helps loosen compacted feces in the bowel so any hidden parasites can be flushed out. If you are taking a liver detox supplement, mix this with a big glass of chilled water.

Lunch

Flaxseed Lemon Drink: 1 glass
Main dish (choose one):
Spicy Green Papaya Salad (anti-parasitic recipe)
Sweet Raspberry, Avocado and Watercress Salad
Tasty Spinach Salad
Tabbouleh (can be used in conjunction with another salad)
Rich Mineral Salad with Papaya, Dill and Baby Spinach
Avocado Dip with Dipping Sticks
Roasted Corn and Cauliflower Soup

Snack (3:00 p.m.)

If you are hungry, try the following alkalizing snacks:
Fresh raw almonds and Brazil nuts (no more than 1 small handful)

> Because most fruit is acidic, it is not permitted during the 3-Day Alkalizing Cleanse, unless it is lemon, lime, avocado, or green papaya. Raspberries are also permitted in one of the recipes.

Avocado: $1/2$, flavored with fresh lemon juice and a pinch of natural sea salt (NOT table salt, as it is acid-forming)
Carrot, celery, and bell pepper sticks
Green Water

Dinner

Green Water: 15 to 30 minutes before dinner, take your probiotic supplement and finish your bottle of Green Water (if you haven't already).
Flaxseed Lemon Drink: Drink the remainder just before dinner. The oil in this drink helps to trigger the satiety response and is wonderful for digestion.
Salad: The 3-day cleanse dinner consists of a light salad with salad dressing containing flaxseed oil, lemon, garlic, and apple cider vinegar.
Main dish (choose one):
Spicy Green Papaya Salad
Roasted Sweet Potato Salad
Sweet Raspberry, Avocado and Watercress Salad
Tasty Spinach Salad
Tabbouleh (in combo with another salad)
Rich Mineral Salad with Papaya, Dill and Baby Spinach
Roasted Corn and Cauliflower Soup

If you are still hungry after dinner, then drink a glass of Skin Juice for Sensitive Skin No. 1 or 2, Spot-Free Skin Juice, or Anti-Aging Broth. You can also have a second serving of salad and 1 small handful of raw almonds or Brazil nuts.

Cold Weather Version
Essential beverages

Spring water: 8 cups (2 L), filtered, sipped throughout the day
Anti-Aging Broth: 1 to 3 cups (250 to 750 mL) per day
Green Water: If you have eczema or salicylate sensitivity, also add glycine to this drink to prevent salicylate reaction.

Optional beverages

Pau d'arco tea; dandelion tea (may stimulate your digestion, which can make you feel hungry); vegetable juices containing cabbage, celery, parsley, carrot, and ginger. NO fruit.

Days 1 to 3
Before breakfast

Green Water: 1 glass with first dosage of probiotics 15 to 30 minutes before breakfast.

Breakfast

Fresh raw almonds: 1 handful

Anti-Aging Broth: 2 cups (500 mL). If you are taking the liver detox supplement, mix it with a big glass of chilled water now.

Lunch

Main dish (choose one):
Roasted Corn and Cauliflower Soup (omit the toast)
Roasted Sweet Potato Salad
Multi-Vitamin Dal (Detox Dal)
Therapeutic Veggie Soup (omit the toast)

Dinner

Fifteen to 30 minutes before dinner, take your probiotic supplement and finish your bottle of Green Water (if you haven't already).

Meal dish (choose one):
Roasted Corn and Cauliflower Soup (omit the toast)
Roasted Sweet Potato Salad
Multi-Vitamin Dal (Detox Dal)
Therapeutic Veggie Soup (omit the toast)

If you are still hungry after dinner, drink a glass of Skin Juice for Sensitive Skin No. 1 or 2, Spot-Free Skin Juice, or Anti-Aging Broth. You can also have a second serving of soup and 1 small handful of raw almonds or Brazil nuts.

Q. Do I need to take supplements during the 3-Day Alkalizing Cleanse?

A. No, supplements aren't essential, but if you have any digestive problems, skin rashes, parasitic infestations, or lowered immunity, it is advisable to take a suitable probiotic supplement. If you are on a special regimen, such as the anti-eczema program or the anti-cellulite program, you can use whatever supplements are specifically recommended for your condition, although I suggest you take less than three types of supplements at a time — you don't want to be popping pills all day! Review Guideline #1 for probiotic information. Probiotics are suitable for all ages, but please use the correct dosage. If you are unsure of the dosage, contact the manufacturer or your doctor for more details. If your rash temporarily worsens during or after the cleanse, it is a sign you may be salicylate sensitive. If so, add glycine to your bottle of Green Water and reduce the amount of chlorophyll and lemon/lime used for the first 2 weeks. See the Eczema Care chapter for glycine dosage (page 217).

Complementary Activities

During the 3-Day Alkalizing Cleanse, get started on the activities that will complement and support your new diet.

- Exercise and sweat three to five times a week for 15 to 30 minutes. Your aim is to sweat for at least 15 minutes each day. This includes doing conventional exercise and having warm baths or saunas once or twice a week. If you are exercising outdoors, remember to wear sunscreen and a hat. However, during the first 3 days, while you are cleansing your body, you should not do any vigorous exercise that will drain your energy. You are eating less food, so you need to rest and relax to promote healing and restoration of vitality.
- Have at least one relaxing warm bath during the 3 days of the cleanse and every week of the 8-week program.
- Avoid caffeine, cigarettes, and alcohol during this period because they are highly acidic and may negate some of the healing effects of the cleanse.
- Relax while you eat and chew your food thoroughly.
- Practice your How to Be Beautiful exercises (page 293).
- Exfoliate your body once or twice a week.
- Relax and make peace with your body.

- Do breathing exercises for at least 5 minutes a day. See the Beauty Breathing chapter (page 281).
- Get plenty of rest. Good-quality sleep is essential to looking good and feeling fabulous. Go to bed by 10:30 p.m. and aim for 8 hours of sleep a night.
- Call a friend or family member for a chat and a laugh (at least once a week).
- Smile and laugh (and make someone else laugh, at least once a day).

Now that you have completed your 3-Day Alkalizing Cleanse, you can plan your meals for an 8-week duration. Follow this program step by step to healthy skin and renewed vitality.

Top 12 Ingredients for the Healthy Skin Diet

But what are the specific foods and liquids that make this diet exceptional? Let's take a quick look at the top 12 ingredients in the Healthy Skin Diet. Stock your shelves and refrigerator with foods containing these ingredients.

1. Apple cider vinegar (ACV)

ACV has an alkalizing effect in the body. This may explain apple cider vinegar's reputation for reducing pain and inflammatory conditions, such as arthritis and eczema. Apple cider vinegar is also anti-fungal, anti-viral, and anti-bacterial, promotes healthy red blood cells, and can help improve digestion if you have low stomach acids. Only use good-quality apple cider vinegar that contains the "mother," the dark cloudy substance that looks like strands linked together, settled at the bottom of the bottle (shake the bottle before use). This indicates that minimal processing has occurred and valuable enzymes and minerals are present. You can eat the mother; it is the most nutritious part. Be sure to consult with your coach or manager if you're an athlete.

> Apple cider vinegar can help improve digestion if you have low stomach acids.

Prescription

For adults with poor digestion: 2 teaspoons (10 mL) daily in a glass of water (in divided doses). Use before meals to increase digestion. For a more pleasant drink, mix ACV in $\frac{1}{2}$ cup (125 mL) of preservative-free apple juice and $\frac{1}{2}$ cup (125 mL) water. Use ACV in salad recipes, such as Tasty Spinach Salad.

> # Caution
>
> Although apple cider vinegar is alkalizing once digested, keep in mind that it is an acid before digestion and acids can aggravate ulcers and slowly strip enamel off teeth (other acids include orange juice, citrus fruits, vitamin C tablets and other types of vinegar). If discomfort occurs, then have Green Water as an alternative. If you have sensitive teeth, you can also rinse your mouth with a bit of baking soda mixed with water or brush your teeth after having ACV.

Avocado improves digestive health, moisturizes the skin, is gluten-free, low on the glycemic index, and highly alkalizing.

2. Avocado

Avocado is a nutrient-dense fruit that is high in monounsaturated fatty acids (omega-9 and some omega-6). Avocado can be used as a nutritious spread and as a healthy alternative to butter and margarine. It contains vitamins B_6, B_3, and C, beta-carotene, folate, copper, magnesium, iron, potassium, amino acids, and antioxidants. Avocado improves digestive health, moisturizes the skin, and is gluten-free, low on the glycemic index, and highly alkalizing.

Prescription

$\frac{1}{4}$ to $\frac{1}{2}$ avocado per day, twice a week. Use avocado as a nutritious spread instead of butter or margarine.

Buckwheat contains the antioxidant quercetin, which has anti-inflammatory properties.

3. Buckwheat

Buckwheat contains the antioxidant quercetin, which has anti-inflammatory properties. It is high in vitamin B_3, folate, calcium, magnesium, potassium, zinc, and antioxidants. Buckwheat is anti-inflammatory and low on the glycemic index. The flour has a higher GI than the grains. Buckwheat is not technically a grain but resembles grain. It is a gluten-free alternative to wheat.

Prescription

Incorporate buckwheat into your weekly diet to increase your intake of anti-inflammatory antioxidants. Buckwheat crêpes make a great breakfast or dessert. Buckwheat grains cook like rice and can be served with curries, fish, or meat.

4. Chlorophyll

Chlorophyll is the green pigment in plants. The green drink called chlorophyll is a combination of green plant pigment and spearmint oil (some brands also contain alfalfa extract). Chlorophyll supplies magnesium needed for cardiovascular and respiratory health, and also contains potassium and iron. Chlorophyll prevents anemia, is highly alkalizing, and is both blood purifying and blood thinning. Chlorophyll increases oxygen-carrying capacity in the blood (so it can increase your energy and stamina); it promotes friendly bacteria in the bowel (so it can reduce harmful bowel microbes); promotes healthy digestion; and prevents bad breath and body odor.

> Chlorophyll prevents anemia, is highly alkalizing, and is both blood purifying and blood thinning.

Prescription

Adult dosage for normal/low strength liquid chlorophyll:
1–2 teaspoons (5–10 mL) diluted in water once or twice a day, beginning on a low dosage. Drink Green Water daily. If you have hypoglycemia or blood sugar level problems (energy crashes/irritability in between meals) mix 2 teaspoons of liquid chlorophyll in a 6-cup (1.5 L) bottle of water and sip throughout the day.

5. Dandelion root

Dandelion root, also known as *Taraxacum officinale* radix, contains bitter compounds called inulin and taraxacin that rapidly improve digestion in people with poor bile secretion. Dandelion root also makes a great morning cup of tea. It is rich in mineral salts and vitamins; activates phase II liver detoxification; prevents constipation; and provides a good tonic for the liver and gallbladder.

> Dandelion root is rich in mineral salts and vitamins, activates phase II liver detoxification, and provides a good tonic for the liver and gallbladder.

Prescription

Enjoy a cup of Soy Dande' from the recipe section up to three times a day (before meals). But be aware that too many cups can overstimulate digestion; if this occurs, reduce dosage and strength.

6. Dark green leafy vegetables

This group includes Chinese greens, kale, dandelion greens, spinach, chicory, beet greens, mustard greens, watercress, and baby spinach. Such vegetables are highly alkalizing to the blood; they deliver more nutrients for fewer calories; and the calcium in kale and watercress is easy for the body to absorb. Greens contain antioxidants, folate, magnesium, calcium, vitamins A and C, B vitamins, potassium, fiber, and cancer-protective phytonutrients. Greens are gluten-free and low on the glycemic index.

> Greens contain antioxidants, folate, magnesium, calcium, vitamins A and C, B vitamins, potassium, fiber, and cancer-protective phytonutrients.

Prescription
Adults: Have 2 handfuls of dark green leafies every day. That's EVERY SINGLE DAY OF YOUR LIFE. **Children:** Have 1 child-sized handful a day.

7. Fish

Oily or deep sea fish contains therapeutic amounts of omega-3 (EPA and DHA) and is a potent anti-inflammatory food. Studies have shown that eating two to three servings of fish a week is good for elevating mood and increasing the health of the brain, skin, and heart. This fish is a good source of protein, vitamin D, and iodine. It boosts metabolism; it is low on the glycemic index; and it is gluten-free. However, avoid raw fish during the 8-week program because it may contain "bad" microbes, but go ahead and eat cooked fish.

> Studies have shown that eating two to three servings of fish a week is good for elevating mood and increasing the health of the brain, skin, and heart.

Prescription
Both adults and children should eat oily fish two to three times a week. Good sources of EPA and DHA include salmon, trout, mackerel, sardines, herring, eel, and salmon and tuna oil supplements. Other minor sources of EPA and DHA include low-fat fish, such as carp, pike, and haddock, and oysters, clams, scallops, and squid. Salmon and trout are commonly farmed in North America, and it has been suggested that these fish contain less omega-3 and less vitamin A and C than fish fresh from the ocean — but any amount of omega-3 is better than none.

8. Flax seeds and flaxseed oil

Flax seeds are anti-inflammatory because they contain a whopping 50% omega-3 essential fatty acids; they also contain omega-6, phytochemicals, silica, mucilage, oleic acid, protein, vitamin E, and fiber. They are a potent bowel cleanser. Flax seeds aid in weight loss and treating constipation. They may improve cardiovascular health and female reproductive health. They are liver protective; stabilize blood sugar levels; and sooth the digestive tract. These seeds and oils are alkalizing and may inhibit tumor formation. Flaxseed oil and ground flax seeds should be refrigerated at all times.

Prescription

Adults: Have 1–2 tablespoons (15–30 mL) of ground flax seeds or flaxseed oil per day — not necessary on the days you eat oily fish. Use flaxseed oil in the Flaxseed Lemon Drink, Skin-Firming Drink, and in homemade salad dressings. Add whole flax seeds to Designer Muesli or grind them in a coffee grinder for use on breakfast cereal or fruit salad. Think of flaxseed oil as a healthy ingredient, not as a supplement: I don't recommend buying flaxseed oil in capsule form because I don't want you popping pills all day. Flax is more beneficial as a food, incorporated into salad dressings and smoothies to increase their nutritional value.

> **Flax seeds are anti-inflammatory because they contain a whopping 50% omega-3 essential fatty acids; they also contain omega-6, phyto-chemicals, silica, mucilage, oleic acid, protein, vitamin E, and fiber.**

9. Lecithin granules

Lecithin is naturally found in soybeans, eggs, beef, and liver. It can also be bought in the form of soy lecithin granules, which kind of look like tiny yellow beads. Lecithin is a special type of lipid that helps break down fats in the body much the same way detergent does when washing greasy dishes. It contains choline for healthy brain neurotransmitters and inositol for healthy cell membranes. Lecithin breaks up cholesterol; helps with weight loss and removal of fats from the body; and aids removal of chemicals and cholesterol from the body. It is low on the glycemic index and gluten-free. Lecithin is considered to be brain food; it enhances phase II liver detoxification; and it improves digestion. Due to inositol content, lecithin may decrease the risk of eczema, hair loss, cellulite, and eye problems.

> **Due to inositol content, lecithin may decrease the risk of eczema, hair loss, cellulite, and eye problems.**

Prescription

Adults: 1 tablespoon (15 mL) of lecithin granules per day
Children aged 1 to 6 years: $^1/_2$ teaspoon (2 mL) per day
Children over 7 years: 1 teaspoon (5 mL) per day
Add lecithin to Papaya Beauty Smoothie, Flaxseed Lemon Drink, and muesli/cereals.

10. Lemons and limes

Lemons and limes contain vitamin C, folate, calcium, and potassium. Lemons and limes enhance phase II liver detoxification and have a strong alkalizing effect. The pectin from the citrus pulp (white part of the fruit) contains valuable flavonoids, and both these fruits aid removal of toxins from the bowel.

Prescription

Adults: Have a squeeze of lemon/lime with the ACV Drink, Tangy Papaya Cups, or Green Water. Drink the Flaxseed Lemon Drink at least once a week; this recipe uses all parts of the lemon, including the skin and pulp. Use lemon/lime in salad dressings, and squeeze lemon/lime onto fish before serving.

11. Seaweed

Certain seaweed, such as kelp and kombu, contains a good dose of metabolism-boosting iodine. Seaweed helps in losing weight and in combating fatigue caused by slow thyroid activity. It helps prevent skin irritations. Seaweed is a good source of iodine, beta-carotene, B vitamins, vitamin A, D, E, and K, folate, calcium, magnesium, potassium, iron, selenium, and zinc. Seaweed is skin-cleansing and good for constipation and arthritis. Seaweed has anti-cancer properties. It is anti-bacterial and anti-viral.

Prescription

Add a sprinkling of kelp or a soaked strip of kombu to soups and stir-fried vegetables. It adds a mild salty flavor. Add kombu seaweed when cooking beans or legumes to make them easier to digest (this helps prevent gas).

12. Turmeric

Turmeric is a spice that contains curcumin, a flavonoid that has an anti-cancer and anti-Alzheimer effect. It contains calcium, magnesium, potassium, and antioxidants, and is anti-inflammatory. Turmeric is low on the glycemic index and gluten-free. Turmeric promotes phase II detoxification; lowers blood sugar levels; and helps prevent blood clotting. It is alkalizing.

Prescription

Adults: Have 2 teaspoons (10 mL) a day in a small amount of water or fresh vegetable juice. It is best used in meals, such as curries or Dal. Add ground black pepper to enhance the absorption of curcumin.

14-Day Healthy Skin Menu & Activity Plan

- -

The **Healthy Skin** Menu and Activity Plan is designed for you if you are looking for a structured approach to this diet. Food and activities are chosen for you from a list of beverages and main dishes. Recipes for preparing these foods and drinks can be found in the recipe section of this book. This menu plan is similar to a rotation diet as you rotate through poultry, fish, vegetarian, and red meat days. However, you do not have to strictly follow this regimen. It is just a guide to help you to monitor, for example, how much fish and red meat you are eating so you can balance acidic and alkaline foods as well as your prostaglandins. Once or twice a week is a gluten-free day.

Of course, if you know you are allergic to something, such as fish or any other ingredient, then substitute the suggested recipe for a suitable alternative. If you have eczema or rosacea, you can choose the recipe that is best suited to you. Read the recipe description with each recipe to see if it is suitable or modifiable.

Complementing the menu plan is a list of activities that promote general good health and skin health. As you change your eating habits to improve your skin condition, work on changing other lifestyle habits based on these physical and breath exercises.

> This menu plan is similar to a rotation diet as you rotate through poultry, fish, vegetarian, and red meat days.

Meal Options for the 14-Day Healthy Skin Diet

In this menu plan, you are at liberty to mix and match the healthy skin recipes listed (see following page). After you have completed the first 14 days of the program, you can plan another 14-day menu substituting these with others listed.

Meal Options for the 14-Day Healthy Skin Diet

Beverages	Breakfast	Lunch
Essential: • Green • ACV drinks **Optional:** • Anti-Aging Broth • Fresh vegetable juice • Herbal teas • Flaxseed Lemon Drink • Pear Flaxseed Drink for Sensitive Skin • Juice for Sensitive Skin No. 1 and No. 2 • Spot-Free Skin Juice • Apple Omega Drink • ACE Smoothie • Soy Dande' • Dandelion Tea • Rosehip tea • Filtered water • Natural mineral water • Skin-Firming Drink	• Berry Beauty Smoothie • Berry Beauty Porridge • Sweet Banana Porridge • Delicious French Toast with Berries and Almonds • Avocado on Toast • Smoked Salmon and Avocado on Toast • Sardines and Lemon on Grainy Toast • Whole Fruit Jam on Toast • Fruit Salad with Flax Seeds • Amine-Free Fruit Salad • Perfect Poached Eggs • Smoked Salmon and Eggs • Egg Soldiers • Tasty Omelet • Designer Muesli • Gluten-Free Muesli • Vitamin E Muesli • Bircher Muesli • Mango and Buckwheat Crêpes • Pear and Buckwheat Crêpes • Boiled Eggs, Vegetables and Rice • Fish and Steamed Vegetables • Anti-Aging Broth with whole-grain toast • Vegetable Hand Rolls and Miso Soup • Beans on Toast • Kids' Scrambled Eggs • Kids' Creamy Beans on Toast *Note: If you have eczema or rosacea, see the individual recipe descriptions, because many of them have modification tips for you.*	• Spicy Green Papaya Salad • Omega Niçoise Salad • Colorful Non-Fried Rice • Annie's Decadent Veggie Bake • Roasted Corn and Cauliflower Soup • Therapeutic Chicken Soup • Roasted Sweet Potato Salad, served with protein • Rich Mineral Salad with Papaya, Dill and Baby Spinach, served with protein • Sweet Raspberry, Avocado and Watercress Salad, with protein (such as Cajun Chicken Breast) • Multi-Vitamin Dal • Tuna and Avocado Wrap • Chickpea Beauty Salad • Chicken and Salad Wrap • Chicken and Salad Sandwich • Tasty Spinach Salad, with protein • Vegetable Hand Rolls • Salad Sandwich with Creamy Mayo • Salmon and Salad Sandwich • Beef Barley Soup • Falafel Wrap • Rich Mediterranean Pasta with a side salad • Steak Sandwich • Healthy Hamburger • Boiled Eggs, Vegetables and Rice • Therapeutic Veggie Soup *Note: Also see under Dinner (page 331) for more meal options.*

Snack	Dinner
• Avocado Dip with Dipping Sticks (equivalent to ½ avocado a day)	• Roasted Corn and Cauliflower Soup
• Avocado Beauty Snack	• Sweet Raspberry, Avocado and Watercress Salad, with protein (such as Cajun Chicken Breast)
• Fresh fruit (1 to 2 servings per day)	• Seafood Hotpot
• Pepitas/green pumpkin seeds (a small handful)	• Beef Barley Soup
• Fresh vegetables (unlimited)	• Kids' Creamy Beans on Toast (or served with pasta)
• Fresh raw oysters (up to 6 per day, once or twice a week)	• Omega Niçoise Salad
• Oysters with Dipping Sauce	• Therapeutic Veggie Soup
• Steamed soybeans, known as edamame (available from Japanese/sushi restaurants)	• Therapeutic Chicken Soup
• Low-GI whole-grain crackers (no more than 6 per day) with avocado and tomato or lemon	• Marinated Whole Steamed Trout
• Fresh raw almonds or Brazil nuts daily (up to 12 nuts per day, or 1 handful)	• Multi-Vitamin Dal
• ½ avocado with fresh lemon juice, diced fresh tomato and sea salt	• Chickpea Beauty Salad
• Vegetable Hand Rolls (raw spring rolls) with Sweet Chile Sauce	• Colorful Non-Fried Rice

Snack column (continued list) and Dinner column:

Snack
- Avocado Dip with Dipping Sticks (equivalent to ½ avocado a day)
- Avocado Beauty Snack
- Fresh fruit (1 to 2 servings per day)
- Pepitas/green pumpkin seeds (a small handful)
- Fresh vegetables (unlimited)
- Fresh raw oysters (up to 6 per day, once or twice a week)
- Oysters with Dipping Sauce
- Steamed soybeans, known as edamame (available from Japanese/sushi restaurants)
- Low-GI whole-grain crackers (no more than 6 per day) with avocado and tomato or lemon
- Fresh raw almonds or Brazil nuts daily (up to 12 nuts per day, or 1 handful)
- ½ avocado with fresh lemon juice, diced fresh tomato and sea salt
- Vegetable Hand Rolls (raw spring rolls) with Sweet Chile Sauce

Dinner
- Roasted Corn and Cauliflower Soup
- Sweet Raspberry, Avocado and Watercress Salad, with protein (such as Cajun Chicken Breast)
- Seafood Hotpot
- Beef Barley Soup
- Kids' Creamy Beans on Toast (or served with pasta)
- Omega Niçoise Salad
- Therapeutic Veggie Soup
- Therapeutic Chicken Soup
- Marinated Whole Steamed Trout
- Multi-Vitamin Dal
- Chickpea Beauty Salad
- Colorful Non-Fried Rice
- Creamy Chickpea Curry
- C-Rich Apricot Chicken
- Creamy Tuna and Mushroom Mornay
- Creamy Salmon Mornay
- Slow-Roasted Lamb with Steamed Greens
- Rich Mediterranean Pasta with Garden Salad
- Salmon Steaks with Peas and Mash
- Rainbow Trout with Honey
- Roasted Vegetables
- Herb and Garlic Chicken Casserole
- Tasty Vegetable Casserole
- Annie's Decadent Veggie Bake with Garden Salad
- Prawn and Sweet Chile Vegetable Stir-Fry
- Lean Meat and Three Veg
- Roasted Sweet Potato Salad with Sweet Chutney
- Thai Baked Fish with Sweet Corn
- Lamb Stir-Fry
- Sweet Chicken Stir-Fry
- Healthy Hamburger
- Chicken and Three Veg
- Tropical Vegetarian Stir-Fry

Note: If not specified, meals can be served with brown rice, basmati rice (occasionally), buckwheat, or quinoa.

Menu & Activity Plan

Day / Time of Day	Menu	Activities
DAY 1 (3-DAY CLEANSE) *The menu plans for the each day of the 3-day cleanse are similar. More recipe options are presented in the instructions for conducting the cleanse. The warm weather and cold weather versions are slightly different.*		
Before Breakfast	Green Water: 1 small glass now and prepare bottle to sip on for the day	• Have a warm bath and exfoliate your skin.
Breakfast	Flaxseed Lemon Drink (warm weather) Anti-Aging Broth (cold weather) Fresh raw almonds (1 small handful) Green pumpkin seeds for parasites (¼ cup/60 mL)	• Practice your breathing exercises for at least 5 minutes.
Lunch	Flaxseed Lemon Drink Anti-Aging Broth Main dish (warm): Spicy Green Papaya Salad (anti-parasitic recipe) Main dish (cold): Multi-vitamin Dal (Detox Dal)	• Master the throat breathing exercises.
Snack	*If you are hungry, try the following alkalizing snacks:* • Fresh raw almonds and Brazil nuts (no more than 1 small handful) • Avocado: ½, flavored with fresh lemon juice and a pinch of natural sea salt (NOT table salt, as it is acid-forming) • Carrot, celery, and bell pepper sticks • Green Water	
Dinner	Green Water: 15 to 30 minutes before dinner, take a probiotic supplement and finish your bottle of Green Water (if you haven't already) Flaxseed Lemon Drink: Drink the remainder just before dinner. The oil in this drink helps to trigger the satiety response and is wonderful for digestion Salad: The 3-day cleanse dinner consists of a light salad with salad dressing containing flaxseed oil, lemon, garlic, and apple cider vinegar Main dish (warm): Roasted Sweet Potato Salad Main dish (cold): Therapeutic Veggie Soup	

Day / Time of Day	Menu	Activities

DAY 2 (3-DAY CLEANSE)

During the second day of the cleanse, you need to eat much the same as you did for the first day, but you have more meal options for lunch and dinner

Day / Time of Day	Menu	Activities
Before Breakfast	See Day 1	• Continue practicing breathing exercises.
Breakfast	See Day 1	
Lunch	Main dish (warm): Tabbouleh Main dish (cold): Roasted Sweet Potato Salad	• Practice the throat breathing exercises.
Snack	See Day 1	• Go for a walk and practice Inner Beauty Exercise Level 1.
Dinner	Main dish (warm): Rich Mineral Salad Main dish (cold): Roasted Corn and Cauliflower Soup	• Optional: Enjoy a sauna.

DAY 3 (3-DAY CLEANSE)

Work ahead. Prepare the Anti-Aging Broth for the Therapeutic Chicken Soup on Day 4 (there is also a non-soup option).

Day / Time of Day	Menu	Activities
Before Breakfast	See Day 1	• Practice your breathing exercises for at least 5 minutes.
Breakfast	See Day 1	
Lunch	Main dish (warm): Sweet Raspberry, Avocado and Watercress Salad Main dish (cold): Tasty Spinach Salad	• Practice Inner Beauty Exercise Levels 2 and 3.
Snack	See Day 1	
Dinner	Main dish (warm): Favorite from Day 1 and Day 2 Main dish (cold): Favorite from Day 1 and Day 2	

DAY 4 (POULTRY DAY)

Ease your way back into having heavier meals, in this case with some soothing chicken soup and sandwiches.

Day / Time of Day	Menu	Activities
Breakfast	Beverage: Drink 1 glass of Green Water on rising (at least 15 minutes before breakfast). Make 1 bottle of Green Water and sip it throughout the day. Main dish: Tasty Omelet or muesli recipe of choice Optional: Skin Juice for Sensitive Skin No. 1 or Anti-Aging Broth	• Exercise until you sweat for at least 15 minutes. • Practice breathing exercises for at least 5 minutes.

Day / Time of Day	Menu	Activities
Lunch	Beverage: Drink 4–8 cups (1–2 L) of water or Green Water in between meals Main dish: Therapeutic Chicken Soup (1 bowl) with 1 to 2 slices of plain whole-grain toast or drizzled with olive oil, no butter or margarine Option: Chicken Salad Sandwich on whole-grain bread	• Grab a piece of paper and list your strengths and positive attributes. Acknowledge your good points on a daily basis to build self-confidence and decrease self-sabotage.
Snack (3:00 p.m.)	10 almonds and 1 pear Option: Skin Juice for Sensitive Skin No. 1	
Dinner	Beverage: Drink 1 glass of ACV Drink 15 to 30 minutes before dinner Main dish: Therapeutic Chicken Soup (1 large bowl) with 1 or 2 slices whole-grain toast [Freeze any leftover soup]	

DAY 5 (FISH AND GLUTEN-FREE DAY)

Even if you are not sensitive to gluten, it is important to have a gluten-free day occasionally to give your digestive system a break from processing gluten and for you to learn how to vary your diet.

Day / Time of Day	Menu	Activities
Breakfast	Beverage: Drink 1 glass of Green Water on rising. Make 1 bottle of Green Water and sip it throughout the day. If you have poor digestion, you may also want to have 1 cup (250 mL) of Soy Dande' before breakfast because it stimulates digestive juices. Use malt-free soy milk (barley malt is a sweetener that contains gluten). Main dish: Fruit Salad with Flax Seeds (if you have eczema), but omit the rolled oats to make it gluten-free Option: Amine-Free Fruit Salad (especially suitable for rosacea), plus 1 glass of Calcium-Rich Smoothie (with malt-free soy milk)	• Exercise until you sweat for 15 minutes. • Do 5 minutes of breathing exercises (a great time for this is after work and before cooking dinner because it relaxes you and helps to restore energy)
Lunch	Main dish: Omega Niçoise Salad Option: Tasty Spinach Salad topped with 1 small tin of tuna (use Omega Salad Dressing because it is gluten-free)	
Snack (3:00 p.m.)	*Choose from the following:* • 1 small handful of pepitas or Brazil nuts • Fresh vegetable sticks (carrot and celery) with Tuna Dip • Soy Dande' • 1 apple	

Day / Time of Day	Menu	Activities
Dinner	Beverage: Drink the last of your Green Water bottle 15 to 30 minutes before dinner (if not already finished) Main dish: Marinated Whole Steamed Trout	

DAY 6 (VEGETARIAN DAY)

Don't drink cold liquids with meals because they dilute digestive acids, whereas drinking Green Water 15 or 20 minutes before a meal improves digestion.

Day / Time of Day	Menu	Activities
Breakfast	Beverage: Drink 1 glass of Green Water on rising. Make 1 bottle of Green Water and sip it throughout the day. Main dish: Avocado on Toast or Beans on Toast	• Rest day, no heavy exercise. • Have a warm bath (or sauna). • Practice abdominal breathing for 5 to 10 minutes.
Lunch	Main dish: Chickpea Beauty Salad	
Snack (3:00 p.m.)	Avocado Beauty Snack and/or Soy Dande'	
Dinner	Beverage: Drink the last of your Green Water bottle 15 to 30 minutes before dinner (if not already finished) Main dish: Tasty Vegetable Casserole Option: Creamy Chickpea Curry	• Have you been grateful today? Show gratitude to others.

DAY 7 (RED MEAT DAY)

Eat only one serving of red meat meal on any given day and only two servings per week in total. Take a break. Don't hesitate to eat leftovers at lunch or dinner from time to time.

Day / Time of Day	Menu	Activities
Breakfast	Beverage: Drink 1 glass of Green Water on rising. Make 1 bottle of Green Water and sip it throughout the day. Main dish: Muesli of choice from recipe section Option: Buy an untoasted oat-based muesli and add ground flax seeds and homemade Almond Milk	• Exercise until you sweat for 15 minutes. • Practice abdominal breathing exercises for 5 minutes.
Lunch	Main dish: Healthy Hamburger or Salad Sandwich with Creamy Mayo	
Snack (3:00 p.m.)	*Choose from the following:* • 4 Brazil nuts • 1 piece of fruit (pear, banana, and papaya are low in salicylates) • Spot-Free Skin Juice • Soy Dande'	
Dinner	Beverage: 1 ACV Drink 15 to 30 minutes before dinner or drink the last of your Green Water bottle 15 to 30 minutes before dinner (if not already finished) Main dish: Lean Meat and Three Veg Options: Lamb Stir-Fry or soup recipe of choice	

Day / Time of Day	Menu	Activities

DAY 8 (POULTRY AND GLUTEN-FREE DAY)

Congratulations on completing your first week of the Healthy Skin Diet. There are more great recipes to try in the second week.

Day / Time of Day	Menu	Activities
Breakfast	Beverage: Drink 1 glass of Green Water on rising. Make 1 bottle of Green Water and sip it throughout the day. Main dish: Boiled Eggs, Vegetables and Rice Option: Gluten-Free Muesli or Mango and Buckwheat Crêpes (or Pear and Buckwheat Crêpes if you have eczema)	• Exercise — sweat for 15 minutes. • Practice breathing exercises for at least 5 minutes. • Count how many times you check your reflection in mirrors. You may need to do your makeup or look to see if your outfit is on properly, but if you glance or gaze at your reflection more than three times a day and criticize your looks/skin/weight, then you need to restrict mirror use.
Lunch	Main dish: Cajun Chicken breast fillet served with Sweet Raspberry, Avocado and Watercress Salad	
Snack (3:00 p.m.)	*Choose from the following:* • 10 almonds and drink recipe of choice • Soy Dande' (with malt-free soy milk) Vegetable sticks with Hummus Dip	
Dinner	Beverage: Drink the last of your Green Water bottle 15 to 30 minutes before dinner (if not already finished) Main dish: C-Rich Apricot Chicken with brown rice or buckwheat or Multi-Vitamin Dal	

DAY 9 (FISH DAY)

Be sure to remain well hydrated. Calculate how many glasses (or quarts) of water you are consuming each day. Is it enough?

Day / Time of Day	Menu	Activities
Breakfast	Beverages: Drink 1 glass of Green Water on rising. Make 1 bottle of Green Water and sip it throughout the day. Main dish: Sardines and Lemon on Grainy Toast Option: Papaya Beauty Smoothie or fruit salad recipe or porridge recipe of choice Option: Soy Dande'	• Sweat without doing high-impact exercise: sauna, warm bath, or go for a walk on a hot day (avoiding the sun between the scorching hours of 10 a.m. and 3 p.m.). • Have you been wearing your hat when outdoors? You may have a cap for exercise/casual attire, but do you need to buy another hat to suit dressier occasions/outfits?
Lunch	Main dish: Tuna and Avocado Wrap or Falafel Wrap	
Snack (3:00 p.m.)	*Choose from the following:* • 2–6 fresh oysters • 6 tinned oysters on 3 to 4 whole wheat/grain crackers • Smoothie recipe of choice	

Day / Time of Day	Menu	Activities
Dinner	Beverage: Drink the last of your Green Water bottle 15 to 30 minutes before dinner Main dish: 2–6 fresh oysters (if you didn't have them earlier) Shrimp and Sweet Chile Vegetable Stir-Fry Option: Thai Baked Fish with Sweet Corn or Roasted Sweet Potato Salad, served with Sweet Chutney	• List your strengths and positive attributes.

DAY 10 (VEGETARIAN DAY)

You can eat an all vegetarian diet from the healthy skin recipes provided in this book, but if you do so, be sure you supplement with vitamin B_{12} and calcium.

Day / Time of Day	Menu	Activities
Breakfast	Beverage: Drink 1 glass of Green Water on rising. Make 1 bottle of Green Water and sip it throughout the day. Main dish: Muesli of choice with Almond Milk or soy milk (containing calcium and whole soybean, not soy isolate) Option: Skin-Firming Drink	• Exercise — sweat for 15 minutes. • In the afternoon or before dinner, lie down and do your breathing exercises for 5 minutes.
Lunch	Main dish: Rich Mediterranean Pasta or Salad Sandwich with Creamy Mayo (if you don't eat egg, substitute Creamy Mayonnaise with Sweet Chutney in this recipe)	
Snack (3:00 p.m.)	*Choose from the following:* • Avocado Salsa (optional: serve with 4 whole wheat/grain crackers) • Fruit • 1 cup (250 mL) of alfalfa tea (add a squeeze of lemon and 2 slices of fresh ginger) or fresh vegetable juice of choice	
Dinner	Beverages: Drink the last of your Green Water bottle 15 to 30 minutes before dinner (if not already finished) Main dish: Creamy Chickpea Curry	

DAY 11 (RED MEAT DAY)

Red meat is a great source of dietary iron that prevents anemia. It is acidic, so try to balance your red meat meals with alkalizing foods.

Day / Time of Day	Menu	Activities
Breakfast	Beverages: Drink 1 glass of Green Water on rising. Make 1 bottle of Green Water and sip it throughout the day. Main dish: Berry Beauty Porridge, served with Almond Milk or soy milk (with added calcium) Option: Fruit salad recipe of choice with smoothie recipe of choice	• Exercise — sweat for 15 minutes. • Practice throat breathing exercises for 5 minutes.

Day / Time of Day	Menu	Activities
Lunch	Main dish: Salad Sandwich with Creamy Mayo (If you are at a café, skip the mayo and have avocado instead) Option: Falafel Wrap or Vegetable Hand Rolls	
Snack (3:00 p.m.)	*Choose from the following:* • A handful of raw almonds and Brazil nuts (for selenium) and a handful of blueberries • 1 cup (250 mL) Soy Dande' and vegetable sticks with Hummus Dip	
Dinner	Beverage: 1 ACV Drink to help with digestion or drink the last of your Green Water bottle 15 to 30 minutes before dinner (if not already finished) Main dish: Slow-Cooked Lamb Casserole Option: Beef Barley Soup	

DAY 12 (POULTRY DAY)

Rotating the daily diet theme through the major protein-rich foods (meat and legumes) insures that you receive adequate micronutrients for digestion.

Day / Time of Day	Menu	Activities
Breakfast	Beverage: Drink 1 glass of Green Water on rising. Make 1 bottle of Green Water and sip it throughout the day. Main dish: Perfect Poached Eggs or Egg Soldiers	• Go for a relaxing walk or stretch for 20 minutes. • Practice breathing exercises for 5 to 10 minutes. • Have a shower or bath and lightly exfoliate your skin (face and body), then moisturize.
Lunch	Main dish: Chicken and Salad Wrap Option: Chicken and salad of choice (e.g., Roasted Sweet Potato Salad)	
Snack (3:00 p.m.)	*Choose from the following:* • Carrot and celery sticks with Hummus Dip • Soy Dande' • Hummus Dip and 4 whole wheat or whole-grain crackers	
Dinner	Beverage: Drink the last of your Green Water bottle 15 to 30 minutes before dinner. Main dish: Sweet Chicken Stir-Fry or Chicken and Three Veg	

DAY 13 (FISH AND GLUTEN-FREE DAY)

Take a break and try the cuisine of another country today. Japanese food is rich in omega-3 fatty acids, but be cautious if you react to gluten — soy sauce contains gluten, so BYO tamari sauce, which tastes the same but is gluten-free.

Day / Time of Day	Menu	Activities
[Day 13] Breakfast	Beverage: Drink 1 glass of Green Water on rising. Make 1 bottle of Green Water and sip it throughout the day Main dish: Mango and Buckwheat Crêpes Option: If you have eczema, go for Pear and Buckwheat Crêpes or Gluten-Free Muesli	• Exercise until you sweat for 15 minutes. • Practice your deep breathing exercises. • Have a relaxing bath before bed. • Make it an early night and get 8 hours of quality sleep.
Lunch	Main dish: Omega Niçoise Salad Option: Gluten-free Japanese sushi rolls. Start with some miso soup (without soy sauce, barley or noodles). Choose from nori rolls with real wasabi (very hot green horseradish paste that can kill microbes in raw fish); salmon, tuna, avocado, cucumber, and other vegetable rolls; and edamame (green soybeans). Garnish with pickled ginger.	
Snack (3:00 p.m.)	*Choose from the following:* • 1 piece of fruit and/or a small handful of raw almonds and Brazil nuts • Fresh vegetable juice or Flaxseed Lemon Drink • Steamed soybeans (edamame).	
Dinner	Beverage: Drink the last of your Green Water bottle 15 to 30 minutes before dinner. Main dish: Seafood Hotpot Option: Salmon Steaks with Peas and Mash	

DAY 14 (VEGETARIAN DAY)

Now that you mastered the 14-day menu plan, you can prepare more plans week by week. Just choose recipes from the Recipe section for each meal. Come back to your favorites.

Day / Time of Day	Menu	Activities
Breakfast	Beverage: Drink 1 glass of Green Water on rising. Make 1 bottle of Green Water and sip it throughout the day. Main dish: Muesli of choice Option: Sweet Banana Porridge with Almond Milk or soy milk (with added calcium and "whole" soybean).	• Exercise until you sweat for 15 minutes. • Practice breathing exercises for 15 minutes. • Do an inner beauty exercise of your choice.
Lunch	Main dish: Choose your favorite vegetarian recipe	
Snack (3:00 p.m.)	*Choose from the following:* • Avocado Dip with Dipping Sticks • 1 cup (250 mL) of Soy Dande' • ¼ avocado with 4 whole-grain crackers	
Dinner	Beverage: Drink the last of your Green Water bottle 15 to 30 minutes before dinner. Main dish: Rich Mediterranean Pasta with Garden Salad or Colorful Non-Fried Rice	

Life after the Healthy Skin Diet

You may have overcome an undesirable skin condition, such as acne or eczema, during the 8-week program, and you might now be wondering, are these results sustainable? The answer is yes and no.

Yes, because you have strengthened your health immensely during the 8 weeks and you have also put into place new habits, many of which you will now automatically follow. For example, you may have found a fab new hat and a good sunscreen, so you can continue with your sun-care program; you might habitually add something green to your lunches and dinners; and as you peek in the mirror you might look for beauty more often than faults. But I'll give you a tip: if you continue to be kind to yourself and speak highly of your strengths and positive attributes, it will be much easier for you to continue to be healthy because your subconscious mind will work with, not against you.

No, because certain conditions are caused by genetics, and although you may have switched off your eczema, psoriasis, or allergic reactions, such as hives, they can reappear if triggered. Triggers include repeated stress, high chemical exposure, illness, a virus, or a return to poor diet and lifestyle habits. However, there are ways to minimize the risk of relapse. On page 341 I have listed the top four things you can do to keep your skin looking good beyond the Healthy Skin Diet. The 4 Healthy Skin Habits can be followed by anyone who wants to maintain healthy skin, vitality, and well-being. I hope you enjoy your new-found vitality and clear skin!

> I'll give you a tip: if you continue to be kind to yourself and speak highly of your strengths and positive attributes, it will be much easier for you to continue to be healthy because your subconscious mind will work with, not against you.

4 Healthy Skin Habits

1. *Think green*

Continue to alkalize your body with green drinks and green foods. Eat two handfuls of dark green leafies every day. You can have a salad or a side of baby spinach leaves, steamed broccoli, and Chinese greens. You should also continue to have a bottle of Green Water daily so you can cleanse your blood and keep track of how much water you consume. Think green for a healthy body and beautiful skin. If you drink alcohol or coffee (caffeine), have one glass of Green Water afterwards to reduce acids in the body.

2. *Moisturize your skin from the inside out*

Eat fish, especially oily deep sea fish, twice a week. Add ground flax seeds or flaxseed oil twice a week. Drink plenty of water. Add lecithin granules to cereals/porridge/smoothies to promote healthy lipid (fat) digestion and hydrated cells.

3. *Be a hat person*

The easiest way to slow down the aging process is to simply wear a hat and apply sunscreen when you go out in the sun.

4. *Think beautiful thoughts to reduce your stress levels*

Stress simply ruins your skin, so you want to reduce its damaging effects as often as possible. The most effective way to cope with daily stress is to spend some time focusing on your good attributes, your strengths, and your beauty. Enjoy your beautiful skin!

Part 7

Healthy Skin Recipes

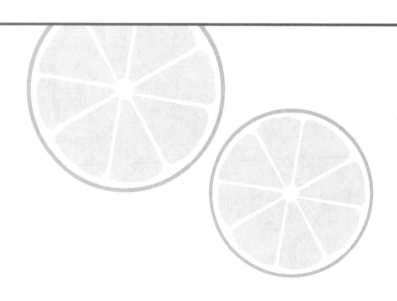

Beverages

Green Water. 344

ACV Drink. 344

Soy Dande'. 345

Dandelion Tea 345

Flaxseed Lemon Drink. 346

Pear Flaxseed Drink for Sensitive Skin. 347

Strawberry Rehydration Water 348

Berry Beauty Smoothie 348

Papaya Beauty Smoothie 349

Skin-Firming Drink. 350

Calcium-Rich Smoothie. 351

Spot-Free Skin Juice 351

Skin Juice for Sensitive Skin No. 1 352

Skin Juice for Sensitive Skin No. 2 353

Apple Omega Drink 354

ACE Smoothie 355

Almond Milk. 356

Green Water

This mild drink is alkalizing and gluten-free. Drink 1 to 2 glasses daily. Use low-strength chlorophyll and begin with 1 tsp (5 mL), working up to 2 to 3 tsp (10 to 15 mL) daily.

Tips

To add more flavor and alkalinity, you can add 1 tsp (5 mL) of fresh lemon juice.

If you have eczema or psoriasis, also add a measured dose of glycine to this drink.

| 1 to 3 tsp | liquid chlorophyll | 5 to 15 mL |
| 1 | glass chilled water or mineral water | 1 |

1. Mix chlorophyll into water and drink.

Variation

If you suffer from blood sugar problems such as hypoglycemia, you could also get a large bottle of filtered water (4 to 6 cups/1 to 1.5 L), add 2 tsp (10 mL) of liquid chlorophyll and sip it throughout the day (don't add lemon juice, as it's no good for the teeth if you're sipping it all day).

NUTRIENTS PER SERVING			
Calories	15	Protein	0 g
Total Fat	0.0 g	Biotin	0 mcg (0% DV)
Saturated Fat	0.0 g	Vitamin C	0 mg (0% DV)
Omega-3	0.0 g	Iron	0.0 mg (0% DV)
Carbohydrate	4 g	Magnesium	2 mg (1% DV)
Fiber	0.0 g (0% DV)	Zinc	0.0 mg (0% DV)

ACV Drink

This alkalizing drink has a mild apple cider taste. It's gluten-free and stimulates digestion, so ideally have it 15 minutes before breakfast or dinner. Drink 1 to 2 glasses daily as an occasional alternative to Green Water (above).

| 1 to 2 cups | chilled water or mineral water | 250 to 500 mL |
| 1 tsp | apple cider vinegar | 5 mL |

1. Mix water and vinegar and drink slowly.

Variation

For a sweeter drink, use $\frac{1}{2}$ cup (125 mL) pure apple juice (sugar- and preservative-free), 1 cup (250 mL) water and 1 to 2 tsp (5 to 10 mL) cider vinegar.

NUTRIENTS PER SERVING			
Calories	2	Protein	0 g
Total Fat	0.0 g	Biotin	0 mcg (0% DV)
Saturated Fat	0.0 g	Vitamin C	0 mg (0% DV)
Omega-3	0.0 g	Iron	0.0 mg (0% DV)
Carbohydrate	1 g	Magnesium	2 mg (1% DV)
Fiber	0.0 g (0% DV)	Zinc	0.0 mg (0% DV)

Soy Dande'

Makes 1 serving

This tasty hot beverage is liver cleansing and caffeine-free, and it stimulates digestive acids for improved digestion. It may overstimulate digestion; if this occurs, reduce dosage.

Tips

Use soy milk that contains "whole" soybean (not isolate).

Favor ground dandelion root if available, as it is better than the instant dandelion root.

½ cup	calcium-fortified soy milk	125 mL
½ cup	boiled water	125 mL
½ to 1 tsp	ground dandelion root	2 to 5 mL
1 tsp	honey (optional) (low GI)	5 mL

1. Heat soy milk in a microwave for 30 seconds, then add boiling water (preheating the soy milk prevents it from curdling). Place the measured amount of ground dandelion root in an enclosed tea strainer, then dunk it into the hot liquid for about 5 to 10 seconds (it should darken the milk quickly). Remove the strainer and discard the contents. Add honey, if desired.

NUTRIENTS PER SERVING			
Calories	54	Protein	3 g
Total Fat	1.8 g	Biotin	7 mcg (2% DV)
Saturated Fat	0.3 g	Vitamin C	0 mg (0% DV)
Omega-3	0.0 g	Iron	0.5 mg (3% DV)
Carbohydrate	6 g	Magnesium	19 mg (5% DV)
Fiber	0.4 g (2% DV)	Zinc	0.3 mg (2% DV)

Dandelion Tea

Makes 1 serving

½ tsp	ground dandelion root	2 mL
1 cup	boiled water	250 mL
1 tsp	honey (optional)	5 mL

1. Place the dandelion root into an enclosed tea strainer. Dunk the tea strainer into boiled water and steep for about 5 seconds, until water is dark brown. Make it weak to begin with, as it can be quite strong in flavor. Add honey, if desired.

NUTRIENTS PER SERVING			
Calories	1	Protein	0 g
Total Fat	0.0 g	Biotin	0 mcg (0% DV)
Saturated Fat	0.0 g	Vitamin C	0 mg (0% DV)
Omega-3	0.0 g	Iron	0.0 mg (0% DV)
Carbohydrate	0 g	Magnesium	2 mg (1% DV)
Fiber	0.1 g (0% DV)	Zinc	0.0 mg (0% DV)

Flaxseed Lemon Drink

**Makes 3 servings
(1 day's supply
for 1 person)**

This special gluten-free therapeutic drink reduces body acidity and may balance weight, improve immune function and alleviate dry skin if consumed on a regular basis. The pectin and oils from lemon peel provide antioxidants, chelate toxins from the bowel and stimulate liver detoxification enzymes. The lecithin aids fat digestion and helps the body use the anti-inflammatory omega-3 oils. If you have eczema, have the Pear Flaxseed Drink (page 347) instead.

Tips

Omit the ginger and add honey if you're making this recipe for children.

Acne-prone people may need to use less or no flaxseed oil.

½	organic lemon, washed, scrubbed	½
2 cups	water	500 mL
1 tbsp	lecithin granules (GMO-free soy)	15 mL
1 tbsp	organic flaxseed oil	15 mL
½	small knob gingerroot, peeled and finely grated	½

1. Finely grate (zest) the peel of the lemon and place in a blender. Add the lemon juice, water, lecithin, oil and ginger and blend for 30 seconds on high. Strain mixture through a fine sieve, if desired.

2. Have this drink throughout the day or before each main meal. Consume within 12 hours.

NUTRIENTS PER SERVING			
Calories	62	Protein	0 g
Total Fat	5.9 g	Biotin	0 mcg (0% DV)
Saturated Fat	0.8 g	Vitamin C	3 mg (5% DV)
Omega-3	2.4 g	Iron	0.1 mg (1% DV)
Carbohydrate	1 g	Magnesium	2 mg (1% DV)
Fiber	0.0 g (0% DV)	Zinc	0.0 mg (0% DV)

Pear Flaxseed Drink for Sensitive Skin

Specially designed for people with eczema, this gluten-free drink contains omega-3 anti-inflammatory oils. Ginger is anti-inflammatory, and lecithin helps your body use the omega-3 oils. This recipe is also fiber-rich if you use ground flax seeds.

Tips

Omit the ginger and add honey if you're making this recipe for children.

Acne-prone people may need to use less or no flaxseed oil.

1 cup	chilled water	250 mL
1 cup	canned pear slices plus natural juice, or freshly juiced pear	250 mL
1 tbsp	lecithin granules (GMO-free soy)	15 mL
1 tbsp	organic ground flax seeds or flaxseed oil	15 mL
½	knob gingerroot, peeled and finely grated	½

1. Combine water, pear and natural juice, lecithin, flax seeds and gingerroot in a blender and blend for 30 seconds on high.

2. Drink one-third before each meal. Consume within 12 hours.

NUTRIENTS PER SERVING			
Calories	86	Protein	0 g
Total Fat	2.3 g	Biotin	1 mcg (0% DV)
Saturated Fat	0.4 g	Vitamin C	1 mg (2% DV)
Omega-3	0.5 g	Iron	0.5 mg (3% DV)
Carbohydrate	15 g	Magnesium	10 mg (3% DV)
Fiber	2.0 g (8% DV)	Zinc	0.1 mg (1% DV)

Strawberry Rehydration Water

This makes a refreshing drink after exercising, as it replenishes electrolytes. Drink within 10 hours of making.

2 cups	water	500 mL
2	fresh strawberries, rinsed and finely diced	2
Pinch	natural sea salt	Pinch

1. Combine water, strawberries and salt in a bottle and shake.

NUTRIENTS PER SERVING			
Calories	12	Protein	0 g
Total Fat	0.1 g	Biotin	0 mcg (0% DV)
Saturated Fat	0.0 g	Vitamin C	21 mg (35% DV)
Omega-3	0.0 g	Iron	0.2 mg (1% DV)
Carbohydrate	3 g	Magnesium	9 mg (2% DV)
Fiber	0.7 g (3% DV)	Zinc	0.1 mg (1% DV)

Berry Beauty Smoothie

This tasty, gluten-free drink contains antioxidants from berries, omega-3s from flax seeds, and protein and calcium from almonds. Plus, coconut oil is anti-fungal.

Tip
Acne-prone people may need to use less or no flaxseed oil.

1 cup	chilled Almond Milk (page 356) or water	250 mL
1 tbsp	organic flaxseed oil or ground flax seeds	15 mL
1 tbsp	lecithin granules (GMO-free soy)	15 mL
½ cup	frozen berries (raspberries or mixed)	125 mL
3 tbsp	coconut milk or coconut water	45 mL

1. Combine almond milk, oil, lecithin, berries and coconut milk in a blender and blend on high until smooth. Consume within 2 hours.

NUTRIENTS PER SERVING			
Calories	468	Protein	9 g
Total Fat	41.3 g	Biotin	23 mcg (8% DV)
Saturated Fat	9.0 g	Vitamin C	9 mg (15% DV)
Omega-3	7.3 g	Iron	3.0 mg (17% DV)
Carbohydrate	17 g	Magnesium	111 mg (28% DV)
Fiber	6.9 g (28% DV)	Zinc	1.3 mg (9% DV)

Papaya Beauty Smoothie

Makes 1 large or 2 small servings

This thick, tropical, gluten-free smoothie is a delicious and refreshing drink. It contains vitamin C–rich papaya, which enhances protein digestion; bananas, which are a great source of fiber; and ginger and lime, which are alkalizing. The only thing missing from this recipe is protein, which is vital for firm skin, so ideally you should use this shake as a digestion-enhancing appetizer and have it 15 to 30 minutes before a protein-rich meal. If consumed before dinner, it may also aid weight loss because flaxseed oil triggers the satiety response.

Tip

Acne-prone people may need to use less or no flaxseed oil.

½ cup	pure apple juice (sugar- and preservative-free)	125 mL
½ cup	water	125 mL
1 cup	chopped papaya (optional: pre-freeze chunks)	250 mL
1	frozen banana (peel and chop before freezing)	1
½	lime, juiced (about 4 tsp/20 mL)	½
¼ tsp	grated gingerroot (optional)	1 mL
1 tbsp	ground flax seeds or flaxseed oil	15 mL
1 tbsp	lecithin granules (GMO-free soy)	15 mL

1. Combine apple juice, water, papaya, banana, lime juice and ginger in a blender and blend on high until smooth. Add flax seeds and lecithin and blend for a further 20 seconds. Serve and drink immediately. For a thinner mixture, add extra water.

NUTRIENTS PER SERVING			
Calories	162	Protein	2 g
Total Fat	3.9 g	Biotin	2 mcg (1% DV)
Saturated Fat	0.8 g	Vitamin C	53 mg (88% DV)
Omega-3	0.9 g	Iron	1.0 mg (6% DV)
Carbohydrate	30 g	Magnesium	50 mg (13% DV)
Fiber	4.3 g (17% DV)	Zinc	0.4 mg (3% DV)

Skin-Firming Drink

Makes 1 serving

This fiber-rich drink helps to promote proper collagen formation and firm skin, as it is high in protein and vitamin C, and is a source of zinc (see tip, below). Lecithin and omega-3 are essential for cell membrane health.

Tips

Choose a glucosamine supplement that also contains copper, zinc and vitamin C, and follow the dosage recommended by manufacturer.

Acne-prone people may need to use less or no flaxseed oil.

1	frozen banana (peel and chop before freezing)	1
1 cup	chilled Almond Milk (page 356) or calcium-fortified soy milk	250 mL
10	blueberries or frozen raspberries	10
	Glucosamine complex supplement (see tip, at left)	
1 tbsp	ground flax seeds or flaxseed oil	15 mL
1 tbsp	lecithin granules (GMO-free soy)	15 mL
2	dashes ground cinnamon	2

1. Combine banana, almond milk, blueberries, glucosamine, flax seeds, lecithin and cinnamon in a blender and blend on high until smooth. Drink immediately.

NUTRIENTS PER SERVING			
Calories	421	Protein	10 g
Total Fat	25.1 g	Biotin	27 mcg (9% DV)
Saturated Fat	2.7 g	Vitamin C	12 mg (20% DV)
Omega-3	1.6 g	Iron	3.0 mg (17% DV)
Carbohydrate	41 g	Magnesium	159 mg (40% DV)
Fiber	10.5 g (42% DV)	Zinc	1.7 mg (11% DV)

Calcium-Rich Smoothie

This drink is a good calcium substitute in a dairy-free diet and is also ideal for eczema sufferers, as it is low in salicylates.

Tip
Banana and papaya contain amines, so use other fruits if you have rosacea or hives.

2 cups	calcium-fortified soy milk	500 mL
1 cup	chopped papaya (or 1 diced banana, pre-frozen)	250 mL
1 tbsp	flaxseed oil or ground flax seeds	15 mL
1 tbsp	lecithin granules (GMO-free soy)	15 mL
1 tbsp	pure maple syrup (optional)	15 mL

1. Combine soy milk, papaya, oil, lecithin and maple syrup (if using) in a blender and blend on high until smooth. Consume within 8 hours.

NUTRIENTS PER SERVING			
Calories	226	Protein	7 g
Total Fat	12.6 g	Biotin	14 mcg (5% DV)
Saturated Fat	1.7 g	Vitamin C	44 mg (73% DV)
Omega-3	3.8 g	Iron	1.4 mg (8% DV)
Carbohydrate	20 g	Magnesium	52 mg (13% DV)
Fiber	1.7 g (7% DV)	Zinc	0.7 mg (5% DV)

Spot-Free Skin Juice

This drink is ideal for anyone who wants clear skin.

4	medium carrots	4
2	apples (leave skin on)	2
1	pear (leave skin on)	1
½ cup	chopped beets	125 mL
½ cup	chopped cabbage	125 mL
	Squeeze of fresh lemon juice	

1. With a juicing machine, juice carrots, apples, pear, beets and cabbage. Mix and add lemon juice. Consume within 8 hours.

NUTRIENTS PER SERVING			
Calories	190	Protein	3 g
Total Fat	0.8 g	Biotin	9 mcg (3% DV)
Saturated Fat	0.1 g	Vitamin C	27 mg (45% DV)
Omega-3	0.0 g	Iron	0.9 mg (6% DV)
Carbohydrate	48 g	Magnesium	27 mg (7% DV)
Fiber	0.0 g (0% DV)	Zinc	0.5 mg (3% DV)

Skin Juice for Sensitive Skin No. 1

Makes 3 servings (1 day's supply for 1 person)

A perfect juice, especially if you have chemical sensitivity or eczema, as it is low in salicylates and rich in anti-inflammatory ingredients.

4	ripe pears	4
3	stalks celery	3
½ cup	chopped cabbage	125 mL
½ cup	water	125 mL
2 tsp	apple cider vinegar	10 mL
½	bunch parsley (including stalks)	½
1	knob gingerroot, peeled	1

1. Wash and scrub pears, celery and cabbage in a bowl of ¼ cup (60 mL) water with apple cider vinegar.

2. With a juicing machine, juice pears, celery, cabbage, parsley and ginger. At the end, run remaining water through machine to flush though remaining juice and dilute drink slightly.

3. Drink 1 glass immediately and consume the rest within 8 hours.

NUTRIENTS PER SERVING			
Calories	83	Protein	2 g
Total Fat	0.5 g	Biotin	1 mcg (0% DV)
Saturated Fat	0.1 g	Vitamin C	24 mg (40% DV)
Omega-3	0.0 g	Iron	0.8 mg (4% DV)
Carbohydrate	21 g	Magnesium	27 mg (7% DV)
Fiber	0.0 g (0% DV)	Zinc	0.2 mg (1% DV)

Skin Juice for Sensitive Skin No. 2

Makes 3 servings (1 day's supply for 1 person)

A great drink, especially if you have chemical sensitivity or eczema, as it is low in salicylates.

4	ripe pears	4
3	stalks celery	3
½ cup	green beans	125 mL
½ cup	chopped cabbage	125 mL
¼ cup	water	60 mL
2 tsp	apple cider vinegar	10 mL
½	bunch parsley (including stalks)	½

1. Wash and scrub pears, celery, green beans and cabbage in a bowl of water with apple cider vinegar.

2. With a juicing machine, juice pears, celery, green beans, cabbage and parsley. Mix and have one glass immediately. Drink the rest within 8 hours.

NUTRIENTS PER SERVING			
Calories	94	Protein	2 g
Total Fat	1.0 g	Biotin	1 mcg (0% DV)
Saturated Fat	0.1 g	Vitamin C	25 mg (42% DV)
Omega-3	0.0 g	Iron	1.0 mg (6% DV)
Carbohydrate	22 g	Magnesium	26 mg (7% DV)
Fiber	0.0 g (0% DV)	Zinc	0.2 mg (1% DV)

Apple Omega Drink

Makes 2 servings

This sweet drink contains omega-3, has a low glycemic index, is gluten-free and anti-inflammatory, and promotes proper fat digestion. Use sugar- and preservative-free apple juice or juice your own apples. Flax seeds make the drink rich in fiber and a bit lumpy, but it is surprisingly delicious.

1 tbsp	flax seeds	15 mL
6 tbsp	water	90 mL
1 cup	pure apple juice (sugar- and preservative-free)	250 mL
½	small knob gingerroot, peeled and finely grated	½
1 tbsp	lecithin granules (GMO-free soy)	15 mL

1. Soak the flax seeds overnight in the water.

2. Place seeds and their water in a blender. Add apple juice, ginger and lecithin and blend on high for 30 seconds. Pour into glasses and serve immediately.

NUTRIENTS PER SERVING			
Calories	105	Protein	1 g
Total Fat	3.5 g	Biotin	1 mcg (0% DV)
Saturated Fat	0.6 g	Vitamin C	1 mg (2% DV)
Omega-3	0.8 g	Iron	0.9 mg (6% DV)
Carbohydrate	15 g	Magnesium	23 mg (6% DV)
Fiber	2.0 g (8% DV)	Zinc	0.3 mg (2% DV)

ACE Smoothie

This tasty drink is rich in vitamin C and also contains vitamins A, E and B complex and chromium.

Tips

To make this drink gluten-free, use rice bran instead of the wheat germ.

Acne-prone people may need to use less or no flaxseed oil.

4	whole raw almonds	4
1 tbsp	wheat germ	15 mL
1 tsp	ground flax seeds or flaxseed oil	5 mL
½	mango, diced (about 1 cup/250 mL), pre-frozen	½
½ cup	sliced peeled papaya, pre-frozen	125 mL
2 cups	chilled plain mineral water	500 mL

1. Soak the almonds in the water overnight (highly recommended but not essential).

2. Combine wheat germ, flax seeds, mango, papaya and water in a blender and blend on high until smooth. Serve immediately.

NUTRIENTS PER SERVING			
Calories	101	Protein	3 g
Total Fat	2.6 g	Biotin	2 mcg (1% DV)
Saturated Fat	0.3 g	Vitamin C	52 mg (87% DV)
Omega-3	0.3 g	Iron	0.6 mg (3% DV)
Carbohydrate	19 g	Magnesium	37 mg (9% DV)
Fiber	3.2 g (13% DV)	Zinc	0.6 mg (4% DV)

Almond Milk

Makes 4 servings

You can use Almond Milk instead of milk in smoothies, on porridge or on cereal. It contains protein. Preferably soak the almonds overnight in water, as this reduces the phytic acid content so you absorb more skin-repairing minerals.

1 cup	whole raw almonds	250 mL
3 cups	water	750 mL
½ tsp	vanilla extract	2 mL
1 tsp	honey or pure maple syrup (optional)	5 mL
Pinch	ground cinnamon or nutmeg	Pinch

1. Soak the almonds in the water overnight (highly recommended but not essential).

2. Combine almonds, water, vanilla, honey and cinnamon in a blender and blend on high for 30 seconds. Strain the liquid. The leftover almond meal can be used on porridge or cereal. Consume within 3 days.

NUTRIENTS PER SERVING			
Calories	208	Protein	8 g
Total Fat	17.7 g	Biotin	23 mcg (8% DV)
Saturated Fat	1.3 g	Vitamin C	0 mg (0% DV)
Omega-3	0 g	Iron	1.4 mg (8% DV)
Carbohydrate	8 g	Magnesium	98 mg (25% DV)
Fiber	4.5 g (18% DV)	Zinc	1.1 mg (7% DV)

Breakfasts

Ground Flax Seeds 358

Berry Beauty Porridge 358

Delicious French Toast with Berries and Almonds 359

Sweet Banana Porridge 360

Avocado on Toast 360

Smoked Salmon and Avocado on Toast 361

Whole Fruit Jam on Toast 361

Sardines and Lemon on Whole-Grain Toast 362

Fruit Salad with Flax Seeds 363

Amine-Free Fruit Salad 363

Perfect Poached Eggs 364

Smoked Salmon and Eggs 365

Egg Soldiers 366

Tasty Omelet 367

Designer Muesli 368

Gluten-Free Muesli 369

Vitamin E Muesli 370

Bircher Muesli 371

Mango and Buckwheat Crêpes 372

Pear and Buckwheat Crêpes 373

Boiled Eggs, Vegetables and Rice 374

Fish and Steamed Vegetables 375

Beans on Toast 376

Kids' Scrambled Eggs 377

Kids' Creamy Beans on Toast 378

Ground Flax Seeds

Flax seeds are available at health food shops and some supermarkets. Add ground flax seeds to breakfast cereals, smoothies and porridge to increase the fiber, calcium and omega-3 content.

1 cup	whole flax seeds	250 mL

1. Grind flax seeds to a fine meal in a clean coffee grinder. Store in an airtight jar in the refrigerator for up to 4 weeks.

NUTRIENTS PER 1 TBSP (15 ML)			
Calories	56	Protein	2 g
Total Fat	4.4 g	Biotin	1 mcg (0% DV)
Saturated Fat	0.4 g	Vitamin C	0 mg (0% DV)
Omega-3	2.4 g	Iron	0.6 mg (3% DV)
Carbohydrate	3 g	Magnesium	41 mg (10% DV)
Fiber	2.9 g (12% DV)	Zinc	0.5 mg (3% DV)

Berry Beauty Porridge

Makes 4 servings

This hearty and warm breakfast is rich in fiber, contains 0.5 g of omega-3, and has a low GI. If you have eczema, have the Sweet Banana Porridge (page 360) instead. If you have gluten intolerance, be sure to purchase certified gluten-free oats.

Tip

Other enzyme-rich options in place of the raspberries are blueberries, chopped papaya, chopped peach, grated apple or strawberries so you have a "living" breakfast fit for a (beauty) queen.

2 cups	large-flake (old-fashioned) rolled oats	500 mL
4 cups	water	1 L
4 tsp	honey or sugar-free jam (optional)	20 mL
1 tbsp	ground flax seeds	15 mL
1 cup	calcium-fortified soy milk	250 mL
1 cup	raspberries, fresh or frozen and thawed	250 mL

1. If possible, soak the oats overnight in the water to germinate the grain, making it more digestible and the nutrients more available.

2. Place oats and their water in a small saucepan. Bring to a boil and simmer for 5 minutes, stirring regularly, until cooked. Serve with honey or jam if extra sweetness is required, then add flax seeds, soy milk and berries.

NUTRIENTS PER SERVING			
Calories	200	Protein	7 g
Total Fat	4.7 g	Biotin	8 mcg (3% DV)
Saturated Fat	0.7 g	Vitamin C	6 mg (10% DV)
Omega-3	0.5 g	Iron	2.3 mg (13% DV)
Carbohydrate	35 g	Magnesium	19 mg (5% DV)
Fiber	4.6 g (18% DV)	Zinc	0.3 mg (2% DV)

Delicious French Toast with Berries and Almonds

This healthy French toast is rich in fiber and protein, is a source of the antioxidant vitamin C, has a low GI and is gluten-free if you use gluten-free bread. Vanilla extract and cinnamon help to keep blood sugar levels steady. If you have eczema, avoid strawberries, cinnamon and jam; use blueberries or banana, and replace the jam with pure maple syrup.

Tip
Use sugar-free berry jam that has been naturally sweetened with grape juice (avoid artificial sweeteners).

3	large free-range eggs	3
¾ cup	calcium-fortified soy milk	175 mL
Pinch	ground cinnamon (optional)	Pinch
1 tsp	vanilla extract	5 mL
8	slices whole-grain bread (preferably low GI)	8
	Extra virgin olive oil	
4 tsp	sugar-free berry jam	20 mL
2 cups	blueberries, raspberries or sliced strawberries (thawed if frozen)	500 mL
⅓ cup	raw almonds, toasted and chopped	75 mL
2 tsp	ground flax seeds	10 mL

1. In a shallow bowl, whisk together eggs, soy milk, cinnamon and vanilla extract. Dip bread slices into liquid, turning to coat.

2. Grease a large skillet with a small amount of olive oil and place over medium heat. Using a spatula, remove bread slices and let excess egg mixture drain off. Cook two slices at a time for about 2 minutes each side, until light golden.

3. Sparingly spread jam onto French toast and top with berries and almonds, then sprinkle with flax seeds. Serve immediately.

NUTRIENTS PER SERVING			
Calories	344	Protein	16 g
Total Fat	12.1 g	Biotin	20 mcg (7% DV)
Saturated Fat	2.0 g	Vitamin C	8 mg (13% DV)
Omega-3	0.5 g	Iron	2.3 mg (13% DV)
Carbohydrate	45 g	Magnesium	102 mg (26% DV)
Fiber	6.0 g (24% DV)	Zinc	2.2 mg (15% DV)

Sweet Banana Porridge

Makes 4 servings

This hearty, warm breakfast is low in salicylates, so it's suitable for eczema sufferers — and children love it. It's rich in fiber, it contains 0.5 g of omega-3, and whole rolled oats have a low GI (instant oats have a high GI and are not suitable). If you have gluten intolerance, be sure to purchase certified gluten-free oats.

2 cups	large-flake (old-fashioned) rolled oats	500 mL
4 cups	water	1 L
4 tsp	pure maple syrup	20 mL
1 tbsp	ground flax seeds	15 mL
1 cup	calcium-fortified soy milk	250 mL
1	ripe banana, thinly sliced	1

1. If possible, soak the oats overnight in the water to germinate the grain, making it more digestible and the nutrients more available.

2. Place oats and their water in a small saucepan. Bring to a boil and simmer for 5 minutes, stirring regularly, until cooked. Serve with maple syrup, flax seeds, soy milk and banana.

NUTRIENTS PER SERVING			
Calories	229	Protein	7 g
Total Fat	4.7 g	Biotin	9 mcg (3% DV)
Saturated Fat	0.7 g	Vitamin C	3 mg (5% DV)
Omega-3	0.5 g	Iron	2.2 mg (12% DV)
Carbohydrate	42 g	Magnesium	28 mg (7% DV)
Fiber	5.4 g (22% DV)	Zinc	0.4 mg (3% DV)

Avocado on Toast

Makes 2 servings

This breakfast is super-quick and rich in iron, magnesium and zinc. However, it is not suitable if you have eczema or gluten intolerance.

4	slices whole-grain bread (soy and flaxseed)	4
½	avocado, mashed or sliced	½
1	banana, thinly sliced (optional)	1

1. Toast bread and add the desired amount of avocado. Top with banana and serve immediately.

NUTRIENTS PER SERVING			
Calories	320	Protein	11 g
Total Fat	12.4 g	Biotin	7 mcg (2% DV)
Saturated Fat	1.7 g	Vitamin C	5 mg (8% DV)
Omega-3	1.7 g	Iron	3.9 mg (22% DV)
Carbohydrate	44 g	Magnesium	135 mg (34% DV)
Fiber	9.4 g (38% DV)	Zinc	2.7 mg (18% DV)

Smoked Salmon and Avocado on Toast

This breakfast is rich in iron, magnesium and zinc, is a source of vitamin C and contains 1.9 grams of omega-3. If you have eczema, omit the avocado and use hummus instead. If you have gluten intolerance, choose gluten-free bread.

4	slices whole-grain bread (soy and flaxseed)	4
½	avocado, mashed or sliced	½
3½ oz	sliced smoked salmon	100 g
	Squeeze of fresh lemon juice	
	Ground black pepper (optional)	
½ cup	baby spinach	125 mL

1. Toast bread and add the desired amount of avocado. Top with smoked salmon, lemon juice (use sparingly) and pepper, and add a side of spinach. Serve immediately.

NUTRIENTS PER SERVING			
Calories	381	Protein	20 g
Total Fat	14.5 g	Biotin	10 mcg (3% DV)
Saturated Fat	2.1 g	Vitamin C	6 mg (10% DV)
Omega-3	1.9 g	Iron	4.5 mg (25% DV)
Carbohydrate	45 g	Magnesium	144 mg (36% DV)
Fiber	9.7 g (39% DV)	Zinc	2.9 mg (19% DV)

Whole Fruit Jam on Toast

This low-GI recipe is suitable as an occasional breakfast. Use sugar-free jam that is full of fruit and sweetened with grape juice (not artificial sweetener). This recipe is not suitable if you have eczema or gluten intolerance. Gluten-free bread is not a good alternative, as it has a high GI and is low in nutrition.

4	slices whole-grain bread (soy and flaxseed)	4
3 tbsp	sugar-free jam	45 mL
1	banana, sliced thinly (optional)	1

1. Toast bread and add the desired amount of jam. Top with banana and serve immediately.

NUTRIENTS PER SERVING			
Calories	293	Protein	10 g
Total Fat	5.0 g	Biotin	5 mcg (2% DV)
Saturated Fat	0.6 g	Vitamin C	2 mg (3% DV)
Omega-3	1.6 g	Iron	3.6 mg (20% DV)
Carbohydrate	60 g	Magnesium	120 mg (30% DV)
Fiber	6.0 g (24% DV)	Zinc	2.4 mg (16% DV)

Sardines and Lemon on Whole-Grain Toast

This breakfast is quick to prepare, has a low GI and contains 2.5 g of omega-3. If you have eczema, use sardines in spring water (not oil) and 1 tbsp (15 mL) of finely chopped flat-leaf (Italian) parsley instead of the greens. If you have gluten intolerance, choose gluten-free bread.

4	slices whole-grain bread (soy and flaxseed)	4
1	can (3.75 oz/106 g) sardines in olive oil or spring water	1
	Squeeze of fresh lemon juice	
	Ground black pepper (optional)	
½ cup	dark green leafy vegetables (arugula, spinach or lettuce)	125 mL

1. Toast bread and spread the desired amount of sardines on toast. Sprinkle with lemon juice and pepper (if using) and add a side of greens (or sprinkle with finely chopped parsley). Serve immediately.

NUTRIENTS PER SERVING			
Calories	352	Protein	23 g
Total Fat	11.1 g	Biotin	7 mcg (2% DV)
Saturated Fat	1.4 g	Vitamin C	1 mg (2% DV)
Omega-3	2.5 g	Iron	5.2 mg (29% DV)
Carbohydrate	40 g	Magnesium	143 mg (36% DV)
Fiber	6.1 g (24% DV)	Zinc	3.1 mg (21% DV)

Fruit Salad with Flax Seeds

Makes 2 servings

This fruit salad is low in salicylates and is suitable for people with eczema. It contains amines, so people with rosacea or hives should choose the Amine-Free Fruit Salad (below) instead. If you have gluten intolerance, be sure to purchase certified gluten-free oats or substitute rice bran.

1	pear, peeled and diced	1
1	ripe banana, chopped	1
1½ cups	diced papaya	375 mL
2 tsp	ground flax seeds	10 mL
4 tsp	rolled oats or rice bran	20 mL

1. Combine pear, banana, papaya, flax seeds and oats. Serve immediately.

NUTRIENTS PER SERVING			
Calories	150	Protein	2 g
Total Fat	1.9 g	Biotin	3 mcg (1% DV)
Saturated Fat	0.3 g	Vitamin C	74 mg (123% DV)
Omega-3	0.6 g	Iron	0.7 mg (4% DV)
Carbohydrate	35 g	Magnesium	53 mg (13% DV)
Fiber	6.6 g (26% DV)	Zinc	0.3 mg (2% DV)

Amine-Free Fruit Salad

Makes 4 servings

This fruit salad is suitable for most people, including those with rosacea or hives. People with eczema should have the Fruit Salad with Flax Seeds (above) instead.

1	red apple, diced	1
½	mango, diced	½
1 cup	strawberries	250 mL
1 cup	blueberries	250 mL
1 cup	diced cantaloupe	250 mL
¼ cup	raw almonds, toasted and chopped	60 mL
4 tsp	ground flax seeds	20 mL

1. Combine apple, mango, strawberries, blueberries and cantaloupe. Sprinkle with almonds and flax seeds.

NUTRIENTS PER SERVING			
Calories	140	Protein	3 g
Total Fat	5.7 g	Biotin	6 mcg (2% DV)
Saturated Fat	0.6 g	Vitamin C	28 mg (47% DV)
Omega-3	0.6 g	Iron	0.8 mg (4% DV)
Carbohydrate	22 g	Magnesium	47 mg (12% DV)
Fiber	3.5 g (14% DV)	Zinc	0.7 mg (5% DV)

Tip

To toast the almonds, place them in a dry skillet over medium heat and cook, stirring, for about 4 minutes or until browned and fragrant. Let cool, then chop.

Perfect Poached Eggs

Makes 2 servings

There is an art to cooking perfect poached eggs, so it may take you a couple of attempts to master the technique, but by following these steps you'll be a pro in no time! Poaching is a much healthier way to cook eggs than frying. This recipe is rich in protein and fiber, is a source of vitamin C and has a low GI. It contains gluten if you use wheat bread. Use antibiotic-free eggs.

2 to 4	large free-range eggs	2 to 4
4 tsp	white vinegar	20 mL
2 to 4	slices whole-grain or sourdough bread	2 to 4
½	avocado, mashed	½
1 tbsp	finely chopped parsley	15 mL
	Natural sea salt and ground black pepper (optional)	

1. Fill a medium-sized saucepan with enough water to cover the eggs. Bring to a boil and add vinegar (the vinegar keeps the egg whites together while cooking).

2. Remove boiling water from heat, so the water ceases movement, then carefully crack the eggs into the water (initially only cook two eggs at a time to ensure correct cooking times). Return saucepan to heat and reduce to a simmer and set timer immediately. A large (2 oz/56 g) egg should take about 4 minutes to cook for a soft yolk.

3. Toast the bread and spread with avocado. After 4 minutes, carefully and swiftly remove eggs with a spatula/slotted spoon and, if desired, rinse off vinegar using slow-running hot water. Drain water off eggs, then place eggs on toast and top with parsley. Sprinkle with salt and pepper, if desired. Serve immediately.

NUTRIENTS PER SERVING			
Calories	224	Protein	11 g
Total Fat	12.3 g	Biotin	13 mcg (4% DV)
Saturated Fat	2.5 g	Vitamin C	8 mg (13% DV)
Omega-3	0.2 g	Iron	2.0 mg (11% DV)
Carbohydrate	17 g	Magnesium	45 mg (11% DV)
Fiber	5.3 g (21% DV)	Zinc	1.4 mg (9% DV)

Smoked Salmon and Eggs

Makes 2 servings

Salmon is a great source of omega-3, and eggs supply a good range of B vitamins and protein. If you have eczema, sparingly use salt-free butter instead of the avocado.

2 to 4	large free-range eggs	2 to 4
4 tsp	white vinegar	20 mL
2 to 4	slices whole-grain or sourdough bread	2 to 4
½	avocado, mashed	½
1 tbsp	finely chopped parsley	15 mL
1¾ oz	sliced smoked salmon	50 g
	Ground black pepper	
	Fresh lemon juice	

1. Follow the Perfect Poached Eggs recipe (page 364) and add smoked salmon on top of the parsley. If desired, sprinkle pepper and a small amount of lemon juice on the fish. Serve immediately.

NUTRIENTS PER SERVING			
Calories	254	Protein	16 g
Total Fat	13.4 g	Biotin	14 mcg (5% DV)
Saturated Fat	2.7 g	Vitamin C	8 mg (13% DV)
Omega-3	0.3 g	Iron	2.3 mg (13% DV)
Carbohydrate	17 g	Magnesium	49 mg (12% DV)
Fiber	5.4 g (22% DV)	Zinc	1.5 mg (10% DV)

Egg Soldiers

Makes 2 servings

This meal is fun for children and grown-ups alike, as it is served in egg cups with toast dipping sticks. It's a healthy way to cook eggs, as no frying is involved. Parsley is alkalizing and supplies chlorophyll. Use antibiotic-free eggs. The vinegar and salt help to prevent the egg shells from cracking during cooking. If you have eczema, omit the olive oil and chutney and use salt-free butter sparingly.

4 tsp	white vinegar	20 mL
Pinch	salt	Pinch
2 to 4	slices whole-grain bread	2 to 4
2 to 4	large free-range eggs	2 to 4
	Extra virgin olive oil, Sweet Chutney (page 384) or mango chutney (optional)	
2 tsp	finely chopped parsley	10 mL

1. Fill a small to medium-sized pot with enough water to cover eggs. Bring to a boil, then add vinegar and salt. Gently spoon the eggs into the water and boil for 5 minutes for a large (2 oz/56 g) egg, turning eggs occasionally to promote even cooking.

2. Toast the bread and cut into strips. If desired, top with a splash of olive oil or chutney. Remove eggs from water. If the egg shell dries immediately, the egg is hard-boiled; if it dries slowly, the egg is soft-boiled.

3. Place eggs in egg cups and cut off the top third. If some of the top egg white is uncooked, scoop the runny whites out or return the top third back onto the egg for 2 minutes to allow the whites to set.

4. Sprinkle with parsley and serve with toast "dipping sticks" and a teaspoon (to eat the cooked whites).

NUTRIENTS PER SERVING			
Calories	144	Protein	10 g
Total Fat	5.0 g	Biotin	11 mcg (4% DV)
Saturated Fat	1.4 g	Vitamin C	2 mg (3% DV)
Omega-3	0.1 g	Iron	1.7 mg (9% DV)
Carbohydrate	13 g	Magnesium	30 mg (8% DV)
Fiber	2.0 g (8% DV)	Zinc	1.1 mg (7% DV)

Tasty Omelet

This omelet is rich in vitamin C and flavor. When choosing a sweet chile sauce, look for one free of artificial flavor enhancers (such as MSG).

- **Preheat broiler**

4	large free-range eggs	4
4 tsp	water	20 mL
½ tsp	tamari or soy sauce	2 mL
1 tsp	sweet chile sauce	5 mL
½	red onion, diced	½
4 tsp	extra virgin olive oil	20 mL
1 cup	baby spinach or chopped Swiss chard	250 mL
1	tomato, diced	1
	Ground black pepper (optional)	

1. Lightly beat the eggs together, then add water, tamari and sweet chile sauce to the eggs and mix.

2. In a small skillet on medium heat, sauté the onion with olive oil for 1 minute, then add spinach and sauté for a further minute or two. Add the tomato and mix, then divide vegetables in two and remove half from the pan (as you want to cook one omelet at a time).

3. Spread vegetables evenly across the pan before adding half the egg mix. Cover pan with a lid and cook for 4 minutes on low heat, being careful not to burn omelet.

4. If egg is still uncooked on top, transfer the pan to the broiler and broil the omelet (keeping the pan's handle away from heat) for 1 minute or until egg is cooked through. Remove omelet from the pan and repeat the process for the second omelet. Add pepper, if desired, and serve immediately.

NUTRIENTS PER SERVING			
Calories	270	Protein	14 g
Total Fat	17.6 g	Biotin	21 mcg (7% DV)
Saturated Fat	3.7 g	Vitamin C	16 mg (27% DV)
Omega-3	0.3 g	Iron	2.5 mg (14% DV)
Carbohydrate	11 g	Magnesium	16 mg (4% DV)
Fiber	1.6 g (7% DV)	Zinc	1.2 mg (8% DV)

Designer Muesli

This is a tasty treat at breakfast time. It is full of fiber, has a low GI and is rich in protein. Use quality soy milk containing added calcium and "whole" soybean (not isolate). If you have gluten intolerance, be sure to purchase certified gluten-free oats.

• **Preheat oven to 400°F (200°C)**

3 cups	large-flake (old-fashioned) or quick-cooking rolled oats	750 mL
2 tbsp	honey	30 mL
½ cup	almonds	125 mL
½ cup	green pumpkin seeds (pepitas)	125 mL
½ cup	whole flax seeds	125 mL
¼ cup	lecithin granules (GMO-free soy)	60 mL
¼ cup	rice bran	60 mL
	Raspberries (thawed if frozen)	
	Almond Milk (page 356) or calcium-fortified soy milk	

1. Combine oats and honey, mixing well. Spread evenly on a large baking sheet. Toast in preheated oven for 6 minutes, checking regularly to avoid burning, then stir and add almonds and pumpkin seeds. Bake for another 2 minutes or until mixture is lightly browned. Let cool.

2. Stir in flax seeds, lecithin and bran. Leftovers can be stored in an airtight container in the pantry for up to 2 weeks.

3. Serve with a small handful of raspberries and almond milk.

NUTRIENTS PER SERVING			
Calories	695	Protein	21 g
Total Fat	38.8 g	Biotin	19 mcg (6% DV)
Saturated Fat	5.2 g	Vitamin C	0 mg (0% DV)
Omega-3	4.8 g	Iron	8.0 mg (44% DV)
Carbohydrate	66 g	Magnesium	201 mg (50% DV)
Fiber	15.7 g (63% DV)	Zinc	1.5 mg (10% DV)

Gluten-Free Muesli

Because gluten-free grains generally have a medium to high GI, so does this recipe. If you have eczema, favor soy milk instead of almond milk. If you have rosacea, use berries instead of banana. If using soy milk, note that barley malt contains gluten, so use gluten-free or malt-free soy milk.

• **Preheat oven to 400°F (200°C)**

¼ cup	almonds	60 mL
1 cup	puffed brown rice cereal	250 mL
1 cup	puffed amaranth cereal	250 mL
½ cup	rice bran	125 mL
¼ cup	green pumpkin seeds (pepitas)	60 mL
½ cup	whole flax seeds	125 mL
¼ cup	lecithin granules (GMO-free soy)	60 mL
	Chilled malt-free soy milk or Almond Milk (page 356)	
	Honey (optional)	
1	banana, sliced	1

1. Spread almonds on a baking sheet and toast in preheated oven for 4 minutes (do not burn them). Remove from heat and let cool.

2. Mix puffed rice, puffed amaranth and rice bran with the almonds, pepitas, flax seeds and lecithin. Store in an airtight container.

3. Serve 1 cup (250 mL) per person and add soy milk, honey and banana.

NUTRIENTS PER SERVING			
Calories	619	Protein	18 g
Total Fat	35.2 g	Biotin	30 mcg (10% DV)
Saturated Fat	4.8 g	Vitamin C	4 mg (7% DV)
Omega-3	6.4 g	Iron	9.4 mg (52% DV)
Carbohydrate	57 g	Magnesium	404 mg (101% DV)
Fiber	15.6 g (63% DV)	Zinc	2.7 mg (18% DV)

Vitamin E Muesli

Makes 1 serving		

If you have eczema, replace the sunflower seeds with 1 tsp (5 mL) flax seeds and use soy milk instead of almond milk. Quality soy milk contains calcium and "whole" soybean (not isolate).

½ cup	large-flake (old-fashioned) rolled oats	125 mL
4 tsp	sunflower seeds	20 mL
1 cup	water	250 mL
4 tsp	wheat germ	20 mL
1 tsp	apple cider vinegar	5 mL
1 cup	Almond Milk (page 356)	250 mL
1 tsp	honey or pure maple syrup	5 mL
	Fruit (raspberries, blueberries and/or sliced banana)	

1. Combine oats, sunflower seeds, water, wheat germ and vinegar in a breakfast bowl and soak overnight.

2. Serve with almond milk, honey and fruit.

NUTRIENTS PER SERVING			
Calories	490	Protein	18 g
Total Fat	27.7 g	Biotin	37 mcg (12% DV)
Saturated Fat	2.4 g	Vitamin C	0 mg (0% DV)
Omega-3	0.0 g	Iron	4.6 mg (26% DV)
Carbohydrate	48 g	Magnesium	165 mg (41% DV)
Fiber	11.5 g (46% DV)	Zinc	2.7 mg (18% DV)

Bircher Muesli

Makes 4 servings

This sweet Bircher muesli recipe is super tasty thanks to the rice bran, fruit and raisins. Soak the grains and seeds overnight to make the nutrients more available. Oats are great for the nerves and skin. Use mango if it's summer and pears if it's winter or if you have eczema. Omit the raisins if you have eczema.

1½ cups	large-flake (old-fashioned) rolled oats	375 mL
½ cup	rice bran or wheat germ	125 mL
4 tsp	whole flax seeds	20 mL
¼ cup	raisins	60 mL
2 cups	pure apple juice (sugar- and preservative-free)	500 mL
1	mango, sliced (or pears or prunes)	1
1	banana, sliced	1
¼ cup	raw almonds, chopped (optional)	60 mL

1. Place oats, bran, flax seeds, raisins and apple juice in a large bowl and soak overnight.

2. The next morning, divide mixture into bowls, add more apple juice if necessary and top with fresh fruit and almonds.

NUTRIENTS PER SERVING			
Calories	340	Protein	8 g
Total Fat	6.6 g	Biotin	8 mcg (3% DV)
Saturated Fat	1.0 g	Vitamin C	8 mg (13% DV)
Omega-3	0.8 g	Iron	5.1 mg (28% DV)
Carbohydrate	66 g	Magnesium	170 mg (43% DV)
Fiber	9.7 g (39% DV)	Zinc	0.4 mg (3% DV)

Mango and Buckwheat Crêpes

This tasty crêpe recipe is gluten-free and rich in flavonoids from buckwheat flour and mango.

2	large free-range eggs	2
3 tbsp	buckwheat flour	45 mL
¼ cup	water	60 mL
1 tsp	ghee, coconut oil or olive oil	5 mL
½	mango, sliced	½
1 to 2 tsp	honey (optional)	5 to 10 mL
1 to 2 tsp	ground flax seeds	5 to 10 mL

1. Beat eggs in a large bowl, and then mix in buckwheat flour until free of lumps. Add water and mix until smooth. The mixture should be runny so you can make thin crêpes.

2. Grease a medium nonstick skillet with ghee and pour in enough batter to make a thin crêpe. Use a spatula to turn over the crêpe once it is lightly cooked. Do not brown the crêpe. Repeat the process until all of the mixture is used.

3. Top the crêpes with mango, honey and flax seeds.

NUTRIENTS PER SERVING			
Calories	335	Protein	16 g
Total Fat	14.6 g	Biotin	22 mcg (7% DV)
Saturated Fat	6.4 g	Vitamin C	9 mg (15% DV)
Omega-3	0.7 g	Iron	2.6 mg (14% DV)
Carbohydrate	32 g	Magnesium	22 mg (6% DV)
Fiber	5.1 g (20% DV)	Zinc	1.2 mg (8% DV)

Pear and Buckwheat Crêpes

Makes 1 serving

This tasty crêpe recipe is low in salicylates, so it's suitable for people with eczema. It's also gluten-free and rich in flavonoids. You can substitute banana for the pear, if desired.

2	large free-range eggs	2
3 tbsp	buckwheat flour	45 mL
¼ cup	water	60 mL
1 tsp	ghee or unsalted butter	5 mL
1	ripe pear, peeled and chopped	1
1 to 2 tsp	pure maple syrup (optional)	5 to 10 mL
1 to 2 tsp	ground flax seeds	5 to 10 mL

1. Beat eggs in a large bowl, and then mix in the buckwheat flour until free of lumps. Add water and mix until smooth. The mixture should be runny so you can make thin crêpes.

2. Grease a medium nonstick skillet with ghee and pour in enough batter to make a thin crêpe. Use a spatula to turn over the crêpe once it is lightly cooked. Do not brown the crêpe. Repeat the process until all of the mixture is used.

3. Top the crêpes with pear, maple syrup and flax seeds and serve immediately.

NUTRIENTS PER SERVING			
Calories	319	Protein	17 g
Total Fat	14.2 g	Biotin	21 mcg (7% DV)
Saturated Fat	5.4 g	Vitamin C	0 mg (0% DV)
Omega-3	0.7 g	Iron	2.6 mg (14% DV)
Carbohydrate	38 g	Magnesium	22 mg (6% DV)
Fiber	4.1 g (16% DV)	Zinc	1.2 mg (8% DV)

Boiled Eggs, Vegetables and Rice

Makes 2 servings			

1 cup	brown rice	250 mL
4 tsp	white vinegar	20 mL
2 to 4	large free-range eggs	2 to 4
4 tsp	extra virgin olive oil	20 mL
½	red or yellow onion, sliced	½
6	mushrooms, sliced	6
½	small zucchini, sliced thinly on the diagonal	½

1. Boil the rice in plenty of water for 15 to 20 minutes or until tender, then drain.

2. In a small saucepan, add enough water to cover eggs and add the vinegar to stop eggs from cracking. Bring water to a boil and add the eggs, cooking on high for 5 minutes for soft-boiled or 7 minutes for a hard-boiled yolk.

3. Heat the oil in a saucepan and sauté the onion and mushrooms on high heat for 2 minutes, stirring often. Then add zucchini and sauté for a further 1 to 2 minutes, mixing constantly. Zucchini should not be overcooked; it should be crisp and slightly browned.

4. Peel the eggs, halve them and place the eggs and rice on a plate. Serve vegetables on top of the rice.

NUTRIENTS PER SERVING			
Calories	296	Protein	11 g
Total Fat	14.5 g	Biotin	12 mcg (4% DV)
Saturated Fat	2.7 g	Vitamin C	9 mg (15% DV)
Omega-3	0.2 g	Iron	1.8 mg (10% DV)
Carbohydrate	29 g	Magnesium	61 mg (15% DV)
Fiber	2.8 g (11% DV)	Zinc	1.6 mg (11% DV)

Fish and Steamed Vegetables

Makes 2 servings

This meal makes a healthy breakfast, lunch or light dinner. Favor the use of omega-3-rich salmon or trout.

- **Steamer basket**

1	large carrot, thinly sliced	1
1 cup	chopped broccoli	250 mL
1½ cups	spinach or chopped Swiss chard	375 mL
2	pieces fish fillet (each 6 oz/175 g)	2
	Juice of ½ lemon (optional)	
	Ground black pepper (optional)	

1. Place some water in a saucepan that has a steamer basket and bring to a boil. Place carrots, broccoli and spinach in the steamer and cook for 2 minutes (maximum of 3 minutes) on high.

2. In a large skillet, cook fish for 2 minutes on each side or until cooked through.

3. Sprinkle fish and vegetables with lemon juice and pepper, if desired. Serve immediately.

NUTRIENTS PER SERVING			
Calories	192	Protein	34 g
Total Fat	2.5 g	Biotin	15 mcg (5% DV)
Saturated Fat	0.5 g	Vitamin C	38 mg (63% DV)
Omega-3	0.5 g	Iron	1.3 mg (7% DV)
Carbohydrate	7 g	Magnesium	53 mg (13% DV)
Fiber	2.9 g (12% DV)	Zinc	0.9 mg (6% DV)

Beans on Toast

This simple and tasty vegetarian breakfast is rich in fiber and vitamin C. If you have eczema, omit the tomatoes and olive oil, and instead use 1 tsp (15 mL) rice bran oil and season with sea salt, if necessary.

1 tsp	extra virgin olive oil	5 mL
½	onion, finely chopped	½
½ tsp	paprika	2 mL
½ cup	drained rinsed canned kidney beans	125 mL
½ cup	drained rinsed canned butter (lima) beans or other white beans	125 mL
½ cup	canned diced tomatoes	125 mL
4 tsp	finely chopped parsley	20 mL
1 tsp	chopped oregano	5 mL
4	slices whole-grain bread, toasted	4
	Ground black pepper (optional)	

1. Heat the oil in a large saucepan on medium heat. Cook the onion and paprika, stirring, for 3 minutes, until onion becomes translucent.

2. Add the kidney beans, butter beans and tomatoes and simmer for 6 to 8 minutes, stirring occasionally, until sauce thickens. Mix in parsley and oregano and serve on toast. Season with pepper, if desired.

NUTRIENTS PER SERVING			
Calories	288	Protein	15 g
Total Fat	5.2 g	Biotin	10 mcg (3% DV)
Saturated Fat	0.8 g	Vitamin C	18 mg (30% DV)
Omega-3	0.1 g	Iron	3.8 mg (21% DV)
Carbohydrate	48 g	Magnesium	46 mg (12% DV)
Fiber	11.1 g (44% DV)	Zinc	1.0 mg (7% DV)

Kids' Scrambled Eggs

Makes 4 servings

Children love fun food, so use low-strength chlorophyll to turn scrambled eggs a pleasant shade of green, then tell the kids you're serving "green eggs" à la Dr. Seuss or "Shrek" eggs.

2	large free-range eggs, lightly beaten	2
4 tsp	calcium-fortified soy milk	20 mL
	Sea salt	
1 tsp	finely chopped parsley	5 mL
½ tsp	low-strength liquid chlorophyll (optional)	2 mL
½ tsp	extra virgin olive oil or rice bran oil	2 mL
4	slices whole-grain bread, toasted	4

1. In a bowl, mix eggs, soy milk, salt, parsley and chlorophyll (if using).

2. Heat the oil in a nonstick skillet on medium heat and add egg mixture. Stir continuously for 2 to 4 minutes, until egg is just cooked. Do not burn or brown eggs. Serve with toast.

NUTRIENTS PER SERVING			
Calories	119	Protein	7 g
Total Fat	4.3 g	Biotin	7 mcg (2% DV)
Saturated Fat	1.0 g	Vitamin C	1 mg (2% DV)
Omega-3	0.1 g	Iron	1.2 mg (7% DV)
Carbohydrate	12 g	Magnesium	24 mg (6% DV)
Fiber	1.9 g (8% DV)	Zinc	0.7 mg (5% DV)

Kids' Creamy Beans on Toast

Makes 2 to 4 servings

This recipe is suitable for children over the age of 1, especially those with eczema and other skin problems. The bean mix can also be puréed for children as young as 8 months old (but leave out the salt and syrup). Make this recipe even more fun for children by coloring it green with low-strength chlorophyll and telling them it's "Shrek Beans on Toast." If your kids are fussy, add the maple syrup; otherwise, omit it, as this meal is also nice when savory. Make sure the bread used is preservative-free. White navy (pea) beans or cannellini (white kidney) beans are best for this meal.

Tip

Children generally prefer a bright green color (the first time I cooked this, my daughter complained that the Shrek Beans weren't green enough).

1/4 to 1/2 cup	calcium-fortified soy milk	60 to 125 mL
1 tsp	whole wheat flour	5 mL
1 to 2 cups	canned white beans, drained and rinsed	250 to 500 mL
Pinch	sea salt	Pinch
1/2 to 1 tsp	pure maple syrup (optional)	2 to 5 mL
1 tsp	finely chopped parsley	5 mL
1/2 to 1 1/2 tsp	low-strength liquid chlorophyll (optional)	2 to 7 mL
2	slices whole-grain bread, toasted and crusts removed	2

1. In a small saucepan, mix soy milk and flour until lump-free, then heat, stirring as it simmers. Add beans, salt, maple syrup and parsley, stirring often. Cook until thickened and beans are soft. Remove from heat.

2. Stir in chlorophyll, 1/2 tsp (2 mL) at a time, until desired color is achieved. Serve warm, on top of toast. Plain butter can be sparingly used on toast.

NUTRIENTS PER SERVING			
Calories	101	Protein	6 g
Total Fat	0.8 g	Biotin	3 mcg (1% DV)
Saturated Fat	0.0 g	Vitamin C	0 mg (0% DV)
Omega-3	0.1 g	Iron	1.4 mg (8% DV)
Carbohydrate	20 g	Magnesium	3 mg (1% DV)
Fiber	5.7 g (23% DV)	Zinc	0.1 mg (1% DV)

Sauces, Dips and Salad Dressings

Creamy Mayonnaise 380

Tartar Sauce 381

Tuna Dip 381

Hummus 382

Aïoli 383

Sweet Chile Sauce 383

Sweet Chutney 384

Tomato Sauce 385

Tasty Salad Dressing 386

Omega Salad Dressing 386

Creamy Mayonnaise

This tasty mayonnaise is unique, as it contains 3.8 g of omega-3. It's free of raw egg white, so it won't cause a biotin deficiency. The apple cider vinegar is not only alkalizing but also works as a natural preservative. The leftover egg whites can be used in an egg white omelet: try the Tasty Omelet recipe (page 367), replacing 2 of the eggs with 3 egg whites. If you have eczema, omit the curry powder and mustard.

Tip

This recipe contains raw egg yolks. If the food safety of raw eggs is a concern for you, look for pasteurized-in-shell eggs, or use 6 tbsp (90 mL) pasteurized liquid whole egg instead.

3	pasteurized-in-shell free-range egg yolks	3
4 tsp	apple cider vinegar	20 mL
4 tsp	lemon juice	20 mL
Pinch	fine sea salt	Pinch
¼ cup	extra virgin olive oil	60 mL
½ cup	flaxseed oil	125 mL
Pinch	finely ground pepper	Pinch
Pinch	curry powder (optional)	Pinch
Dash	Dijon mustard (optional)	Dash

1. Using a wooden spoon, a whisk or a small food processor, beat together the egg yolks, vinegar, lemon juice and salt until smooth. Gradually add olive oil, 1 tbsp (15 mL) at a time, and beat very well after each addition. Add flaxseed oil, 1 tbsp (15 mL) at a time, and beat until thick and creamy.

2. Adjust the taste to your liking: you can add another 4 tsp (20 mL) lemon juice or more curry powder or Dijon mustard, and salt and pepper. Store in a sterilized jar and keep refrigerated (see tips, page 384). Will keep for 1 week.

NUTRIENTS PER 1 TBSP (15 ML)			
Calories	103	Protein	0 g
Total Fat	11.4 g	Biotin	2 mcg (1% DV)
Saturated Fat	1.4 g	Vitamin C	1 mg (2% DV)
Omega-3	3.8 g	Iron	0.1 mg (1% DV)
Carbohydrate	0 g	Magnesium	0 mg (0% DV)
Fiber	0.0 g (0% DV)	Zinc	0.1 mg (1% DV)

Tartar Sauce

Makes 1 cup (250 mL)

This healthy and tasty tartar sauce is a great addition to steamed or pan-fried fish.

1 tsp	capers, finely chopped	5 mL
1 tsp	finely chopped parsley	5 mL
1 tsp	minced green onion or onion	5 mL
1	recipe Creamy Mayonnaise (page 380)	1

1. Add capers, parsley and green onion to mayonnaise and mix.

NUTRIENTS PER 1 TBSP (15 ML)			
Calories	7	Protein	0 g
Total Fat	0.7 g	Biotin	0 mcg (0% DV)
Saturated Fat	0.1 g	Vitamin C	0 mg (0% DV)
Omega-3	0.2 g	Iron	0.0 mg (0% DV)
Carbohydrate	0 g	Magnesium	0 mg (0% DV)
Fiber	0.0 g (0% DV)	Zinc	0.0 mg (0% DV)

Tuna Dip

Makes 2 cups (500 mL)

This delicious dip is perfect for serving guests and goes well with plain crackers, sourdough bread and chopped vegetable sticks. Use quality chunky-style tuna in spring water or olive oil.

Tip

For presentation, top with a sprig of parsley or a few chopped green onions.

2½	cans (each 6 oz/170 g) chunky-style tuna, drained well	2½
1	recipe Creamy Mayonnaise (page 380)	1
¼ cup	finely chopped green onions (green parts only)	60 mL
4 tsp	lemon juice	20 mL
1	large clove garlic, minced	1
	Sea salt and ground black pepper (optional)	

1. Mash the tuna in a bowl and add mayonnaise (there should be no dry or chunky bits of tuna). Mix in green onions, lemon juice and garlic. Add salt and pepper, if desired.

NUTRIENTS PER ¼ CUP (60 ML)			
Calories	70	Protein	10 g
Total Fat	2.7 g	Biotin	0 mcg (0% DV)
Saturated Fat	0.5 g	Vitamin C	3 mg (5% DV)
Omega-3	0.9 g	Iron	0.5 mg (3% DV)
Carbohydrate	1 g	Magnesium	14 mg (4% DV)
Fiber	0.0 g (0% DV)	Zinc	0.2 mg (1% DV)

Hummus

This gluten-free dip is a source of protein and contains alkalizing lemon and garlic. If you have eczema, or if you want this dip to contain omega-3, use flaxseed oil or rice bran oil instead of olive oil. Serve with carrot, celery and bell pepper sticks.

Tips

If you have a larger can of chickpeas, use 1½ cups (375 mL), drained and rinsed. Refrigerate any extra in an airtight container for up to 5 days.

If refrigerated, hummus will stay fresh for up to 1 week.

1	can (14 oz/398 mL) chickpeas	1
3	cloves garlic, minced	3
6 tbsp	tahini (sesame seed paste)	90 mL
	Juice of 2 lemons	
¼ cup	extra virgin olive oil or flaxseed oil	60 mL
	Sea salt and ground black pepper	
	Paprika	
	Chopped parsley	

1. Drain and rinse the chickpeas and discard any discolored ones, then place in a food processor. Add garlic, tahini, lemon juice and oil and blend on high speed for up to 5 minutes, until puréed. Add extra lemon juice if the dip is too thick. Taste the mixture and season with salt and pepper, if necessary. Garnish with paprika and parsley.

NUTRIENTS PER ¼ CUP (60 ML)			
Calories	195	Protein	5 g
Total Fat	13.7 g	Biotin	5 mcg (2% DV)
Saturated Fat	1.9 g	Vitamin C	7 mg (12% DV)
Omega-3	0.1 g	Iron	1.2 mg (7% DV)
Carbohydrate	15 g	Magnesium	26 mg (7% DV)
Fiber	2.8 g (11% DV)	Zinc	1.1 mg (7% DV)

Aïoli

Makes 1 cup (250 mL)

Aïoli is a delicious garlic dipping sauce suitable for fish and for vegetable sticks such as carrots and green beans.

2	cloves garlic, minced	2
1 tsp	finely chopped parsley	5 mL
1	recipe Creamy Mayonnaise (page 380)	1

1. Add garlic and parsley to mayonnaise and mix.

NUTRIENTS PER 1 TBSP (15 ML)			
Calories	7	Protein	0 g
Total Fat	0.7 g	Biotin	0 mcg (0% DV)
Saturated Fat	0.1 g	Vitamin C	0 mg (0% DV)
Omega-3	0.2 g	Iron	0.0 mg (0% DV)
Carbohydrate	0 g	Magnesium	0 mg (0% DV)
Fiber	0.0 g (0% DV)	Zinc	0.0 mg (0% DV)

Sweet Chile Sauce

Makes about 6 tbsp (90 mL)

This sauce is not your traditional sweet chili, as it is runny like a gourmet Thai dipping sauce. Delish with Vegetable Hand Rolls (page 388), spring rolls or Shrimp and Sweet Chile Vegetable Stir-Fry (page 418), it's gluten-free if you use tamari.

1	small red chile pepper, thinly sliced	1
4 tsp	honey, melted	20 mL
3 tbsp	lime juice	45 mL
4 tsp	apple cider vinegar	20 mL
½ tsp	tamari or soy sauce	2 mL

1. Mix together chile pepper, honey, lime juice, vinegar and tamari and let stand for at least 30 minutes before serving. Keeps for 1 week if refrigerated.

NUTRIENTS PER 1 TBSP (15 ML)			
Calories	22	Protein	0 g
Total Fat	0.0 g	Biotin	0 mcg (0% DV)
Saturated Fat	0.0 g	Vitamin C	12 mg (20% DV)
Omega-3	0.0 g	Iron	0.1 mg (1% DV)
Carbohydrate	6 g	Magnesium	2 mg (1% DV)
Fiber	0.1 g (0% DV)	Zinc	0.0 mg (0% DV)

Sweet Chutney

Makes about 4½ cups (1.125 L)

This gluten-free mango chutney contains less than half the sugar of store-bought chutneys, but tastes just as sweet. It can be served on curries or mixed into Roasted Sweet Potato Salad (page 434), and is wonderful for marinating fish. Not suitable for children with eczema.

Tips

After cooking chutneys, jams and sauces, immediately store them in hot sterilized jars. Scoop the mixture into these jars with a sterilized metal spoon or measuring cup. To sterilize jars, their lids and utensils, boil them for 5 to 10 minutes in a very large pot with enough water to cover them. To remove equipment, use tongs (remembering to sterilize the ends only). Seal jars with lids while hot.

This recipe is not safe for home canning and must be stored in the refrigerator (not at room temperature).

- **Hot sterilized jars with lids (see tip, at left)**

2 tsp	extra virgin olive oil	10 mL
2 tsp	cumin seeds	10 mL
1 tsp	mustard seeds	5 mL
4	cloves garlic, finely diced or minced	4
1	large onion, chopped	1
2 tsp	grated gingerroot	10 mL
2 tsp	ground coriander	10 mL
1 tsp	ground turmeric	5 mL
½ cup	apple cider vinegar	125 mL
¼ cup	white vinegar	60 mL
¾ cup	packed brown sugar	175 mL
3 to 4	large mangos (about 3 lbs/1.5 kg), diced	3 to 4
½ cup	raisins, chopped	125 mL
1 tsp	finely ground sea salt	5 mL

1. In a large saucepan, heat the oil on medium and cook cumin seeds and mustard seeds, stirring, until they pop. Add the garlic, onion and ginger. Mix until onion is translucent, then add the coriander and turmeric and cook until the spices are fragrant, stirring regularly.

2. In a bowl, mix the cider vinegar, white vinegar and sugar, then add to the saucepan. Stir in mangos, raisins and salt. Simmer, uncovered, for 1 hour, stirring regularly to prevent the bottom of the chutney from burning.

3. Pour the chutney into prepared jars and seal while hot (see tip, at left). Let cool, then store in the refrigerator for up to 1 month.

Variation

Add 1 small red chile pepper, finely chopped.

NUTRIENTS PER 1 TBSP (15 ML)			
Calories	27	Protein	0 g
Total Fat	0.2 g	Biotin	0 mcg (0% DV)
Saturated Fat	0.0 g	Vitamin C	7 mg (12% DV)
Omega-3	0.0 g	Iron	0.1 mg (1% DV)
Carbohydrate	6 g	Magnesium	3 mg (1% DV)
Fiber	0.4 g (2% DV)	Zinc	0.0 mg (0% DV)

Tomato Sauce

**Makes about
3½ cups
(875 mL)**

This sauce is rich in vitamin C, bursting with tangy tomato flavor and gluten-free if the mustard used is free of wheat gluten. To make a darker red sauce, add 1 chopped red bell pepper in the initial cooking phase. Not suitable for people with eczema.

- **Muslin bag or cheesecloth**
- **Hot sterilized jars (see tip, page 384) or airtight containers (optional)**

2 lbs	ripe Roma (plum) tomatoes, roughly chopped	1 kg
1	large red onion, diced	1
6 tbsp	apple cider vinegar	90 mL
3 tbsp	packed brown sugar	45 mL
1 tsp	fine sea salt	5 mL
½ to 1 tsp	Dijon mustard (to taste)	2 to 5 mL
½ tsp	paprika (or to taste)	2 mL
1	cinnamon stick	1
1 tsp	whole allspice	5 mL
1 tsp	celery seeds	5 mL
1 tsp	black peppercorns	5 mL

1. In a large saucepan, combine the tomatoes and onion, and cook on medium heat for 15 minutes or until very soft, stirring occasionally. Remove and briefly purée in batches in a blender (if the mixture is too thick to purée, add the vinegar during this step). Then push through a coarse-mesh sieve or a food mill to remove seeds and skin.

2. Return to a smaller pot and add the vinegar, sugar, salt, mustard and paprika. Place the cinnamon stick, allspice, celery seeds and peppercorns in the muslin bag and secure the bag tightly. Add the bag to the sauce and bring to a boil.

3. Reduce to a simmer, stirring often, and cook for 20 to 40 minutes, until the mixture reduces and thickens. Taste the mixture and add more mustard and paprika, if necessary. Remove muslin bag.

4. Pour the tomato sauce into prepared jars or containers, if desired. Store in the refrigerator for up to 1 week or in the freezer for up to 6 months.

NUTRIENTS PER ½ CUP (125 ML)			
Calories	69	Protein	1 g
Total Fat	0.6 g	Biotin	6 mcg (2% DV)
Saturated Fat	0.0 g	Vitamin C	23 mg (38% DV)
Omega-3	0.0 g	Iron	0.7 mg (4% DV)
Carbohydrate	16 g	Magnesium	5 mg (1% DV)
Fiber	1.5 g (6% DV)	Zinc	0.1 mg (1% DV)

Tasty Salad Dressing

This healthy salad dressing is the star ingredient of the Tasty Spinach Salad (page 432), but it can be used with any lettuce-based salad. You can even use it to flavor salad in wraps or burgers. This recipe is only gluten-free if the chutney, sweet chile sauce and mustard are gluten-free.

Tip

The dressing keeps in the refrigerator for weeks.

6 tbsp	flaxseed oil	90 mL
1/3 cup	apple cider vinegar	75 mL
3 tbsp	Sweet Chutney (page 384) or mango chutney	45 mL
2 tsp	grainy mustard	10 mL
2 tsp	sweet chile sauce (page 383 or store-bought)	10 mL
1/2 tsp	mild curry powder	2 mL
	Salt and ground black pepper	

1. Blend oil, vinegar, chutney, mustard, chile sauce, curry powder, salt and pepper together and let stand for at least 30 minutes before serving.

NUTRIENTS PER 1 TBSP (15 ML)			
Calories	60	Protein	0 g
Total Fat	5.2 g	Biotin	0 mcg (0% DV)
Saturated Fat	0.5 g	Vitamin C	3 mg (5% DV)
Omega-3	2.7 g	Iron	0.1 mg (1% DV)
Carbohydrate	3 g	Magnesium	2 mg (1% DV)
Fiber	0.2 g (1% DV)	Zinc	0.0 mg (0% DV)

Omega Salad Dressing

This sweet, gluten-free, therapeutic salad dressing is specifically designed for people with eczema, but anyone can enjoy it.

Tip

The dressing keeps in the refrigerator for weeks.

1/4 cup	flaxseed oil	60 mL
1/4 cup	apple cider vinegar	60 mL
1	clove garlic, crushed and finely diced	1
2 tbsp	pure maple syrup	30 mL

1. Combine oil, vinegar, garlic and maple syrup and serve on your favorite salad.

NUTRIENTS PER 1 TBSP (15 ML)			
Calories	63	Protein	0 g
Total Fat	5.5 g	Biotin	0 mcg (0% DV)
Saturated Fat	0.5 g	Vitamin C	0 mg (0% DV)
Omega-3	2.9 g	Iron	0.0 mg (0% DV)
Carbohydrate	4 g	Magnesium	1 mg (0% DV)
Fiber	0.0 g (0% DV)	Zinc	0.1 mg (1% DV)

Snacks

Vegetable Hand Rolls 388

Miso Soup 389

Avocado Salsa 390

Avocado Beauty Snack 390

Avocado Dip with Dipping Sticks. 391

Anti-Aging Broth 392

Oysters with Dipping Sauce 394

Vegetable Hand Rolls

Raw spring rolls are a healthy snack or light meal. Bean sprouts are rich in enzymes, and this meal is vegetarian if you use tofu and gluten-free if you use gluten-free sauce. The Sweet Chile Sauce (page 383) makes a perfect dipping sauce to serve with this dish.

Tip

You can use store-bought sweet chile sauce if it is free of artificial preservatives.

3 tbsp	apple cider vinegar	45 mL
2 cups	bean sprouts	500 mL
3	medium carrots, grated	3
3	green onions, ends removed and green parts sliced thinly on the diagonal	3
1 cup	fresh mint or cilantro leaves, chopped	250 mL
4 tsp to 3 tbsp	Sweet Chile Sauce (page 383)	20 to 45 mL
12 oz	firm tofu or cooked chicken, cut into thin strips	375 g
20	round rice paper wrappers	20

1. Add the vinegar to a bowl of water and wash the bean sprouts in the water. Drain and dry with a clean tea towel.

2. In a small bowl, combine carrots, green onions, mint and sweet chile sauce. Wet another tea towel, wring out excess water and place flat on bench. Then soften rice paper (two at a time) in a large bowl of very warm water, soaking each for 10 seconds. Remove and place flat on damp tea towel.

3. Put about 2 tbsp (30 mL) of carrot mixture on the rice paper near the end closest to you; add slices of tofu and bean sprouts on top, then roll up, tucking the ends in about halfway so they look like cylinders. Serve immediately or store in plastic wrap in the refrigerator for up to 6 hours.

NUTRIENTS PER ROLL			
Calories	58	Protein	3 g
Total Fat	1.0 g	Biotin	1 mcg (0% DV)
Saturated Fat	0.1 g	Vitamin C	3 mg (5% DV)
Omega-3	0.0 g	Iron	0.5 mg (3% DV)
Carbohydrate	10 g	Magnesium	5 mg (1% DV)
Fiber	0.7 g (3% DV)	Zinc	0.1 mg (1% DV)

Miso Soup

Makes 4 servings

This vegetarian soup is a quick and tasty snack, and goes well as a side dish to the Vegetable Hand Rolls (page 388).

¼	sheet kombu (seaweed), cut into small, thin strips (about 4 tsp/20 mL)	¼
4 cups	water	1 L
½ cup	finely chopped green onions	125 mL
3½ oz	soft silken tofu, diced	100 g
3 tbsp	miso paste	45 mL
	Tamari (optional)	

1. Boil kombu in the water for 10 minutes or until seaweed becomes soft, then remove from heat.

2. Add green onions and tofu; stir in the miso paste (miso should not be boiled). Add a dash of tamari if extra saltiness is desired.

NUTRIENTS PER SERVING			
Calories	37	Protein	3 g
Total Fat	1.3 g	Biotin	1 mcg (0% DV)
Saturated Fat	0.1 g	Vitamin C	6 mg (10% DV)
Omega-3	0.1 g	Iron	0.7 mg (4% DV)
Carbohydrate	4 g	Magnesium	12 mg (3% DV)
Fiber	0.6 g (2% DV)	Zinc	0.2 mg (1% DV)

Avocado Salsa

Makes 4 servings

This tangy salsa is alkalizing. Perfect as a snack on sourdough bread or served alongside fish. Not suitable if you have eczema.

1	large avocado, diced	1
1/2	red onion, finely diced	1/2
1	vine-ripened tomato, seeds removed and diced	1
1 1/2 cups	flat-leaf (Italian) parsley leaves, finely chopped	375 mL
	Juice of 1 lime	
	Ground black pepper	
8	slices sourdough bread, toasted	8

1. Combine avocado, onion, tomato, parsley, lime juice and pepper and serve on sourdough toast.

NUTRIENTS PER SERVING			
Calories	329	Protein	11 g
Total Fat	9.1 g	Biotin	4 mcg (1% DV)
Saturated Fat	1.5 g	Vitamin C	44 mg (73% DV)
Omega-3	0.1 g	Iron	4.7 mg (26% DV)
Carbohydrate	53 g	Magnesium	50 mg (13% DV)
Fiber	6.5 g (26% DV)	Zinc	1.3 mg (9% DV)

Avocado Beauty Snack

Makes 2 servings

This healthy snack is rich in vitamin C. For the tuna, choose the type packed in spring water or olive oil.

1	large avocado, halved lengthwise, seed carefully removed	1
2 tbsp	drained chunky-style tuna	30 mL
	Juice of 1/2 lemon	
	Ground black pepper	

1. Top each avocado half with tuna, lemon juice and pepper.

NUTRIENTS PER SERVING			
Calories	176	Protein	4 g
Total Fat	15.1 g	Biotin	4 mcg (1% DV)
Saturated Fat	2.2 g	Vitamin C	15 mg (25% DV)
Omega-3	0.2 g	Iron	0.7 mg (4% DV)
Carbohydrate	10 g	Magnesium	33 mg (8% DV)
Fiber	6.8 g (27% DV)	Zinc	0.7 mg (5% DV)

Avocado Dip with Dipping Sticks

Makes 4 servings

This quick and healthy gluten-free snack is also ideal for serving at casual social functions. For extra spice, add a dash of cayenne pepper and one-quarter of a red onion, finely diced. Not suitable for those with eczema.

2	large ripe avocados, mashed	2
1/4 to 1/3 cup	lemon juice (from 1 large lemon)	60 to 75 mL
	Sea salt and ground black pepper	
3 to 4	large carrots	3 to 4
6	stalks celery	6
2	red bell peppers	2
	Parsley sprig (optional)	

1. Blend together the avocado, lemon juice, salt and pepper until smooth. Taste the dip and adjust the seasoning if necessary.

2. Peel the carrots, then halve them lengthwise and cut into sticks. Remove the strings from the celery with a potato peeler, then cut into sticks. Cut the bell peppers into sticks. Put vegetables on a platter and place dip beside them. Garnish with a sprig of parsley, if desired.

NUTRIENTS PER SERVING			
Calories	218	Protein	4 g
Total Fat	15.2 g	Biotin	4 mcg (1% DV)
Saturated Fat	2.2 g	Vitamin C	127 mg (212% DV)
Omega-3	0.2 g	Iron	1.2 mg (7% DV)
Carbohydrate	21 g	Magnesium	52 mg (13% DV)
Fiber	10.5 g (42% DV)	Zinc	1.1 mg (7% DV)

Anti-Aging Broth

This tasty, alkalizing, gluten-free broth is fantastic for bone, liver and skin health. It is rich in glycine and gelatin, which makes the broth thick and jelly-like when cold. Use this broth as a drink or as a tasty stock in casseroles and soups. Make it 1 day in advance, as it is important to refrigerate it overnight before use.

- **Preheat the oven to 400°F (200°C)**
- **Roasting pan**

2	large beef bones with a little meat on them	2
16 cups	filtered water (room temperature, not heated)	4 L
1	large free-range chicken carcass	1
1 tbsp	apple cider vinegar or lemon juice	15 mL
3	stalks celery (including tops)	3
1	large leek (white part only)	1
1	large carrot	1
1	large red onion	1
1	small knob fresh gingerroot	1
4	cloves garlic	4
1 tsp	good-quality sea salt (optional)	5 mL

1. Place beef bones in a roasting pan and roast in preheated oven for 30 minutes or until deliciously fragrant and browned. Remove from the oven and add them to a stockpot or very large saucepan, along with the water, chicken carcass and vinegar. Cover and bring to a boil, then simmer on low heat for 1 to 2 hours.

2. Meanwhile, wash, scrub and chop the celery, leek, carrot and onion into small pieces. Finely chop the ginger and garlic.

3. Break apart the chicken carcass with tongs to allow more of the minerals to be extracted from the bones. Add the chopped vegetables and the salt. Simmer for 6 hours. The broth should be reduced by half (add more water if it reduces more than this).

4. Use tongs to remove the larger bones. Place a strainer over a large bowl, then pour the broth through the strainer, pressing out as much liquid as possible as you strain the broth (you can use a measuring cup and press on the cooked meat and vegetables to squeeze out the remaining liquid). Discard the boiled bones and vegetables.

Tip

This broth will last for 1 week if refrigerated in an airtight container. If you plan to freeze it, ladle it into small containers — 1 cup (250 mL) per container is ideal — and write the volume on the container. You can also freeze 1-tbsp (15 mL) portions in ice cube trays, then transfer the frozen cubes to freezer bags, to use in pasta dishes and casseroles.

5. Store the broth in a sealed container in the refrigerator overnight so the fat has time to solidify. The next day, carefully lift or skim off the layer of fat (this saturated fat is no good for your skin). If your broth is thick and jelly-like, it means it's rich in gelatin.

NUTRIENTS PER 1 CUP (250 ML)			
Calories	27	Protein	3 g
Total Fat	0.5 g	Biotin	0 mcg (0% DV)
Saturated Fat	0.3 g	Vitamin C	1 mg (2% DV)
Omega-3	0.0 g	Iron	0.5 mg (3% DV)
Carbohydrate	3 g	Magnesium	8 mg (2% DV)
Fiber	0.5 g (2% DV)	Zinc	0.2 mg (1% DV)

Oysters with Dipping Sauce

Oysters are extra-special with this decorative dipping sauce. Oysters are rich in zinc, which is vital for healthy, acne-free skin. For presentation, line your platter with crushed ice before serving. Suitable for all skin conditions.

¼ cup	lemon juice	60 mL
1 cup	apple cider vinegar	250 mL
2 tbsp	finely sliced green onions	30 mL
2	cloves garlic, minced	2
½ tsp	sea salt	2 mL
1 tbsp	finely chopped parsley	15 mL
24	fresh oysters, on the half shell	24
1	lemon, sliced into wedges	1

1. Mix together the lemon juice, vinegar, green onions, garlic and salt and let stand for 30 minutes before serving.

2. Just before serving, mix in the parsley and taste to see if it needs seasoning or more lemon.

3. Arrange the oysters on a platter and decorate the platter with lemon wedges. Spoon a teaspoon (5 mL) of the lemon juice mixture on each oyster if desired and place the dipping bowl on the platter beside the oysters.

NUTRIENTS PER SERVING			
Calories	57	Protein	4 g
Total Fat	1.3 g	Biotin	0 mcg (0% DV)
Saturated Fat	0.3 g	Vitamin C	8 mg (13% DV)
Omega-3	0.0 g	Iron	2.8 mg (16% DV)
Carbohydrate	9 g	Magnesium	1 mg (0% DV)
Fiber	0.1 g (0% DV)	Zinc	22.0 mg (147% DV)

Chicken Lunches and Dinners

Therapeutic Chicken Soup 396

Chicken and Salad Sandwich 397

Chicken and Salad Wrap. 398

Herb and Garlic Chicken Casserole 399

Sweet Chicken Stir-Fry 400

C-Rich Apricot Chicken. 402

Cajun Chicken 404

Chicken and Three Veg. 406

Therapeutic Chicken Soup

This soup is fantastic for the immune system. Chicken contains cysteine, which helps to reduce mucus associated with colds and flu; garlic and vegetables contain flavonoids; and the broth is rich in glycine and gelatin. Leftovers can be frozen in serving-sized containers for up to 2 months. Cayenne pepper gives the soup a hint of spice, so omit it if serving to children. If you have eczema, omit the cayenne and mushrooms.

Tip

If using dried mushrooms, soak them for 5 minutes in boiling water, remove and chop into strips. Then add mushrooms and their soaking water to soup.

4 cups	Anti-Aging Broth (page 392)	1 L
4 cups	water	1 L
1	large red onion, finely diced	1
3	stalks celery, finely chopped	3
½ cup	finely chopped cabbage or cauliflower	125 mL
1	carrot, diced	1
2	cloves garlic, smashed and finely chopped	2
½	small knob gingerroot, peeled and finely grated	½
1	strip kombu (seaweed), cut into ½ inch (1 cm) pieces	1
4	chicken drumsticks (preferably free-range), skin removed	4
4	shiitake mushrooms, chopped (optional)	4
Pinch	cayenne pepper (optional)	Pinch
	Good-quality sea salt (optional)	

1. In a large pot, combine broth, water, onions, celery, cabbage, carrot, garlic, ginger, kombu, chicken and mushrooms. Bring to a boil. Cook for 30 minutes, then remove chicken and let cool slightly. If necessary, add more water.

2. Cut chicken from bones, discard gristle and bones (or freeze them for the next broth), and dice chicken. Return meat to the soup and cook for longer, if necessary. Add a pinch (up to 1/8 tsp/0.5 mL) of cayenne pepper to add extra flavor and spice to soup (not suitable for small children). Season with salt, if desired. Serve with whole-grain bread.

NUTRIENTS PER SERVING			
Calories	88	Protein	11 g
Total Fat	2.6 g	Biotin	3 mcg (1% DV)
Saturated Fat	0.0 g	Vitamin C	4 mg (7% DV)
Omega-3	0.0 g	Iron	0.4 mg (2% DV)
Carbohydrate	4 g	Magnesium	12 mg (3% DV)
Fiber	1.1 g (4% DV)	Zinc	0.2 mg (1% DV)

Chicken and Salad Sandwich

This sandwich has a perfect balance of alkalizing vegetables, dietary fiber and protein. If you would like to make home-cooked chicken, follow the Cajun Chicken recipe (page 404).

1	medium avocado, mashed	1
8	slices spelt bread (or spelt sourdough)	8
10 oz	cooked chicken breast (free-range, no additives), sliced	300 g
1	large carrot, grated	1
2½ cups	mixed salad greens (arugula, baby spinach, romaine)	625 mL

1. Spread the avocado over the bread. On top of the avocado, place chicken, carrot and greens. Close the sandwiches and serve.

NUTRIENTS PER SERVING			
Calories	397	Protein	27 g
Total Fat	12.6 g	Biotin	11 mcg (4% DV)
Saturated Fat	1.4 g	Vitamin C	9 mg (15% DV)
Omega-3	0.1 g	Iron	3.3 mg (18% DV)
Carbohydrate	47 g	Magnesium	37 mg (9% DV)
Fiber	10.5 g (42% DV)	Zinc	1.0 mg (7% DV)

Chicken and Salad Wrap

Makes 2 servings

This wrap gets a healthy hand from the addition of alkalizing greens, avocado, lime and beets.

½	large avocado, mashed	½
1 tsp	fresh lime juice (¼ lime)	1
2¼ tsp	Cajun seasoning (page 405 or store-bought, optional), divided	11 mL
2 to 4	spelt flour tortillas or wraps (additive-free)	2 to 4
1 cup	mixed salad leaves or baby spinach	250 mL
½	beet, peeled and grated	½
2	boneless skinless chicken thighs (free-range), fat trimmed	2
½ tsp	extra virgin olive oil	2 mL

1. Mix the avocado with the lime juice and ¼ tsp (1 mL) of the Cajun seasoning, and spread over the tortillas. Then at one end, arrange the salad leaves and grated beet.

2. Cut the chicken into 1-inch (2.5 cm) slices and season with the remaining Cajun seasoning if spicy chicken is desired. Heat oil in a skillet on high heat and cook chicken for 5 minutes, turning once, until completely cooked through. Remove from pan.

3. Place chicken on top of the salad and roll up the tortillas. Cut each wrap in half before serving.

NUTRIENTS PER SERVING			
Calories	333	Protein	20 g
Total Fat	18.5 g	Biotin	7 mcg (2% DV)
Saturated Fat	4.5 g	Vitamin C	8 mg (13% DV)
Omega-3	0.2 g	Iron	1.9 mg (11% DV)
Carbohydrate	26 g	Magnesium	43 mg (11% DV)
Fiber	7.0 g (28% DV)	Zinc	1.8 mg (12% DV)

Herb and Garlic Chicken Casserole

Makes 4 servings

This vitamin C–rich casserole is gluten-free if the stock is free of wheat or gluten. If you have eczema, omit the eggplant and cauliflower, and use cabbage and celery instead.

- **Preheat oven to 350°F (180°C)**
- **Large casserole dish with a lid**

1 lb	boneless skinless chicken thighs (free-range), fat removed, chicken chopped into ½-inch (1 cm) strips	500 g
1 tbsp	brown rice flour	15 mL
1 tsp	ground cinnamon	5 mL
½ tsp	extra virgin olive oil	2 mL
1 tsp	grated peeled gingerroot	5 mL
3	cloves garlic, minced	3
1 cup	finely diced eggplant	250 mL
2 cups	chopped cauliflower	500 mL
2 cups	chopped sweet potato	500 mL
3 cups	Anti-Aging Broth (page 392) or vegetable stock (organic or additive-free)	750 mL
½ tsp	dried basil	2 mL
½ cup	flat-leaf (Italian) parsley leaves, chopped	125 mL
2 cups	cooked basmati rice	500 mL

1. Place the chicken, flour and cinnamon in a plastic bag, seal and shake to coat the chicken. Heat the oil in a skillet and quickly fry the chicken pieces for 1 to 2 minutes so they're partially cooked. Remove and place in casserole dish.

2. Add ginger, garlic, eggplant, cauliflower, sweet potato and broth to the dish. Sprinkle with basil, then cover with the lid.

3. Bake for 40 minutes or until the chicken is cooked through. Stir a couple of times during cooking.

4. Remove from heat and stir in parsley. Serve with warm rice in large bowls.

NUTRIENTS PER SERVING			
Calories	375	Protein	32 g
Total Fat	7.0 g	Biotin	9 mcg (3% DV)
Saturated Fat	1.6 g	Vitamin C	40 mg (67% DV)
Omega-3	0.2 g	Iron	3.6 mg (20% DV)
Carbohydrate	45 g	Magnesium	114 mg (29% DV)
Fiber	6.7 g (27% DV)	Zinc	3.7 mg (25% DV)

Sweet Chicken Stir-Fry

This tasty stir-fry is rich in vitamin C, protein and cancer-protective indoles, and it's gluten-free. If you have eczema or salicylate sensitivity, leave out the mango.

1 tsp	garlic powder	5 mL
2 tbsp	brown rice flour	30 mL
½ tsp	ground cinnamon	2 mL
1 lb	boneless skinless chicken thighs (free-range), fat trimmed, chicken thinly sliced	500 g
1 tsp	rice bran oil	5 mL
½ cup	Anti-Aging Broth (page 392)	125 mL
2 cups	finely chopped red cabbage (about 7 oz/210 g)	500 mL
2 cups	thinly sliced green onions (sliced on the diagonal)	500 mL
4	large stalks celery, finely chopped	4
	Good-quality sea salt	
1	medium mango, peeled and diced (or 1 small papaya, cut into chunks)	1
1½ cups	basmati rice, cooked	375 mL

1. Mix together the garlic powder, rice flour and cinnamon and place in a plastic bag. Add the chicken, seal the bag and shake to coat the chicken pieces.

2. Heat half the oil in a large skillet on medium to high heat, and cook the chicken for 5 minutes or until it is cooked through. Do not let the rice flour burn. Remove the chicken and set aside. Add the broth to the pan and mix with the rice flour remaining in the pan. Once it has thickened, pour the broth onto the cooked chicken and set aside. Clean the pan in preparation for stir-frying the vegetables.

3. Heat $\frac{1}{2}$ tsp (2 mL) of the oil in the skillet and quickly stir-fry the red cabbage, green onions and celery on high heat, adding a sprinkle of salt. Continuously stir the vegetables for 1 minute, then add the chicken and broth and cook for 1 to 2 minutes or until heated through. Cook the vegetables for no longer than 3 minutes, as you want them to be crisp and tasty. Remove from the heat and stir in half the mango slices.

4. Serve stir-fry on a bed of rice and garnish with the remaining mango.

NUTRIENTS PER SERVING			
Calories	315	Protein	26 g
Total Fat	6.8 g	Biotin	7 mcg (2% DV)
Saturated Fat	1.6 g	Vitamin C	55 mg (92% DV)
Omega-3	0.2 g	Iron	3.7 mg (21% DV)
Carbohydrate	37 g	Magnesium	77 mg (19% DV)
Fiber	4.0 g (16% DV)	Zinc	2.9 mg (19% DV)

C-Rich Apricot Chicken

Makes 4 servings

This unique apricot chicken recipe is rich in vitamin C, and is gluten-free if the stock cube does not contain gluten. Not suitable for people with eczema.

- Preheat oven to 350°F (180°C)
- Large casserole dish with lid

1 tsp	ground turmeric	5 mL
1 tsp	ground ginger	5 mL
1 tsp	ground cinnamon	5 mL
1 tsp	Cajun seasoning (page 405 or store-bought)	5 mL
1 lb	boneless skinless chicken thighs (free-range), fat trimmed, chicken cut into 1/2 inch (1 cm) pieces	500 g
1/2 tsp	extra virgin olive oil	2 mL
1	vegetable bouillon cube (organic or no artificial additives)	1
2 cups	boiling water (filtered)	500 mL
6	ripe apricots, halved and pitted	6
1 tsp	finely grated peeled gingerroot	5 mL
2	cloves garlic, crushed and diced	2
1	large red onion, sliced chunky-style	1
2	medium carrots, sliced	2
1	medium red bell pepper, thinly sliced	1
1 1/2 cups	basmati rice (or 2 cups/500 mL long-grain brown rice)	375 mL
2 tsp	brown rice flour (optional)	10 mL
1/4 cup	cold water	60 mL
1/2 cup	chopped cilantro or flat-leaf (Italian) parsley	125 mL

1. Place the turmeric, ground ginger, cinnamon and Cajun seasoning in a plastic bag. Add the chicken, seal the bag and shake to coat the chicken pieces with the spices.

2. In a skillet, heat the oil on high heat and quickly brown chicken pieces, 1 minute each side, but do not cook right through. Transfer chicken to the casserole dish.

3. Dissolve bouillon cube in boiling water, then add to casserole.

Tip

If fresh apricots are not in season, you can use 1 can (14 to 15 oz/398 to 425 mL) apricot halves in juice (no added sugar), juice drained.

4. Add apricots, gingerroot, garlic, onion, carrots and red pepper to the casserole and mix. Cover with lid and bake for 40 minutes, stirring occasionally.

5. Meanwhile, bring a large pot of water to a boil and cook the rice. Boil basmati for 10 minutes and brown rice according to package instructions (about 20 minutes), then drain.

6. Remove the casserole from the oven and stir. If you would like to thicken the liquid, mix brown rice flour with cold water, stirring until lump-free, and add to the casserole. Replace the lid and bake for a further 10 minutes or until the chicken is cooked through. Remove the casserole dish from the heat and stir in the cilantro. Serve with the rice.

NUTRIENTS PER SERVING			
Calories	301	Protein	25 g
Total Fat	6.6 g	Biotin	9 mcg (3% DV)
Saturated Fat	1.4 g	Vitamin C	63 mg (105% DV)
Omega-3	0.1 g	Iron	2.5 mg (14% DV)
Carbohydrate	32 g	Magnesium	71 mg (18% DV)
Fiber	4.7 g (19% DV)	Zinc	2.9 mg (19% DV)

Cajun Chicken

Makes 4 to 5 servings

Serve with a side salad such as Garden Salad (page 437); Sweet Raspberry, Avocado and Watercress Salad (page 431) or vegetables and rice.

1¼ lbs	boneless skinless chicken breasts or thighs (free-range), fat trimmed	625 g
2 tbsp	Cajun seasoning (see opposite or store-bought)	30 mL
2 tsp	extra virgin olive oil	10 mL

1. Slice the chicken pieces in half (or smaller pieces for faster cooking). Place the chicken pieces and Cajun seasoning in a plastic bag, seal and shake to coat the chicken.

2. Heat the oil in a large skillet or grill on medium to high heat and cook the chicken for 3 to 5 minutes per side or until cooked right through.

NUTRIENTS PER SERVING			
Calories	165	Protein	29 g
Total Fat	4.1 g	Biotin	5 mcg (2% DV)
Saturated Fat	0.8 g	Vitamin C	2 mg (3% DV)
Omega-3	0.0 g	Iron	1.0 mg (6% DV)
Carbohydrate	2 g	Magnesium	39 mg (10% DV)
Fiber	0.9 g (4% DV)	Zinc	1.1 mg (7% DV)

Cajun Seasoning

This spicy seasoning
makes chicken and fish
delicious.

⅓ cup	sweet paprika	75 mL
4 tsp	garlic powder	20 mL
2 tsp	dried oregano	10 mL
2 tsp	dried thyme	10 mL
1 tsp	ground cinnamon	5 mL
1 tsp	ground black pepper	5 mL
1 tsp	finely ground sea salt	5 mL
½ tsp	cayenne pepper	2 mL

1. Mix together paprika, garlic powder, oregano, thyme, cinnamon, black pepper, salt and cayenne. Store in an airtight jar.

NUTRIENTS PER 1 TSP (5 ML)			
Calories	7	Protein	0 g
Total Fat	0.2 g	Biotin	0 mcg (0% DV)
Saturated Fat	0.0 g	Vitamin C	0 mg (0% DV)
Omega-3	0.0 g	Iron	0.4 mg (2% DV)
Carbohydrate	1 g	Magnesium	3 mg (1% DV)
Fiber	0.7 g (3% DV)	Zinc	0.1 mg (1% DV)

Chicken and Three Veg

Makes 4 servings

This is a tasty way to serve chicken, and it's accompanied by specially selected vegetables for maximum nutrition and flavor. The meal is gluten-free if you use malt-free soy milk. If you have eczema, omit the Cajun seasoning, cook with rice bran oil and use green beans and cabbage instead of broccoli and snow peas.

1¼ lbs	sweet potatoes (about 2 medium), peeled and diced	625 g
¼ cup	organic soy milk	60 mL
	Ground cinnamon	
1 lb	boneless skinless chicken thighs (free-range), fat trimmed, chicken sliced	500 g
2 tbsp	Cajun Seasoning (page 405 or store-bought)	30 mL
1 tsp	extra virgin olive oil	5 mL
10 oz	frenched green beans or snow peas, trimmed	300 g
2 cups	chopped broccoli (about 10 oz/300 g)	500 mL

1. In a saucepan, bring some water to a boil and cook the sweet potato for 10 minutes or until very soft, then strain and return the sweet potato to the saucepan. Mash until lump-free, then stir in soy milk and a sprinkle of cinnamon. Keep the mixture in the saucepan.

2. Place the chicken and Cajun seasoning in a plastic bag, seal and shake to coat the chicken. Heat the oil in a large skillet or grill on medium to high heat and cook the chicken for 3 to 4 minutes per side or until cooked right through.

3. In a steamer, steam the beans and broccoli for 2 to 3 minutes (maximum) — do not overcook the vegetables, as they must be slightly crisp. Reheat the mash on the stovetop if necessary.

NUTRIENTS PER SERVING			
Calories	331	Protein	30 g
Total Fat	6.9 g	Biotin	12 mcg (4% DV)
Saturated Fat	1.6 g	Vitamin C	61 mg (102% DV)
Omega-3	0.2 g	Iron	4.1 mg (23% DV)
Carbohydrate	38 g	Magnesium	74 mg (19% DV)
Fiber	7.9 g (32% DV)	Zinc	3.0 mg (20% DV)

Fish and Seafood

Omega Niçoise Salad 408

Tuna and Avocado Wrap. 409

Salmon and Salad Sandwich. 410

Thai Fish with Corn 411

Rainbow Trout with Honey-Roasted Vegetables. 412

Marinated Whole Steamed Trout. 414

Salmon Steaks with Peas and Mash. 416

Shrimp and Sweet Chile Vegetable Stir-Fry 418

Seafood Hotpot. 420

Omega Niçoise Salad

<table>
<tr><td>Makes 4 servings</td></tr>
</table>

This delicious salad is best when you use quality chunky-style tuna or freshly baked trout or salmon. It's gluten-free if the mustard is free of wheat products.

4	large free-range eggs	4
2	cans (each 6 oz/170 g) quality chunky-style tuna, drained well	2
1¼ lbs	baby potatoes, scrubbed and quartered	625 g
10 oz	baby green beans, ends trimmed, halved	300 g
2 cups	grape tomatoes, halved	500 mL
½ cup	small black olives	125 mL
¼	red onion, sliced into thin rings	¼

Anchovy Dressing

6	anchovy fillets, drained	6
⅓ cup	flaxseed oil or extra virgin olive oil	75 mL
4 tsp	Dijon mustard	20 mL
¼ cup	apple cider vinegar	60 mL

1. Place the eggs in a small saucepan and cover with water. Cover with a lid and bring to a boil. Cook the eggs for 8 minutes, then remove from the heat and immediately place the eggs in cold water. After a minute or so, remove the shells, then cut the eggs in half and set aside.

2. Boil the potatoes for 3 minutes, then add the beans and blanch for 1 minute only. Remove from heat and place the beans in ice cold water (to keep their color vivid). Potato can be served warm or cold.

3. *Dressing:* Blend anchovies, oil, mustard and vinegar in a small food processor until combined.

4. Combine eggs, potatoes, beans, tomatoes, olives and onion in a large bowl, cover with half the dressing, then mix gently. Then place chunks of tuna on top, and mix if necessary. Serve, then drizzle with the remaining dressing. Use within 12 hours and refrigerate if not serving immediately.

NUTRIENTS PER SERVING			
Calories	505	Protein	33 g
Total Fat	26.2 g	Biotin	12 mcg (4% DV)
Saturated Fat	3.9 g	Vitamin C	23 mg (38% DV)
Omega-3	10.2 g	Iron	3.7 mg (21% DV)
Carbohydrate	35 g	Magnesium	77 mg (19% DV)
Fiber	5.5 g (22% DV)	Zinc	1.7 mg (11% DV)

Tuna and Avocado Wrap

Spelt wraps are similar to the wheat ones, but spelt is easier to digest and better for the skin. If you have eczema, omit the avocado, red onion, olives and lime juice, and instead use romaine or iceberg lettuce, green onions, grated carrot and celery.

2	cans (each 6 oz/170 g) quality chunky-style tuna, drained well	2
1	avocado, sliced and diced	1
¼ cup	finely diced red onion	60 mL
4 tsp	finely chopped kalamata olives	20 mL
2 tsp	fresh lime juice	10 mL
	Ground black pepper (optional)	
4	large spelt tortillas or wraps (preservative-free)	4
2 cups	shredded mixed salad greens	500 mL

1. In a bowl, combine tuna, avocado, onion, olives, lime juice and pepper, and mix gently.

2. Lay the tortillas out flat and arrange the lettuce on them, then spoon a quarter of the mixture onto each. Roll the wraps into cylinders and cut each wrap in half before serving.

NUTRIENTS PER SERVING			
Calories	239	Protein	28 g
Total Fat	14.8 g	Biotin	17 mcg (6% DV)
Saturated Fat	2.5 g	Vitamin C	8 mg (13% DV)
Omega-3	0.9 g	Iron	3.0 mg (17% DV)
Carbohydrate	34 g	Magnesium	48 mg (12% DV)
Fiber	6.9 g (28% DV)	Zinc	0.8 mg (5% DV)

Salmon and Salad Sandwich

Makes 4 servings		

Salmon is full of omega-3, and you can use freshly cooked salmon or trout if desired. If you have eczema, use iceberg or romaine lettuce and omit the avocado and lime.

1	can (14.75 oz/418 g) salmon (or two 6 to 7.5 oz/170 to 213 g cans), drained	2
1	avocado, diced	1
½ cup	thinly sliced green onions	125 mL
1	carrot, grated	1
4 tsp	fresh lime juice	20 mL
½ tsp	Cajun seasoning (page 405 or store-bought, optional)	2 mL
2 cups	leafy greens or lettuce of choice, shredded	500 mL
8	slices spelt sourdough or whole-grain bread (preservative-free)	8

1. In a bowl, combine salmon, avocado, green onions, carrot, lime juice and Cajun seasoning, and mix gently.

2. Lay the bread flat and arrange lettuce on four of the slices, then spoon a quarter of the mixture onto each. Close each sandwich and cut in half before serving.

NUTRIENTS PER SERVING			
Calories	354	Protein	25 g
Total Fat	16.1 g	Biotin	6 mcg (2% DV)
Saturated Fat	2.9 g	Vitamin C	15 mg (25% DV)
Omega-3	1.4 g	Iron	2.9 mg (16% DV)
Carbohydrate	30 g	Magnesium	66 mg (17% DV)
Fiber	7.9 g (32% DV)	Zinc	1.4 mg (9% DV)

Thai Fish with Corn

- **Preheat oven to 375°F (190°C)**
- **Baking dish, lined with parchment paper**

2	pieces salmon fillet (about 14 oz/400 g total) (or fish of choice)	2
4 tsp	chopped lemongrass	20 mL
2	cloves garlic, crushed and chopped	2
½	small red chile pepper, finely sliced	½
1	lime	1
2 tbsp	tamari	30 mL
8	cobs baby corn, halved lengthwise	8
10	grape tomatoes (or cherry tomatoes)	10
½	red bell pepper, finely sliced	½
1 tbsp	sesame seeds	15 mL
1 cup	bean sprouts, washed in apple cider vinegar and water	250 mL
1	green onion, finely sliced on the diagonal	1
1 cup	cooked brown or basmati rice (optional)	250 mL

1. Place the fish in prepared baking dish and garnish with lemongrass, garlic and chile pepper.

2. Zest the lime and sprinkle ½ tsp (2 mL) over the fish. Juice the lime, mix the juice with the tamari, and pour over the fish. Place the baby corn, tomatoes and red pepper around the fish. Bake in preheated oven for about 12 minutes, depending on fish thickness. (Note that salmon is beginning to overcook if small white clumps appear on the flesh.)

3. In a skillet, toast the sesame seeds for 2 minutes, stirring regularly, being careful not to burn them. Remove seeds from the heat, transfer to a bowl and set aside.

4. Garnish the fish with bean sprouts, green onion and sesame seeds. Place vegetables on top of rice (if using).

NUTRIENTS PER SERVING			
Calories	632	Protein	51 g
Total Fat	24.6 g	Biotin	14 mcg (5% DV)
Saturated Fat	6.3 g	Vitamin C	103 mg (172% DV)
Omega-3	5.1 g	Iron	2.6 mg (14% DV)
Carbohydrate	52 g	Magnesium	229 mg (57% DV)
Fiber	8.3 g (33% DV)	Zinc	1.6 mg (11% DV)

Rainbow Trout with Honey-Roasted Vegetables

Makes 2 servings

This is the perfect way to roast vegetables with minimal oil and maximum flavor. If you have eczema, roast potato, sweet potato, carrot and rutabaga. This recipe is gluten-free if the bouillon powder does not contain gluten.

- **Preheat oven to 400°F (200°C)**
- **Shallow baking pan or dish**
- **Large steamer**

1 tbsp	honey, melted	15 mL
2 tsp	extra virgin olive oil	10 mL
½ to 1 tsp	vegetable bouillon powder	2 to 5 mL
1	medium parsnip, sliced into long, thin pieces	1
2	medium zucchini, sliced chunky on the diagonal	2
1	large carrot, sliced chunky on the diagonal	1
1	small sweet potato, peeled and sliced chunky-style	1
1	onion, halved	1
2	cloves garlic	2
	Ground black pepper	
¼ cup	fresh thyme leaves, chopped (plus extra for garnish)	60 mL
2	rainbow trout fillets (about 14 oz/400 g total), skin removed if desired	2
½	lime	½

1. In a large bowl, mix honey, olive oil and bouillon powder, making sure honey is runny. Combine parsnip, zucchini, carrot, sweet potato, onions and garlic and coat with the honey mixture, then transfer to baking pan. Season with pepper and some of the thyme. Bake in preheated oven for 20 to 30 minutes, checking regularly to avoid burning.

Make sure the stock is free of artificial additives.

2. Place the fish in steamer, garnish with thyme and steam above rapidly boiling water for 5 minutes or until cooked. Remove from heat and serve alongside roasted vegetables. Squeeze lime juice over fish and vegetables, and garnish with thyme.

NUTRIENTS PER SERVING			
Calories	486	Protein	43 g
Total Fat	17.4 g	Biotin	12 mcg (4% DV)
Saturated Fat	3.5 g	Vitamin C	40 mg (67% DV)
Omega-3	1.9 g	Iron	2.4 mg (13% DV)
Carbohydrate	38 g	Magnesium	84 mg (21% DV)
Fiber	6.0 g (24% DV)	Zinc	1.5 mg (10% DV)

Marinated Whole Steamed Trout

Makes 2 servings

Steaming the fish whole is the best way to retain most of the omega-3s. You need a large steamer for this recipe. If you have eczema, omit the sauce and season with sea salt.

- **Large steamer**
- **Small steamer**

1	whole rainbow trout (about 1¼ lbs/625 g dressed)	1
	Sea salt	
½	lime, cut into thin rounds	½
1	knob gingerroot, peeled and finely sliced	1
1	clove garlic, minced	1
1 cup	basmati rice	250 mL
1	bunch Chinese greens of choice	1
8	pieces broccolini or broccoli (2 small florets per person)	8
4	green onions, thinly sliced on the diagonal	4

Sauce

1	small knob gingerroot, peeled and grated	1
1	clove garlic, minced	1
¼ cup	tamari or soy sauce	60 mL
¼ cup	fresh lime juice	60 mL
1 tsp	honey	5 mL
4 tsp	water	20 mL
½	small red chile pepper, thinly sliced (optional)	½

1. Rinse the fish and dry with absorbent paper towels, then sprinkle generously with salt to firm up the skin, leaving salt on for 30 minutes.

2. *Sauce:* Meanwhile, place ginger, garlic, tamari, lime juice, honey, water and chile pepper (if using) in a small saucepan and simmer for 5 minutes, then set aside.

3. Wipe the salt off the trout and place lime slices, ginger and garlic inside the fish.

Tip

I use a large steel vegetable steamer, and it works just as well as the traditional Japanese basket steamers.

4. In a saucepan large enough to accommodate the large steamer, bring a small amount of water to a boil. Place the fish in the steamer and place the steamer in the saucepan. Cover with a lid and steam for 10 to 15 minutes, depending on size of fish. Do not overcook. When cooked, eyes will be white and insides will be lighter in color.

5. Boil the rice for 10 minutes, then drain.

6. In a smaller steamer, steam the greens and broccolini for 2 to 3 minutes only; they should be slightly undercooked to retain their brilliant color and crispness.

7. Reheat the sauce if necessary, then place the fish in a large dish, pour the sauce over top and garnish with green onions. Serve with rice and greens.

NUTRIENTS PER SERVING			
Calories	587	Protein	46 g
Total Fat	14.0 g	Biotin	10 mcg (3% DV)
Saturated Fat	2.0 g	Vitamin C	51 mg (85% DV)
Omega-3	2.0 g	Iron	4.0 mg (22% DV)
Carbohydrate	74 g	Magnesium	77 mg (19% DV)
Fiber	6.2 g (25% DV)	Zinc	1.0 mg (7% DV)

Salmon Steaks with Peas and Mash

Makes 2 servings

Baking the salmon steaks ensures they remain tender, and the presentation is beautiful. This recipe is gluten-free. If you have eczema, omit the chile pepper, corn and olive oil, and use rice bran oil for cooking and red cabbage instead of corn.

- **Preheat oven to 400°F (200°C)**

1	very large sweet potato, peeled and diced	1
¼ cup	organic soy milk	60 mL
	Ground black pepper (optional)	
	Extra virgin olive oil	
2	salmon steaks, with or without skin (about 14 oz/400 g total)	2
1	large clove garlic, crushed and finely chopped	1
½	small red chile pepper, finely sliced into rings	½
	Grated zest and juice of 1 lime	
2	cobs corn	2
1 cup	frozen green peas	250 mL

1. In a small saucepan, bring some water to a boil, then boil the sweet potato for 10 minutes or until very soft. Strain and return the sweet potato to the saucepan. Mash until lump-free, then stir in soy milk and pepper (if using) to make a creamy mash. Keep the mixture in the saucepan.

2. Cut two 12-inch (30 cm) long sheets of foil and cut two 11-inch (28 cm) long sheets of parchment paper. Place one sheet of parchment on top of each piece of foil and set aside.

3. Heat a dash of olive oil in a skillet on high heat and quickly fry the fish to brown the outer layer, for 1 minute each side (if the salmon steaks are very thick, cut them in half lengthwise to speed up cooking time). Remove the fish, place one steak in the middle of each sheet of parchment and fold up the edges of the foil and parchment so they cup the salmon (so the marinade does not spill out).

4. Top the fish with the garlic, chile pepper, a pinch of lime zest and the lime juice. Close the ends of the foil over the fish to make parcels and set aside on a baking sheet.

5. In a medium-sized saucepan, bring some water to a boil and cook the corn for 15 minutes. After the corn has been boiling for 10 minutes, add peas and simmer for 3 to 4 minutes, then drain.

6. Bake the fish parcels in the preheated oven for 8 to 10 minutes. Check to see if the fish is cooked to your liking. If you would like to cook the fish for longer, keep the parcels open and cook for another 2 minutes, then check again and cook for longer if necessary. If fish develops white clumps on the sides, then it is well done or overcooked; however, this cooking method should preserve its tenderness.

7. Reheat the mash on the stovetop and serve on plates with corn and peas, leaving room for the fish parcels. You can either serve the fish inside their parcels for guests to open, or take out of parcels and pour a little of the lime marinade over top.

NUTRIENTS PER SERVING			
Calories	583	Protein	48 g
Total Fat	22.3 g	Biotin	16 mcg (5% DV)
Saturated Fat	6.4 g	Vitamin C	52 mg (87% DV)
Omega-3	5.1 g	Iron	2.6 mg (14% DV)
Carbohydrate	46 g	Magnesium	239 mg (60% DV)
Fiber	9.1 g (36% DV)	Zinc	1.8 mg (12% DV)

Shrimp and Sweet Chile Vegetable Stir-Fry

This fresh-tasting stir-fry can be made with homemade or store-bought sweet chile sauce (choose one that is free of artificial additives). The recipe is gluten-free if the sauce is free of gluten. Not suitable if you have eczema.

1	clove garlic, minced	1
1/2	small red chile pepper, sliced	1/2
1/2 tsp	extra virgin olive oil	2 mL
	Juice of 1/2 lime	
1 lb	large shrimp, peeled and deveined	500 g
1¾ cups	long-grain brown rice	425 mL
	Ground cinnamon	
1 tsp	extra virgin olive oil	5 mL
1	red onion, sliced	1
2	medium zucchini, thinly sliced on the diagonal	2
1 cup	finely chopped red cabbage	250 mL
1	medium red bell pepper, thinly sliced	1
2 cups	bean sprouts, washed in water and apple cider vinegar	500 mL
1 cup	fresh cilantro leaves, chopped	250 mL
2 tbsp	sweet chile sauce (page 383 or store-bought)	30 mL

1. In a cup, mix the garlic, chile pepper, olive oil and lime juice, then pour over the shrimp.

2. In a large skillet, cook shrimp in their marinade for 2 to 3 minutes, then remove from the heat, placing both the shrimp and the juices aside.

3. Bring plenty of water to a boil and cook the rice for 20 minutes (or according to package instructions), then drain and sprinkle with cinnamon.

4. Meanwhile, clean the pan, add the oil and heat briefly, being careful not to smoke the oil, then, on high heat, cook the onion and zucchini for 1 minute only, stirring constantly. Add the cabbage and red pepper and stir-fry for 1 minute, then add the shrimp and leftover juices and stir-fry for 1 more minute, mixing constantly to prevent burning. Use a timer and do not overcook.

Tips

Chop the veggies as thin as possible to ensure a quick cooking time.

If you don't like cilantro, use flat-leaf (Italian) parsley or Thai basil.

5. If using store-bought sweet chile sauce, stir it in now. Turn off the heat and stir in the bean sprouts and coriander. Remove from the heat to prevent further cooking, as you want the vegetables to be slightly crisp and tasty.

6. Portion the rice into large bowls, then top with stir-fry. If using homemade Sweet Chile Sauce, sprinkle over each dish.

NUTRIENTS PER SERVING			
Calories	467	Protein	27 g
Total Fat	5.7 g	Biotin	5 mcg (2% DV)
Saturated Fat	0.9 g	Vitamin C	91 mg (152% DV)
Omega-3	0.2 g	Iron	2.5 mg (14% DV)
Carbohydrate	77 g	Magnesium	170 mg (43% DV)
Fiber	5.8 g (23% DV)	Zinc	3.4 mg (23% DV)

Seafood Hotpot

Makes 4 servings		

A winter treat. Choose a low-mercury fish such as salmon, trout, flathead or hake (see page 90 for a list of fish to avoid). This recipe is gluten-free if the stock and laksa are free of gluten. A side of toasted sourdough bread or basmati rice goes nicely with this meal.

1 tsp	extra virgin olive oil	5 mL
2	medium red onions, coarsely chopped	2
½	small knob gingerroot, peeled and finely chopped	½
2	cloves garlic, minced	2
1 to 2 tbsp	laksa paste	15 to 30 mL
½ cup	coconut milk	125 mL
3 cups	Anti-Aging Broth (page 392) or vegetable stock (organic or additive-free)	750 mL
1 lb	fish fillets, skin removed and cubed	500 g
10 oz	shelled mussels	300 g
10 oz	shrimp, peeled and deveined	300 g
1	red bell pepper, thinly sliced	1
1 cup	bean sprouts, washed in vinegar and water	250 mL
½ cup	fresh cilantro leaves	125 mL

1. Heat the oil in a large saucepan and sauté the onions, ginger and garlic until the onions are translucent. Stir in the laksa paste and coconut milk. Add stock and bring to a boil.

2. Add fish, mussels, shrimp and red pepper, and add extra water if desired. Cover and simmer for 8 to 10 minutes or until the seafood is cooked. Before serving, stir in the bean sprouts and cilantro.

NUTRIENTS PER SERVING			
Calories	322	Protein	37 g
Total Fat	12.0 g	Biotin	17 mcg (6% DV)
Saturated Fat	6.5 g	Vitamin C	67 mg (112% DV)
Omega-3	0.8 g	Iron	4.9 mg (27% DV)
Carbohydrate	15 g	Magnesium	94 mg (24% DV)
Fiber	2.3 g (9% DV)	Zinc	2.8 mg (19% DV)

Beef
and Lamb

Healthy Hamburger. 422

Steak Sandwiches 424

Beef Barley Soup 425

Lean Lamb and Three Veg 426

Slow-Cooked Lamb Casserole 427

Lamb Stir-Fry 428

Healthy Hamburger

Hamburgers are much healthier if made at home, as you can choose quality ground beef and use whole-grain buns. These burgers are also delish with the addition of a slice of fresh pineapple, and arugula can be used instead of romaine lettuce.

1 lb	extra-lean ground beef	500 g
½	medium red onion, finely diced	½
1	large carrot, grated, divided	1
2	slices whole-grain bread, lightly toasted and made into bread crumbs	2
3	cloves garlic, minced	3
1	vegetable bouillon cube, crumbled	1
1 tsp	mixed dried herbs	5 mL
¼ cup	parsley leaves, finely chopped	60 mL
1	large free-range egg, lightly beaten	1
4 tsp	extra virgin olive oil	20 mL
½	medium onion, cut into rings	½
4	large whole-grain hamburger buns (preservative-free)	4
3 tbsp	Sweet Chutney (page 384) or Tomato Sauce (page 385)	45 mL
4	leaves romaine lettuce, halved	4
1	tomato, sliced (optional)	1
1	beet, grated (or 8 slices canned beets)	1

1. Combine the beef, diced onion, ¼ cup (60 mL) of the carrot, bread crumbs, garlic, bouillon cube, dried herbs, parsley and egg (and add 4 tsp/20 mL of water, if necessary) and mix.

2. Form 4 large meat patties and cook on medium heat for 4 to 5 minutes each side, using a skillet, grill pan or barbecue grill greased with olive oil. At the same time, sauté the onion rings for 2 to 3 minutes, until translucent.

Tips

Use a coffee or seed grinder to make the bread crumbs.

Use a bouillon cube that is either organic or free of artificial additives.

3. Split the buns in half and, if desired, toast the insides for 1 to 2 minutes, until slightly browned, then remove and spread buns with chutney. Put two layers of lettuce on each bun, plus a meat patty, onion rings, remaining carrot, tomato and beet. Close the buns and serve immediately.

NUTRIENTS PER SERVING			
Calories	409	Protein	31 g
Total Fat	13.1 g	Biotin	8 mcg (3% DV)
Saturated Fat	2.9 g	Vitamin C	15 mg (25% DV)
Omega-3	0.1 g	Iron	4.5 mg (25% DV)
Carbohydrate	44 g	Magnesium	53 mg (13% DV)
Fiber	6.2 g (25% DV)	Zinc	5.8 mg (39% DV)

Steak Sandwiches

Makes 2 servings

This steak sandwich gets its healthy status from my nutritious version of Aïoli (page 383) and spelt bread. To increase the meal size, serve the sandwiches with a side salad such as Garden Salad (page 437).

1 tsp	extra virgin olive oil	5 mL
1	small red onion, sliced into rings	1
2	boneless beef fast-frying steaks (thin slices of sirloin or tenderloin) (about 7 oz/210 g total)	2
	Sea salt and ground black pepper (optional)	
4	slices spelt bread, toasted	4
3 tbsp	Aïoli (page 383) or Tomato Sauce (page 385)	45 mL
1 cup	mixed salad leaves or lettuce of choice	250 mL
1	medium carrot, grated	1
1	vine-ripened tomato, sliced	1

1. Heat the oil in a large skillet and cook the onion on medium heat for 2 minutes, until slightly translucent, then remove from heat and transfer to a bowl.

2. Increase the heat to high. When pan is hot, quickly cook the steaks, adding salt and pepper, if desired. Depending on the thickness of the steaks, cooking time will be about 1 minute or less for each side.

3. Spread the toast with aïoli. Place salad greens on two slices, then add carrot, tomato, steak and onion, and close the sandwiches. Cut in half before serving.

NUTRIENTS PER SERVING			
Calories	524	Protein	41 g
Total Fat	17.1 g	Biotin	12 mcg (4% DV)
Saturated Fat	4.1 g	Vitamin C	19 mg (32% DV)
Omega-3	0.5 g	Iron	4.8 mg (27% DV)
Carbohydrate	52 g	Magnesium	40 mg (10% DV)
Fiber	8.6 g (34% DV)	Zinc	6.0 mg (40% DV)

Beef Barley Soup

Makes 4 servings

This soup is for meat lovers and is ideal for a cold winter's night. Barley contains gluten.

1 tsp	extra virgin olive oil	5 mL
8 oz	boneless stewing beef, fat trimmed, cut into chunks	250 g
1	medium red onion, diced	1
2	carrots, thinly sliced	2
2	stalks celery, finely chopped	2
2	cloves garlic, crushed and finely diced	2
6 cups	Anti-Aging Broth (page 392) or vegetable stock	1.5 L
½ cup	barley, rinsed	125 mL

1. Add the oil to a large saucepan and cook the meat on high heat until browned, for 3 to 5 minutes. Then transfer to paper towels to drain.

2. Add the onion, carrots, celery, garlic, broth and barley to the saucepan and bring to a boil. Reduce heat to low. Return the meat to the pan and simmer for 40 to 50 minutes, until meat is tender and barley is cooked.

NUTRIENTS PER SERVING			
Calories	279	Protein	20 g
Total Fat	8.4 g	Biotin	4 mcg (1% DV)
Saturated Fat	2.6 g	Vitamin C	8 mg (13% DV)
Omega-3	0.0 g	Iron	2.8 mg (16% DV)
Carbohydrate	31 g	Magnesium	39 mg (10% DV)
Fiber	6.5 g (26% DV)	Zinc	3.6 mg (24% DV)

Lean Lamb and Three Veg

<table>
<tr><td>Makes 4 servings</td></tr>
</table>

This tasty lamb dish is balanced with specially selected vegetables. It's gluten-free if you use malt-free soy milk. If you have eczema, exclude the tamari, broccoli and Swiss chard, and use sea salt and chopped cabbage.

- **Preheat barbecue grill to high**
- **Shallow baking dish**
- **Steamer**

2	medium sweet potatoes (about 1 lb/500 g total), peeled and diced	2
⅓ cup	organic soy milk	75 mL
	Ground black pepper	
1 lb	lean lamb loin chops or leg cutlets, fat trimmed	500 g
1 tsp	dried rosemary	5 mL
10 oz	yellow wax beans or frenched green beans	300 g
3 cups	chopped broccoli	750 mL

1. In a saucepan, bring some water to a boil and cook the sweet potato for 10 minutes or until very soft, then drain and return the sweet potato to the saucepan. Mash the sweet potato until lump-free, then stir in soy milk and pepper. Keep the mixture in the saucepan.

2. Place the lamb on the preheated grill and sprinkle with rosemary. Grill for about 5 minutes per side or until cooked to your liking.

3. In a steamer, cook the beans and broccoli for 2 to 3 minutes (maximum). Set the timer so you don't overcook the vegetables; they must be slightly crisp.

4. Reheat the mash if necessary and serve immediately with lamb and vegetables.

NUTRIENTS PER SERVING			
Calories	484	Protein	35 g
Total Fat	23.9 g	Biotin	9 mcg (3% DV)
Saturated Fat	9.9 g	Vitamin C	75 mg (125% DV)
Omega-3	0.4 g	Iron	4.1 mg (23% DV)
Carbohydrate	31 g	Magnesium	45 mg (11% DV)
Fiber	7.4 g (30% DV)	Zinc	4.4 mg (29% DV)

Slow-Cooked Lamb Casserole

Makes 4 servings

Slow cooking makes lamb tender and tasty. This vitamin C–rich casserole is gluten-free if you use Anti-Aging Broth. If you have eczema, omit the eggplant and cauliflower, and use cabbage and celery instead.

- **Preheat oven to 325°F (160°C)**
- **Large casserole dish with a lid**

4	small boneless lamb steaks, fat removed, lamb chopped into 1-inch (2.5 cm) thick strips	4
1 tbsp	brown rice flour	15 mL
1 tsp	ground cinnamon	5 mL
1 tsp	extra virgin olive oil	5 mL
1 tsp	grated peeled gingerroot	5 mL
3	cloves garlic, minced	3
1 cup	finely diced eggplant	250 mL
2 cups	chopped cauliflower	500 mL
2 cups	chopped sweet potato	500 mL
3 cups	hot Anti-Aging Broth (page 392) or vegetable stock (organic or additive-free)	750 mL
½ cup	flat-leaf (Italian) parsley leaves, chopped	125 mL
2 cups	cooked basmati rice	500 mL

1. Place the lamb, flour and cinnamon in a plastic bag, seal and shake to coat the lamb.

2. Heat the oil in a skillet and quickly fry the lamb strips for 1 to 2 minutes so they're partially cooked. Remove and place in casserole dish.

3. Add ginger, garlic, eggplant, cauliflower, sweet potato and broth to the dish, then cover with the lid.

4. Bake in preheated oven for 1 to 1½ hours, until the lamb is cooked through and tender. Stir a couple of times during cooking. Remove from heat and stir in parsley.

5. Serve with warm rice in large bowls.

NUTRIENTS PER SERVING			
Calories	352	Protein	24 g
Total Fat	8.6 g	Biotin	9 mcg (3% DV)
Saturated Fat	2.7 g	Vitamin C	40 mg (67% DV)
Omega-3	0.0 g	Iron	3.7 mg (21% DV)
Carbohydrate	45 g	Magnesium	100 mg (25% DV)
Fiber	6.3 g (25% DV)	Zinc	3.8 mg (25% DV)

Lamb Stir-Fry

This crispy and tasty stir-fry is gluten-free and has a slightly nutty taste from the toasted sesame seeds. Thinly slice the vegetables for best effect. You can serve each portion with ½ cup (125 mL) of cooked brown rice if you want more carbs.

- **Preheat oven to 480°F (250°C)**
- **Shallow baking dish**

4 tsp	sesame seeds	20 mL
2	boneless lean lamb loin chops, fat trimmed	2
1 tsp	dried mint	5 mL
1 tsp	extra virgin olive oil	5 mL
1 cup	thinly sliced mushrooms	250 mL
1½ cups	finely chopped cabbage	375 mL
3	green onions, sliced on the diagonal	3
1	small red bell pepper, thinly sliced	1
1	large carrot, halved lengthwise and thinly sliced	1
1 cup	bean sprouts, rinsed in vinegar and water	250 mL

1. In a skillet, toast the sesame seeds on high, stirring constantly, for 2 minutes, until slightly browned, then remove from heat.

2. Place the lamb chops in baking dish and sprinkle with mint. Bake in preheated oven for 8 to 10 minutes per side. Transfer the lamb to paper towels to drain.

3. Heat the oil in the skillet and stir-fry the mushrooms, cabbage, green onions, red pepper and carrot for no more than 2 minutes (vegetables must be slightly crisp). Stir in the bean sprouts and top with sesame seeds.

4. Slice lamb and place on top of stir-fried vegetables.

NUTRIENTS PER SERVING			
Calories	331	Protein	22 g
Total Fat	20.4 g	Biotin	6 mcg (2% DV)
Saturated Fat	6.7 g	Vitamin C	121 mg (202% DV)
Omega-3	0.3 g	Iron	3.3 mg (18% DV)
Carbohydrate	17 g	Magnesium	53 mg (13% DV)
Fiber	5.1 g (20% DV)	Zinc	3.2 mg (21% DV)

Vegetable Main Courses and Side Dishes

Not all of these meals are strictly vegetarian or vegan. Some contain Anti-Aging Broth (page 392), made with chicken bones, or Creamy Mayonnaise (page 380), made with egg yolk. See the notes in each recipe for vegetarian meal descriptions if you are a strict vegetarian.

Chickpea Beauty Salad 430

Sweet Raspberry, Avocado and Watercress Salad 431

Tasty Spinach Salad 432

Roasted Sweet Potato Salad 434

Rich Mineral Salad with Papaya, Dill and Baby Spinach 435

Spicy Green Papaya Salad 436

Garden Salad 437

Therapeutic Veggie Soup 438

Roasted Corn and Cauliflower Soup 439

Detox Dal 440

Creamy Chickpea Curry 441

Salad Sandwiches with Creamy Mayo 442

Falafel 443

Falafel Wraps 444

Tabbouleh 446

Tropical Vegetarian Stir-Fry 447

Rich Mediterranean Pasta 448

Colorful Non-Fried Rice 449

Tasty Vegetable Casserole 450

Chickpea Beauty Salad

Makes 2 main-dish servings

This tasty vegetarian meal is gluten-free if you use chutney without gluten, is rich in vitamin C and is a source of fiber and protein. If you don't have time to make my delicious Sweet Chutney (page 384), use a good-quality mango chutney that's free of artificial additives.

Tips

To cook dried chickpeas, soak ¾ cup (175 mL) dried chickpeas overnight in water. Drain and rinse, then simmer in fresh water for 1½ to 2 hours or until tender. Let cool in the cooking water, if time permits. Drain and rinse chickpeas. If you have trouble digesting beans, add ½ strip of kombu (seaweed) during the simmering process.

As a side dish, this salad serves 4 people.

1 tsp	extra virgin olive oil	5 mL
2	zucchini, thinly sliced on the diagonal	2
1½ cups	cooked chickpeas (see tip, at left) or rinsed drained canned chickpeas	375 mL
½	small red onion, thinly sliced into rings	½
½ cup	flat-leaf (Italian) parsley leaves, chopped	125 mL
1 tbsp	Sweet Chutney (page 384) or mango chutney	15 mL
1 tbsp	fresh lemon juice	15 mL
1	small clove garlic, minced	1
½ tsp	ground cumin	2 mL
½ tsp	ground coriander	2 mL
Pinch	cayenne pepper	Pinch

1. Heat the olive oil in a skillet over high heat, quickly add zucchini and cook, turning often, for 2 minutes, until slightly browned. Transfer to paper towels to drain.

2. In a large salad bowl, combine the zucchini, chickpeas, onion and parsley.

3. In a small bowl, combine chutney, lemon juice, garlic, cumin, coriander and cayenne pepper, then mix this dressing into the salad just before serving.

NUTRIENTS PER SERVING			
Calories	105	Protein	5 g
Total Fat	2.5 g	Biotin	9 mcg (3% DV)
Saturated Fat	0.2 g	Vitamin C	17 mg (28% DV)
Omega-3	0.0 g	Iron	1.5 mg (8% DV)
Carbohydrate	17 g	Magnesium	8 mg (2% DV)
Fiber	3.8 g (15% DV)	Zinc	0.2 mg (1% DV)

Sweet Raspberry, Avocado and Watercress Salad

Makes 4 side-dish servings

This gluten-free vegetarian side dish salad is bursting with skin-loving antioxidants. Watercress is highly alkalizing and is a good vegetable source of calcium.

2	firm ripe avocados, diced	2
1½ cups	raspberries (about 8 oz/250 g)	375 mL
1 tbsp	apple cider vinegar	15 mL
1 tbsp	extra virgin olive oil	15 mL
2 tsp	honey, heated slightly so it's runny	10 mL
6 cups	lightly packed watercress sprigs, trimmed	1.5 L

1. Place the avocado and raspberries in a bowl.

2. Make the dressing in a separate bowl by whisking together the vinegar, olive oil and honey, and spoon over the fruit. Toss gently to avoid squashing the avocado and raspberries.

3. Line a platter with watercress and pile the fruit on top.

NUTRIENTS PER SERVING			
Calories	230	Protein	4 g
Total Fat	18.3 g	Biotin	4 mcg (1% DV)
Saturated Fat	2.6 g	Vitamin C	41 mg (68% DV)
Omega-3	0.2 g	Iron	0.8 mg (4% DV)
Carbohydrate	19 g	Magnesium	28 mg (7% DV)
Fiber	7.0 g (28% DV)	Zinc	0.7 mg (5% DV)

Tasty Spinach Salad

This alkalizing salad is rich in both vitamin C and flavor. It's perfect as a side dish with meat, tofu or fish. (Thanks to Elaine Read and Kerry Meates for this recipe.)

2 tbsp	sesame seeds	30 mL
2 tbsp	pine nuts	30 mL
4 oz	baby spinach (or half arugula and half spinach)	125 g
2	red apples, peeled and grated	2
½	red onion, thinly sliced	½
1	large carrot, grated	1
½ cup	chopped raisins	125 mL
¼ cup	Sweet Chutney Dressing (see recipe, opposite)	60 mL

1. In a small skillet, toast the sesame seeds and pine nuts, stirring constantly, until lightly browned. Remove and let cool.

2. Mix spinach, apples, onion, carrot and raisins. Top with sesame seeds and pine nuts. Do not add the dressing until you are ready to serve the salad. Gradually add dressing, using less if necessary, and lightly mix.

NUTRIENTS PER SERVING			
Calories	198	Protein	4 g
Total Fat	5.5 g	Biotin	4 mcg (1% DV)
Saturated Fat	0.3 g	Vitamin C	17 mg (28% DV)
Omega-3	0.0 g	Iron	2.1 mg (12% DV)
Carbohydrate	38 g	Magnesium	27 mg (7% DV)
Fiber	4.9 g (20% DV)	Zinc	0.5 mg (3% DV)

Sweet Chutney Dressing

This alkalizing dressing keeps in the refrigerator for up to 2 weeks and goes with most lettuce-based salads. It is gluten-free if the chutney is gluten-free. If you have acne or oily skin, omit the oil or use olive oil instead of flaxseed oil.

1 tbsp	flaxseed oil or extra virgin olive oil	15 mL
1 tbsp	apple cider vinegar	15 mL
2 tsp	Sweet Chutney (page 384) or store-bought mango chutney	10 mL
2 tsp	fresh lime juice	10 mL
2 tsp	honey	10 mL
¼ tsp	mild yellow curry powder	1 mL
	Sea salt and pepper (optional)	

1. Blend oil, vinegar, chutney, lime juice, honey and curry powder together. Taste and season with salt and pepper, if desired. Store in a jar.

NUTRIENTS PER 1 TBSP (15 ML)			
Calories	49	Protein	0 g
Total Fat	3.5 g	Biotin	0 mcg (0% DV)
Saturated Fat	0.3 g	Vitamin C	2 mg (3% DV)
Omega-3	1.8 g	Iron	0.0 mg (0% DV)
Carbohydrate	5 g	Magnesium	1 mg (0% DV)
Fiber	0.1 g (0% DV)	Zinc	0.0 mg (0% DV)

Roasted Sweet Potato Salad

This gluten-free, hearty, alkalizing salad can be served on its own or as a side dish.

Tip

As a side dish, this salad serves 4 people.

• **Preheat oven to 350°F (180°C)**

1	large sweet potato, peeled if desired and diced into bite-size chunks	1
1 tsp	extra virgin olive oil	5 mL
2 tsp	fresh lemon juice	10 mL
1 tsp	honey	5 mL
½ tsp	flaxseed oil or extra virgin olive oil	2 mL
Pinch	sea salt	Pinch
	Ground black pepper	
4 oz	mixed salad leaves (about 4 cups/1 L)	125 g

1. Place the sweet potato in a bowl and mix with the olive oil, then place on a baking sheet and bake in preheated oven for 30 minutes or until pieces are soft and browned (not mushy). Remove from the oven and set aside.

2. In a large bowl, combine the lemon juice, honey, flaxseed oil, salt and pepper. Then add the sweet potato and salad leaves and mix gently.

NUTRIENTS PER SERVING			
Calories	140	Protein	3 g
Total Fat	3.6 g	Biotin	6 mcg (2% DV)
Saturated Fat	0.5 g	Vitamin C	38 mg (63% DV)
Omega-3	0.6 g	Iron	1.4 mg (8% DV)
Carbohydrate	25 g	Magnesium	25 mg (6% DV)
Fiber	4.0 g (16% DV)	Zinc	0.3 mg (2% DV)

Rich Mineral Salad with Papaya, Dill and Baby Spinach

Makes 2 side-dish servings

This gluten-free vegetarian salad is rich in nutrients: each serving supplies 204 mg of magnesium (51% DV), 7.6 mg of iron (42% DV) and 62 mg of vitamin C (103% DV). Serve with a protein, such as steamed white fish.

- **Preheat oven to 400°F (200°C)**

½ cup	green pumpkin seeds (pepitas)	125 mL
1 cup	buckwheat groats	250 mL
1 tsp	extra virgin olive oil	5 mL
½	small red onion, finely chopped	½
1	clove garlic, minced	1
½	papaya, chopped into small chunks	½
4 cups	baby spinach, finely chopped	1 L
	Juice of 2 limes	
½ cup	fresh dill fronds, finely chopped	125 mL
Pinch	natural sea salt	Pinch

1. Spread the pumpkin seeds on a baking sheet and toast in preheated oven for 2 to 4 minutes, until slightly browned, then set aside.

2. In a saucepan, bring some water to a boil, then add the buckwheat and simmer for 5 minutes. Drain and set aside to cool.

3. In a small saucepan, heat the oil and lightly sauté the onions and garlic, being careful not to brown or burn them. Remove from the heat and set aside.

4. In a mixing bowl, combine pumpkin seeds, buckwheat, onion mixture, papaya, spinach, lime juice, dill and salt.

NUTRIENTS PER SERVING			
Calories	633	Protein	22 g
Total Fat	26.2 g	Biotin	21 mcg (7% DV)
Saturated Fat	4.2 g	Vitamin C	62 mg (103% DV)
Omega-3	0.1 g	Iron	7.6 mg (42% DV)
Carbohydrate	85 g	Magnesium	204 mg (51% DV)
Fiber	14.2 g (57% DV)	Zinc	2.2 mg (15% DV)

Spicy Green Papaya Salad

Makes 3 servings

This spicy, gluten-free vegetarian salad is anti-parasitic and rich in digestive enzymes, so it's great for improving gut health. Green papaya is usually sold at Chinese markets. If you can't handle the heat, omit the chile pepper.

Tip

This salad will last for 2 days if stored in the refrigerator without the dressing. The dressing will last for at least a week in the refrigerator.

Dressing

½	small red chile pepper, finely chopped	½
1	clove garlic, crushed and chopped	1
¼ cup	tamari	60 mL
	Juice of 2 limes	
1 tbsp	apple cider vinegar	15 mL

Salad

2 cups	chopped trimmed long beans or green beans (1¼-inch/3 cm pieces)	500 mL
1	medium green papaya, grated (about 6 cups/1.5 L)	1
2 cups	bean sprouts, washed in apple cider vinegar and water	500 mL
1 cup	fresh mint leaves	250 mL
½ cup	fresh cilantro leaves	125 mL
½ cup	roasted cashews, chopped	125 mL
½	small red chile pepper, finely chopped (optional)	½
8 oz	cherry tomatoes (about 1½ cups/375 mL)	250 g
	Roasted cashews	

1. *Dressing:* Mix the chile pepper, garlic, tamari, lime juice and apple cider vinegar in a medium screw-top jar or container, then set aside.

2. *Salad:* Boil some water in a small pot and blanch the beans for 1 minute, then drain and transfer to a bowl filled with ice cold water and soak for 1 to 2 minutes (this helps to preserve the beans' color). Drain and put beans in a large bowl.

3. Add papaya, bean sprouts, mint, cilantro, cashews, chile pepper and tomatoes to beans in bowl. Toss lightly. Stir in 3 to 4 tbsp (45 to 60 mL) of the dressing just before serving. Serve in large bowls and garnish with cashews.

NUTRITIENTS PER SERVING	
Calories	239

Total Fat
  Saturated Fat
  Omega-3
	11.3 g
	2.3 g
	0.2 g

Carbohydrate	30 g
Fiber	6.7 g (27% DV)
Protein	11 g
Biotin	7 mcg (2% DV)
Vitamin C	83 mg (138% DV)
Iron	4.2 mg (23% DV)
Magnesium	130 mg (33% DV)
Zinc	2.2 mg (15% DV)

Garden Salad

**Makes 4 side-
dish servings**

This simple, stylish, gluten-free vegetarian salad will not steal the limelight from your main meal. If you have eczema, omit the red pepper, olive oil and tomato, and replace them with celery, grated carrot and more flaxseed oil.

4 cups	mixed lettuce leaves, torn into bite-size pieces	1 L
1 cup	finely shredded red cabbage	250 mL
1	small red bell pepper, finely sliced	1
2	ripe tomatoes, sliced	2
2	green onions, thinly sliced on the diagonal	2
1 tsp	extra virgin olive oil	5 mL
4 tsp	fresh lime juice	20 mL
	Ground black pepper	

1. In a large bowl, mix the lettuce, cabbage, red pepper, tomatoes and green onions.

2. In a cup or jar, mix the olive oil, lime juice and pepper. Add the dressing to the salad just before serving.

NUTRIENTS PER SERVING			
Calories	52	Protein	2 g
Total Fat	1.7 g	Biotin	4 mcg (1% DV)
Saturated Fat	0.2 g	Vitamin C	56 mg (93% DV)
Omega-3	0.1 g	Iron	1.3 mg (7% DV)
Carbohydrate	9 g	Magnesium	15 mg (4% DV)
Fiber	2.2 g (9% DV)	Zinc	0.2 mg (1% DV)

Therapeutic Veggie Soup

Makes 6 servings

This soup is fantastic for the immune system. Garlic and vegetables are rich in flavonoids, and the broth is rich in glycine and gelatin. Cayenne pepper gives the soup a hint of spice, so omit it if serving to children. If you have eczema, avoid corn, cauliflower and cayenne, and add cabbage. Serve with spelt bread, if desired.

Tips

If you're a vegetarian, use vegetarian stock instead of the Anti-Aging Broth.

Leftovers can be frozen in serving-sized containers for up to 2 months.

1⅓ cups	dried red lentils (8 oz/250 g)	325 mL
8 cups	Anti-Aging Broth (page 392) or organic vegetable stock	2 L
1 to 2	red onions, finely diced	1 to 2
3	stalks celery, finely chopped	3
2 cups	chopped cauliflower	500 mL
1	carrot, diced	1
2	cloves garlic, minced	2
½ tsp	finely grated peeled gingerroot	2 mL
Pinch	cayenne pepper (optional)	Pinch

1. Rinse the lentils and discard any that are discolored. Boil the lentils in a saucepan with plenty of water for 30 minutes. Strain the lentils, rinse and set aside.

2. Meanwhile, in a large pot, bring the broth to a boil. Then add onions, celery, cauliflower, carrot, garlic and ginger and simmer for 20 minutes.

3. Add the lentils and simmer for an additional 10 minutes, if necessary. Stir in cayenne pepper (if using).

NUTRIENTS PER SERVING			
Calories	213	Protein	17 g
Total Fat	1.5 g	Biotin	2 mcg (1% DV)
Saturated Fat	0.1 g	Vitamin C	23 mg (38% DV)
Omega-3	0.0 g	Iron	3.4 mg (19% DV)
Carbohydrate	35 g	Magnesium	20 mg (5% DV)
Fiber	8.7 g (35% DV)	Zinc	0.4 mg (3% DV)

Roasted Corn and Cauliflower Soup

Makes 6 servings

This creamy soup is great for detoxification, thanks to the indole-rich cauliflower. Seaweed, such as kombu, supplies iodine, which can boost metabolism. The soup is gluten-free if the stock is gluten-free. Cauliflower and corn are not suitable for those with eczema. Omit the cayenne if you're serving the soup to small children.

- **Preheat oven to 400°F (200°C)**
- **Rimmed baking sheet**

2	cobs corn	2
2	red onions, finely diced	2
2	cloves garlic, minced	2
1	large leek (white part only), thinly sliced	1
8 cups	Anti-Aging Broth (page 392) or organic vegetable stock	2 L
1	large (or 2 small) cauliflower, cut into small chunks	1
4	bay leaves	4
1	sheet kombu (seaweed), cut into pieces (optional)	1
1/8 tsp	cayenne pepper (optional)	0.5 mL
	Chopped fresh parsley (optional)	
	Ground black pepper (optional)	

1. Shave the kernels off the corn cobs, place them on the rimmed baking sheet and roast in preheated oven for about 5 minutes, until slightly browned. Remove from the oven and set aside.

2. Add the onion, garlic and leek to a large pot and add 2 to 3 tbsp (30 to 45 mL) of water. Cook on a medium heat for 2 to 4 minutes, until translucent, stirring often. Add broth, corn, cauliflower, bay leaves and kombu (if using). Cover the pot and bring to a boil. Reduce the heat and simmer for 30 minutes, stirring occasionally.

3. Remove from heat and discard bay leaves. Stir in cayenne pepper (if using). Working in small batches, purée soup in a blender or food processor. Serve garnished with chopped parsley and pepper, if desired.

Variation

To make this a true vegetarian meal, replace the Anti-Aging Broth with 3 cups (750 mL) vegetable stock and 5 cups (1.25 L) water.

NUTRIENTS PER SERVING	
Calories	89
Total Fat	0.8 g
Saturated Fat	0.1 g
Omega-3	0.0 g
Carbohydrate	15 g
Fiber	2.6 g (10% DV)
Protein	6 g
Biotin	2 mcg (1% DV)
Vitamin C	19 mg (32% DV)
Iron	1.0 mg (6% DV)
Magnesium	19 mg (5% DV)
Zinc	0.4 mg (3% DV)

Detox Dal

This gluten-free vegetarian meal contains turmeric, which is rich in flavonoids, and the addition of black pepper enhances the flavonoids' cancer-protective abilities. Kombu also promotes proper digestion of legumes, and it may boost metabolism due to its iodine content.

1 tsp	extra virgin olive oil	5 mL
1	red onion, finely chopped	1
2 tsp	ground turmeric	10 mL
2 tsp	ground coriander	10 mL
1 tsp	ground cinnamon	5 mL
2	cloves garlic, minced	2
½ tsp	hot pepper flakes (optional)	2 mL
2⅔ cups	dried red lentils (1 lb/500 g)	650 mL
4 cups	water	1 L
½	sheet kombu (seaweed), cut into thin strips	½
2	stalks celery, finely chopped	2
	Fresh cilantro or parsley	
	Ground black pepper	

1. Heat the oil in a large saucepan on medium heat, add the onion and sauté until translucent, about 4 minutes. Add the turmeric, coriander, cinnamon, garlic and hot pepper flakes (if you want a hot and spicy dal) and sauté for a further 2 minutes.

2. Rinse the lentils and discard any that are discolored. Add the lentils, water, kombu and celery to the saucepan and bring to a boil. Reduce the heat and simmer for 25 minutes, stirring occasionally, until lentils and kombu are soft and dal is smooth in consistency, adding extra water if necessary (but do not make the dal runny).

3. Serve dal garnished with cilantro and pepper.

NUTRIENTS PER SERVING			
Calories	650	Protein	47 g
Total Fat	5.3 g	Biotin	39 mcg (13% DV)
Saturated Fat	0.3 g	Vitamin C	7 mg (12% DV)
Omega-3	0.0 g	Iron	10.8 mg (60% DV)
Carbohydrate	107 g	Magnesium	15 mg (4% DV)
Fiber	27.0 g (108% DV)	Zinc	0.2 mg (1% DV)

Creamy Chickpea Curry

This tasty vegetarian curry is rich in cancer-protective flavonoids, enhanced by the addition of black pepper. Curry is not suitable for people with eczema or rosacea.

1 tsp	extra virgin olive oil	5 mL
1 tbsp	mild yellow curry powder	15 mL
1 tsp	garam masala	5 mL
½ tsp	ground cinnamon	2 mL
2	cloves garlic, minced	2
1 cup	finely diced eggplant	250 mL
1 tsp	grated gingerroot	5 mL
2 cups	chopped cauliflower	500 mL
1½ cups	cooked chickpeas (or one 14-oz/398 mL can, drained and rinsed)	375 mL
½ cup	coconut milk	125 mL
½	sheet kombu (seaweed), cut into ½-inch (1 cm) lengths (optional)	½
2 cups	organic vegetable stock	500 mL
1 cup	long-grain brown rice	250 mL
½ cup	fresh cilantro leaves, chopped	125 mL
	Ground black pepper	
	Chopped cilantro	

1. Heat the oil in a large saucepan and sauté the curry powder, garam masala, cinnamon and garlic for 1 minute. Add the eggplant, ginger, cauliflower, chickpeas, coconut milk, kombu and stock. Bring to a boil, then simmer on low heat for 30 minutes, stirring occasionally.

2. Meanwhile, in a saucepan, bring plenty of water to a boil and cook the rice according to package instructions (about 20 minutes). Drain.

3. Mix cilantro into the curry and serve curry on a bed of rice. Sprinkle with pepper and garnish with extra cilantro.

NUTRIENTS PER SERVING			
Calories	691	Protein	19 g
Total Fat	20.2 g	Biotin	44 mcg (15% DV)
Saturated Fat	11.7 g	Vitamin C	55 mg (92% DV)
Omega-3	0.1 g	Iron	6.7 mg (37% DV)
Carbohydrate	113 g	Magnesium	194 mg (49% DV)
Fiber	14.2 g (57% DV)	Zinc	2.8 mg (19% DV)

Salad Sandwiches with Creamy Mayo

This sandwich is rich in skin-protective antioxidants, thanks to the purple lettuce leaves, carrot and beet. The mayonnaise contains egg yolk, so omit it if you are vegan. If you have eczema, skip the avocado and use iceberg lettuce.

1	medium avocado, mashed	1
8	slices spelt bread	8
1 tbsp	Creamy Mayonnaise (page 380) (optional)	15 mL
1	large carrot, grated	1
1	small beet, peeled and grated	1
2½ cups	mixed salad leaves or iceberg lettuce, shredded	625 mL
1	green onion, sliced thinly on the diagonal	1
	Ground black pepper (optional)	

1. Spread avocado on four slices of bread and mayonnaise on the other four (or just use avocado). On top of the avocado, place carrot, beet, salad leaves and green onion. Season with pepper, if desired. Close the sandwiches and cut in half before serving.

NUTRIENTS PER SERVING			
Calories	347	Protein	10 g
Total Fat	14.4 g	Biotin	9 mcg (3% DV)
Saturated Fat	1.5 g	Vitamin C	9 mg (15% DV)
Omega-3	1.1 g	Iron	3.2 mg (18% DV)
Carbohydrate	49 g	Magnesium	26 mg (7% DV)
Fiber	10.9 g (44% DV)	Zinc	0.5 mg (3% DV)

Falafel

Makes 12 falafel

This recipe is gluten-free and vegetarian. If you have eczema, omit the broad beans, cayenne pepper and olive oil, as they are rich in salicylates, and use chickpeas and rice bran oil instead.

Tips

If you prefer to use fresh broad beans, buy about 2 lbs (1 kg) if they are in their pods (about 1 lb/500 g once pods are removed). Remove pods and boil the beans for up to 1 minute to loosen the skins. Submerge in cold water to stop the cooking process, then remove skins.

If you cannot find broad beans or if you have eczema, use 1 cup (250 mL) dried chickpeas (soaked for 6 hours, then boiled in plenty of water for 1½ to 2 hours).

If you want to make falafels in a hurry, you can use rinsed drained canned chickpeas and skip step 1.

- **Preheat oven to 350°F (180°C)**
- **Food processor**
- **Baking sheet, lined with parchment paper**

2 cups	frozen broad (fava or lima) beans, thawed (see tips, at left)	500 mL
½ cup	fresh flat-leaf (Italian) parsley leaves, finely chopped	125 mL
½ cup	fresh cilantro leaves, chopped	125 mL
1	clove garlic, minced	1
	Sea salt	
¼ tsp	cayenne pepper	1 mL
1 tsp	ground cumin	5 mL
1 to 2 tsp	brown rice flour	5 to 10 mL
1 tbsp	rice bran oil or extra virgin olive oil	15 mL

1. Remove the skins of the broad beans by pinching them, and discard the shells. Rub beans dry on a clean tea towel.

2. In a food processor, process the beans, parsley, cilantro, garlic, ½ tsp (2 mL) salt, cayenne and cumin until the paste is soft and sticks together. Mix in 1 tsp (5 mL) rice flour to thicken the mix. Add more flour if necessary.

3. Using a spoon, form paste into twelve 1¼-inch (3 cm) balls. Place on prepared baking sheet and flatten balls slightly. Brush both sides with oil and sprinkle with salt, if desired.

4. Bake in preheated oven for 20 to 30 minutes or until golden brown. Drain on absorbent paper towels.

NUTRIENTS PER SERVING			
Calories	92	Protein	7 g
Total Fat	0.8 g	Biotin	4 mcg (1% DV)
Saturated Fat	0.1 g	Vitamin C	4 mg (7% DV)
Omega-3	0.0 g	Iron	1.9 mg (11% DV)
Carbohydrate	15 g	Magnesium	50 mg (13% DV)
Fiber	6.4 g (26% DV)	Zinc	0.8 mg (5% DV)

Falafel Wraps

These wraps make a healthy lunchtime meal rich in vitamin C. It's easiest to buy your falafel pre-made, but if this isn't possible, follow the delicious recipe on page 443. If you have eczema, omit the tomato (in the tabbouleh), as it is high in salicylates, and use grated carrot and iceberg lettuce instead of the cucumber and romaine lettuce.

1	small Lebanese cucumber (or $\frac{1}{2}$ English cucumber)	1
1	avocado, mashed	1
2 tsp	fresh lime juice	10 mL
4	large spelt tortillas or wraps	4
8	leaves red romaine lettuce or iceberg lettuce, shredded	8
2 cups	Tabbouleh (page 446)	500 mL
12	falafel balls (page 443 or store-bought), heated and halved	12

1. Using a vegetable peeler, thinly slice the cucumber into long strips.

2. Mix the avocado and lime juice and spread over the tortillas.

3. Arrange the cucumber, lettuce, tabbouleh and falafel on the tortillas. Roll up tortillas.

Variation
In place of the Tabbouleh, you can use 1 diced large ripe tomato and $\frac{1}{2}$ diced onion.

NUTRIENTS PER SERVING			
Calories	544	Protein	27 g
Total Fat	14.5 g	Biotin	10 mcg (3% DV)
Saturated Fat	2.5 g	Vitamin C	19 mg (32% DV)
Omega-3	0.1 g	Iron	7.7 mg (43% DV)
Carbohydrate	80 g	Magnesium	171 mg (43% DV)
Fiber	26.2 g (105% DV)	Zinc	2.9 mg (19% DV)

Spelt Wraps

> **Makes four
> 9-inch (23 cm)
> wraps**

Spelt contains gluten
and is similar to wheat,
but it is easier to digest
and is better for your
waistline.

1¼ cups	spelt flour (or 1 cup/250 mL whole-grain spelt flour)	300 mL
¾ tsp	finely ground sea salt	3 mL
	Ground cinnamon	
1 tbsp	rice bran oil	15 mL
⅔ cup	boiling water	150 mL

1. In a bowl, mix the spelt flour, salt and a sprinkle of cinnamon. Add the oil and boiling water and mix with a knife.

2. Lightly flour a cutting board and knead the dough for about 3 minutes, until smooth and elastic. Cut into 4 balls. Place onto a plate, cover with plastic wrap and rest for 30 minutes.

3. On a floured board, roll out each ball with a rolling pin to make large, thin circles (make them as thin as possible) about 9 inches (23 cm) in diameter.

4. Heat a large nonstick skillet over high heat. Cook each flatbread for 1 minute per side or until bubbles appear and the bread becomes browned in spots. Use immediately.

NUTRIENTS PER SERVING			
Calories	168	Protein	6 g
Total Fat	4.7 g	Biotin	7 mcg (2% DV)
Saturated Fat	0.7 g	Vitamin C	0 mg (0% DV)
Omega-3	0.1 g	Iron	1.4 mg (8% DV)
Carbohydrate	29 g	Magnesium	0 mg (0% DV)
Fiber	2.5 g (10% DV)	Zinc	0.0 mg (0% DV)

Tabbouleh

This is a vegetarian cracked wheat salad with parsley, onion and tomatoes. It is highly alkalizing and a source of vitamin C. To make it gluten-free, exclude the bulgur. If you have eczema, leave out the tomato.

Tip

Serve in wraps, burgers and sandwiches, or as a side salad.

3 tbsp	fine bulgur (cracked wheat)	45 mL
3	firm ripe tomatoes (about 8 oz/250 g total), diced	3
2 to 3 tsp	fresh lemon juice	10 to 15 mL
1	bunch flat-leaf (Italian) parsley (about 8 oz/250 g), finely chopped	1
1 tsp	extra virgin olive oil	5 mL

1. Soak the bulgur in hot water for 10 minutes, then drain and blot with paper towels.

2. Mix the bulgur with the tomato and lemon juice and let stand for 20 minutes to absorb the juices. Then mix in the parsley and oil.

NUTRIENTS PER SERVING			
Calories	45	Protein	1 g
Total Fat	1.4 g	Biotin	4 mcg (1% DV)
Saturated Fat	0.2 g	Vitamin C	11 mg (18% DV)
Omega-3	0.0 g	Iron	0.4 mg (2% DV)
Carbohydrate	8 g	Magnesium	18 mg (5% DV)
Fiber	2.0 g (8% DV)	Zinc	0.3 mg (2% DV)

Tropical Vegetarian Stir-Fry

This colorful stir-fry is rich in vitamin C and is gluten-free if you use tamari instead of soy sauce. Not suitable if you have eczema.

Tips

Leftovers can be added to a salad or chicken wrap the next day.

10 oz	firm or extra-firm tofu, diced	300 g
¼ cup	tamari or soy sauce	60 mL
3	slices pineapple, core removed, cut into chunks	3
1 cup	basmati rice	250 mL
1 tsp	extra virgin olive oil	5 mL
1	small knob gingerroot, grated	1
1	clove garlic, minced	1
2 cups	snow peas, strings removed	500 mL
1	small red bell pepper, thinly sliced	1
1 cup	finely shredded red cabbage	250 mL
1	medium carrot, peeled and thinly sliced	1
2 cups	chopped green onions	500 mL
¼ cup	unsalted roasted cashews	60 mL

1. In a small bowl, marinate the tofu in tamari for at least 20 minutes. Drain off excess tamari and reserve to add at end of cooking.

2. Place the pineapple chunks on absorbent paper towels and blot to remove excess moisture.

3. In a saucepan, bring plenty of water to a boil and simmer the rice for 8 minutes. Drain.

4. In a large skillet or wok, heat the oil over high heat and stir-fry the tofu, ginger and garlic for 1 minute. Add the snow peas, red pepper, cabbage and carrot, and stir-fry for 1 minute only. Vegetables must remain crisp.

5. Add the pineapple, green onions and cashews, and stir-fry for a further 1 minute only, stirring constantly to avoid burning.

6. Serve stir-fry on a bed of rice and top with the desired amount of tamari.

NUTRIENTS PER SERVING			
Calories	711	Protein	32 g
Total Fat	21.7 g	Biotin	20 mcg (7% DV)
Saturated Fat	3.0 g	Vitamin C	137 mg (228% DV)
Omega-3	0.1 g	Iron	10.0 mg (56% DV)
Carbohydrate	105 g	Magnesium	78 mg (20% DV)
Fiber	12.3 g (49% DV)	Zinc	1.4 mg (9% DV)

Rich Mediterranean Pasta

Makes 4 servings

This fresh, decorative, satisfying Mediterranean pasta is vegetarian and rich in low-GI carbohydrates. Not suitable if you have eczema.

- **Preheat oven to 425°F (220°C)**
- **Large shallow baking dish**

1 tbsp	apple cider vinegar	15 mL
2 tbsp	extra virgin olive oil, divided	30 mL
6	plum (Roma) tomatoes, halved	6
	Sea salt	
1	large red onion, cut into chunks	1
6	whole cloves garlic, peeled	6
2	medium zucchini, thinly sliced on the diagonal	2
1	red bell pepper, sliced	1
1 to 2 tsp	dried basil	5 to 10 mL
	Ground black pepper	
1 lb	spelt pasta (or colored vegetable pasta)	500 g
3 tbsp	finely chopped parsley	45 mL
½ cup	kalamata olives	125 mL
⅓ cup	fresh lemon juice	75 mL

1. Place the vinegar and 1 tsp (5 mL) of oil in a bowl and mix before adding the tomatoes and a sprinkle of salt. Toss to coat, then place the tomatoes in baking dish and roast in preheated oven for 10 minutes.

2. Place the onion, garlic, zucchini and red pepper in a bowl, then drizzle with 2 tsp (10 mL) of olive oil and sprinkle with basil and pepper. Mix, then add the vegetables to the same dish as the tomato (pushing the tomatoes to one side, so as not to combine juices). Roast for a further 20 to 25 minutes, until the vegetables are soft and turning slightly golden, stirring occasionally to promote even cooking. Once cooked, remove from the oven.

3. Cook the pasta in a large saucepan of boiling salted water (add salt to pasta now instead of salting the meal later). Boil the pasta for the time recommended by the manufacturer or until al dente.

4. Drain the pasta and gently mix in the remaining olive oil. Place on top of cooked vegetables and toss to coat. Stir in parsley, olives, lemon juice and pepper. Serve hot.

NUTRITIENTS PER SERVING	
Calories	553

Total Fat
  Saturated Fat
  Omega-3
	12.5 g
	1.3 g
	0.1 g

Carbohydrate	101 g
Fiber	14.3 g (57% DV)
Protein	20 g
Biotin	9 mcg (3% DV)
Vitamin C	82 mg (137% DV)
Iron	5.5 mg (31% DV)
Magnesium	26 mg (7% DV)
Zinc	0.5 mg (3% DV)

Colorful Non-Fried Rice

Makes 4 servings

Fried rice is just as tasty when you skip the frying part. This recipe is gluten-free if you use tamari. If you are a vegetarian, see the variation below.

Variation

Instead of the eggs, you can use 8 oz (250 g) firm tofu, diced. Marinate the tofu in tamari for at least 10 minutes, then briefly heat it in the microwave or fry it without oil for 2 to 4 minutes before adding it to the rice in Step 4.

2 cups	basmati rice	500 mL
4 cups	water	1 L
4	large free-range eggs, lightly beaten	4
1 cup	frozen peas	250 mL
1	large carrot, diced	1
1 cup	cooked corn kernels	250 mL
3	green onions (green and white parts), chopped	3
1	small red bell pepper, diced	1
2 tbsp	finely chopped fresh parsley	30 mL
	Tamari or soy sauce	
3 tbsp	sweet chile sauce (page 383 or store-bought; optional)	45 mL
	Ground black pepper (optional)	

1. Boil the rice in the water, simmering on low for 8 to 10 minutes or until rice boils dry. Check the rice regularly while cooking: once water is absorbed, switch off heat, stir and cover with a lid for the remaining cooking time. The rice needs to end up cooked but partially dry so it's not sticky. If, after 10 minutes of cooking, there is water left in the rice, drain it and set aside on a tray to air-dry.

2. Cook the eggs in batches in a small nonstick skillet — you want each portion to look like a flat pancake or crêpe. Flip the egg and briefly cook the second side, being careful not to burn. Remove, cut 1¼-inch (3 cm) strips and set aside.

3. In a small pot, boil the peas for 2 minutes, then add carrots and blanch for 1 minute. Drain and add the vegetables to the rice.

4. Add cooked egg or tofu, corn, green onions, red pepper, parsley and tamari to taste. Mix in sweet chile sauce and ground black pepper, if desired.

NUTRIENTS PER SERVING			
Calories	449	Protein	16 g
Total Fat	7.5 g	Biotin	16 mcg (5% DV)
Saturated Fat	1.2 g	Vitamin C	46 mg (77% DV)
Omega-3	0.1 g	Iron	3.5 mg (19% DV)
Carbohydrate	83 g	Magnesium	26 mg (7% DV)
Fiber	8.2 g (33% DV)	Zinc	1.0 mg (7% DV)

Tasty Vegetable Casserole

Makes 2 servings

This soupy vegetarian casserole is suitable for everyone — including those with eczema or gluten intolerance (but check to make sure the stock you use is gluten-free).

- **Preheat oven to 350°F (180°C)**
- **Large casserole dish with a lid**

2 cups	chopped cauliflower	500 mL
½ cup	sliced shiitake mushrooms (optional)	125 mL
½ cup	finely diced red cabbage	250 mL
2 cups	chopped sweet potato	500 mL
1 tbsp	brown rice flour	15 mL
3 cups	organic vegetable stock, divided	750 mL
2	cloves garlic, minced	2
	Mixed dried herbs (such as basil and oregano)	
	Ground cinnamon	
¼ cup	fresh parsley leaves, finely chopped	60 mL

1. Place cauliflower, mushrooms, cabbage and sweet potato in large casserole dish.

2. In a bowl, mix the flour with ¼ cup (60 mL) of cold stock until lump-free. Add the remaining stock and the garlic, mix, then pour over the casserole. Sprinkle with mixed herbs and cinnamon, then cover with a lid.

3. Bake in preheated oven for 30 to 40 minutes or until the vegetables are softened. Stir a couple of times during cooking.

4. Remove from the oven and stir in the parsley.

NUTRIENTS PER SERVING			
Calories	192	Protein	5 g
Total Fat	0.6 g	Biotin	8 mcg (3% DV)
Saturated Fat	0.1 g	Vitamin C	79 mg (132% DV)
Omega-3	0.0 g	Iron	2.3 mg (13% DV)
Carbohydrate	44 g	Magnesium	64 mg (16% DV)
Fiber	7.3 g (29% DV)	Zinc	1.0 mg (7% DV)

Desserts and Sweet Treats

Stewed Pears with Vanilla Soy Custard 452

Poached Apple Surprise 453

Tangy Papaya Cups 454

Mango Ice 454

Sweet Banana and Carob Spread 455

Rhubarb Crumble 456

Carrot Cake 457

Banana Cake 458

Stewed Pears with Vanilla Soy Custard

Makes 4 servings

This dessert is delicious, sophisticated and easy to make. It's suitable for people with eczema (preferably use pear juice), and is gluten-free if the soy milk is malt-free. The soy custard contains calcium. If you have blood sugar issues, sprinkle this dessert with cinnamon, as maple syrup has a high GI.

Tip

You can use the leftover egg whites in an omelet (modify the Tasty Omelet recipe on page 367).

2 cups	apple or pear juice (sugar- and preservative-free)	500 mL
2 cups	water	500 mL
6	pears, peeled, halved lengthwise and cored	6

Vanilla Soy Custard

5	large free-range egg yolks	5
¼ cup	pure maple syrup	60 mL
2 cups	organic soy milk	500 mL
1	vanilla bean, split	1
3	cardamom pods, crushed	3
	Ground cinnamon	

1. Place the apple juice and water in a large saucepan and bring to a boil. Add the pears and simmer for 10 minutes, until soft. Remove the pears, place three halves in each dessert bowl and set aside.

2. *Custard:* In a small bowl, lightly beat the egg yolks, then add the maple syrup, mix and set aside.

3. In a small saucepan, combine the soy milk, vanilla bean and cardamom pods. Bring to a boil and simmer for 5 minutes, stirring continuously. While mixing, gradually add the egg yolks and stir until the custard thickens (this should take less than 1 minute). Remove from the heat before curdling occurs. Remove cardamom pods and vanilla bean.

4. Pour custard over the pears. For presentation, sprinkle a tiny amount of cinnamon over each dessert before serving.

NUTRIENTS PER SERVING			
Calories	401	Protein	13 g
Total Fat	7.6 g	Biotin	19 mcg (6% DV)
Saturated Fat	1.8 g	Vitamin C	11 mg (18% DV)
Omega-3	0.2 g	Iron	2.5 mg (14% DV)
Carbohydrate	73 g	Magnesium	66 mg (17% DV)
Fiber	8.1 g (32% DV)	Zinc	1.4 mg (9% DV)

Poached Apple Surprise

The surprise is that this gluten-free recipe is so simple and tasty. If you have blood sugar issues, sprinkle the dessert with cinnamon.

2 cups	apple juice (sugar- and preservative-free)	500 mL
2 cups	water	500 mL
2	green apples, peeled, cored and halved	2
1 tsp	pure maple syrup	5 mL
	Ground cinnamon	

1. Place the apple juice and water in a saucepan and bring to a boil. Add the apples and simmer for 15 minutes, until soft. Remove the apples and place in dessert bowls. Decorate with maple syrup and cinnamon.

Variation

Pour Vanilla Soy Custard (page 452) over the apples in place of the maple syrup and flax seeds. Serve warm.

NUTRIENTS PER SERVING			
Calories	227	Protein	1 g
Total Fat	0.6 g	Biotin	4 mcg (1% DV)
Saturated Fat	0.1 g	Vitamin C	11 mg (18% DV)
Omega-3	0.0 g	Iron	0.5 mg (3% DV)
Carbohydrate	58 g	Magnesium	24 mg (6% DV)
Fiber	3.4 g (14% DV)	Zinc	0.2 mg (1% DV)

Tangy Papaya Cups

This healthy, light, gluten-free dessert (or snack) tastes fantastic and contains alkalizing lime, banana and flax seeds. If you have eczema, omit the lime juice.

1	large ripe papaya, halved lengthwise and seeds removed	1
1	ripe banana, sliced	1
	Juice of 1 lime	
2 tsp	ground flax seeds	10 mL

1. Fill the papaya halves with chopped banana and sprinkle with lime juice and flax seeds.

NUTRIENTS PER SERVING			
Calories	234	Protein	3 g
Total Fat	2.2 g	Biotin	2 mcg (1% DV)
Saturated Fat	0.4 g	Vitamin C	244 mg (407% DV)
Omega-3	0.2 g	Iron	1.1 mg (6% DV)
Carbohydrate	57 g	Magnesium	98 mg (25% DV)
Fiber	8.7 g (35% DV)	Zinc	0.4 mg (3% DV)

Mango Ice

Mangos are rich in vitamin C and make a great frozen dessert.

Tip

Frozen mango can also be used in smoothies.

| 2 | large ripe mangos, sliced | 2 |
| 4 tsp | ground flax seeds | 20 mL |

1. Divide the mango slices into four small containers and freeze. Before serving, sprinkle with flax seeds.

NUTRIENTS PER SERVING			
Calories	114	Protein	2 g
Total Fat	1.6 g	Biotin	1 mcg (0% DV)
Saturated Fat	0.2 g	Vitamin C	61 mg (102% DV)
Omega-3	0.1 g	Iron	0.3 mg (2% DV)
Carbohydrate	26 g	Magnesium	17 mg (4% DV)
Fiber	3.1 g (12% DV)	Zinc	0.2 mg (1% DV)

Sweet Banana and Carob Spread

Makes 2 servings

A fab children's snack or dessert. Spread it on French Toast (page 359) or Banana Cake (page 458), or drizzle it over fruit. You can also double or triple the recipe and freeze it in ice pop molds, or freeze it for 30 minutes to make a light "pudding." It's very suitable for people with eczema. (Thanks to Lynda Spencely for this modified recipe.)

- **Electric mixer**

2	large ripe bananas, mashed	2
1 to 2 tsp	carob powder (less is best)	5 to 10 mL
2 tsp	pure maple syrup	10 mL
Dash	vanilla extract	Dash

1. Combine bananas, carob powder, maple syrup and vanilla and, using an electric mixer, mix on high speed until smooth and creamy.

Variation

Banana Cake Filling: Use 6 bananas, $1/4$ cup (60 mL) pure maple syrup, 4 tsp (20 mL) carob powder and vanilla extract to taste.

NUTRIENTS PER SERVING			
Calories	126	Protein	1 g
Total Fat	0.4 g	Biotin	3 mcg (1% DV)
Saturated Fat	0.1 g	Vitamin C	10 mg (17% DV)
Omega-3	0.0 g	Iron	0.3 mg (2% DV)
Carbohydrate	32 g	Magnesium	33 mg (8% DV)
Fiber	3.2 g (13% DV)	Zinc	0.3 mg (2% DV)

Rhubarb Crumble

Makes 6 servings	

This dessert is just gorgeous, and it has half the sugar of regular crumbles. If you have eczema, modify this recipe to use sliced or canned pears instead of rhubarb. Cinnamon assists with keeping blood sugar levels steady.

- **Preheat oven to 350°F (180°C)**
- **8-inch (20 cm) square glass baking dish**

3 to 4 cups	chopped rhubarb	750 mL to 1 L
¼ cup	fresh lemon juice	60 mL
4 tsp	packed brown sugar	20 mL
4 tsp	water	20 mL
½ tsp	ground cinnamon	2 mL

Topping

½ cup	spelt flour	125 mL
2 tbsp	oat bran or rice bran	30 mL
¼ tsp	baking soda	1 mL
1 cup	large-flake (old-fashioned) rolled oats	250 mL
4 tsp	packed brown sugar	20 mL
4 tsp	whole flax seeds	20 mL
¼ cup	extra virgin olive oil (approx.)	60 mL
	Ground cinnamon (optional)	

1. Arrange the rhubarb in the baking dish and sprinkle with lemon juice, brown sugar, water and cinnamon.

2. *Topping:* In a bowl, combine the flour, oat bran and baking soda. Add oats, brown sugar, flax seeds and oil, and mix until crumbly. Add another 4 tsp (20 mL) oil if the mixture looks too dry. Spread evenly over the rhubarb and top with a sprinkling of cinnamon, if desired.

3. Bake in preheated oven for 30 minutes or until rhubarb is soft and topping is light golden. Serve warm.

NUTRIENTS PER SERVING			
Calories	223	Protein	5 g
Total Fat	11.6 g	Biotin	7 mcg (2% DV)
Saturated Fat	1.5 g	Vitamin C	9 mg (15% DV)
Omega-3	0.1 g	Iron	1.3 mg (7% DV)
Carbohydrate	28 g	Magnesium	13 mg (3% DV)
Fiber	3.9 g (16% DV)	Zinc	0.1 mg (1% DV)

Carrot Cake

Makes 8 servings

This cake is dairy-free and full of carrot goodness. To counteract some of the acid effect produced by ingesting sugar and flour, have a glass of Green Water (page 344) afterwards.

Tip

Store in an airtight container in the refrigerator.

- **Preheat oven to 300°F (150°C)**
- **9- by 5-inch (23 by 12.5 cm) metal loaf pan, greased**

1 cup	spelt flour or whole wheat flour	250 mL
½ cup	packed brown sugar	125 mL
1 tsp	baking soda	5 mL
1 tsp	baking powder	5 mL
1 tsp	ground cinnamon	5 mL
½ cup	extra virgin olive oil	125 mL
2	large free-range eggs, lightly beaten	2
1 tsp	vanilla extract	5 mL
2 cups	grated carrots	500 mL
1	grated peeled green apple	1
3 tbsp	water (if necessary)	45 mL

1. In a mixing bowl, combine the flour, sugar, baking soda, baking powder and cinnamon. Stir in the oil, eggs and vanilla and beat well until smooth. Add the carrot and apple, and water if mixture is not quite wet enough. Mix well.

2. Pour into prepared loaf dish. Bake on the lower rack of the preheated oven for 20 to 30 minutes or until a tester inserted in the center comes out clean. Let cool slightly before removing the cake from the dish.

NUTRIENTS PER SERVING			
Calories	277	Protein	4 g
Total Fat	15.6 g	Biotin	9 mcg (3% DV)
Saturated Fat	2.3 g	Vitamin C	3 mg (5% DV)
Omega-3	0.1 g	Iron	1.1 mg (6% DV)
Carbohydrate	31 g	Magnesium	7 mg (2% DV)
Fiber	2.5 g (10% DV)	Zinc	0.2 mg (1% DV)

Banana Cake

This cake is a party treat or a suitable birthday cake for children with eczema. To counteract some of the acid effect produced by ingesting sugar, flour and saturated fat, have a glass of Green Water (page 344) afterwards.

Tip

You can add a sprinkling of confectioners' (icing) sugar on top of the cooled cake if serving it as a birthday cake.

- **Preheat oven to 350°F (180°C)**
- **Electric mixer**
- **Two 8- by 4-inch (20 by 16 cm) metal loaf pans, greased and floured**

2 cups	spelt flour or whole wheat flour	500 mL
1 tbsp	baking powder	15 mL
1/2 tsp	ground cinnamon	2 mL
1/2 tsp	baking soda	2 mL
1/2 cup	packed brown sugar	125 mL
1/2 cup	unsalted butter, softened	125 mL
2	large free-range eggs, lightly beaten	2
3	medium very ripe bananas, mashed	3
1/4 cup	organic soy milk	60 mL
	Banana Cake Filling (variation, page 455; optional)	

1. In a bowl, combine flour, baking powder, cinnamon and baking soda, and mix.

2. In a separate bowl, beat the brown sugar and butter with an electric mixer to cream. Add the eggs and beat well, then beat in the mashed banana. Fold in the flour mixture. Add soy milk and mix to form a soft dough.

3. Divide the mixture between prepared loaf pans. Bake for 20 minutes or until a tester inserted in the center comes out clean. Let cool on a wire rack.

4. If desired, turn one cake upside down and top with Banana Cake Filling, then place the other cake on top (right side up).

Variation

Instead of the loaf pans, you can divide the batter among 12 lined or greased cups of a muffin pan and reduce the baking time to about 10 minutes.

NUTRIENTS PER SERVING			
Calories	328	Protein	8 g
Total Fat	13.8 g	Biotin	12 mcg (4% DV)
Saturated Fat	7.7 g	Vitamin C	4 mg (7% DV)
Omega-3	0.1 g	Iron	1.8 mg (10% DV)
Carbohydrate	48 g	Magnesium	14 mg (4% DV)
Fiber	3.3 g (13% DV)	Zinc	0.2 mg (1% DV)

Appendix

Additives to Avoid

The following food additives may cause adverse skin reactions.

Type of additive	Additive name	Used in
Preservatives	Sorbates	Some processed fruits and vegetables, and wines
	Benzoates	Most soft drinks, diet drinks, cordials, juices
	Sulfites	Wine, beer, processed meats, sausages, dried fruit
	Nitrates, nitrites	Processed meats, such as ham and salami
	Propionates (especially calcium propionate)	Breads
	Antioxidants (not the natural kind)	Oils, margarines, french fries, fried snack foods, fast foods
Flavor enhancers	Monosodium glutamate	Flavored noodles, flavored chips and crackers, sauces, fast foods, traditional Chinese cooking
Artificial sweeteners	Aspartame (NutraSweet, Equal)	Diet and "sugar-free" products
	Saccharin	Diet and "sugar-free" products
Artificial colors	FD&C Yellow #5 and #6	
	FD&C Red #2, #3, #8, #10, #40	
	FD&C Blue #1	

Acknowledgments

Many people have helped me to fine-tune this book, and I am very grateful for their time, wisdom, and assistance. Firstly, I'd love to say a huge thank you to my writer's agent, Selwa Anthony, and also Exisle Publishing for believing in me and my book — I could not have completed this project without your support. I'd like to thank my editors, Anouska Jones and Karen Gee, for doing a great job editing *The Healthy Skin Diet*. I also had some early editing assistance from Sue Tierney, Joy Fischer, Alice Hocking, Katie Ashton, and Louise Roberts — thanks, guys; I really appreciate your invaluable advice! Sophie Gabriel, author of *Breathe for Life*, put a lot of time and effort into fine-tuning Beauty Breathing, and I am forever grateful that she freely shared her extensive knowledge on breathing training with me. It has made a huge difference to my own health and stamina. Thanks to my biochemistry teacher, Helen Stevenson, for her information on prostaglandins, which I've included in Guideline #2. I also received valuable skin-care information from cosmetic physician Dr Van Huynh-Park, Snezna Kerekovic, Bahar Etminan, and Ray Thatcher. There are hundreds of awesome scientific studies on skin care and skin health and I really appreciate the scientific researchers who have allowed their findings to be published on the net. I'd also like to thank author Tara Moss for forwarding my book "aspirations" on to her writer's agent, Selwa. And I'd love to thank Jon, Ayva, Jack, and the rest of my family for your patience and infinite support.

For Mom and Dad, thanks for everything.

Resources

Health Before Beauty
(my free health information website)
For skin-care and product reviews, log on to www.healthbeforebeauty.com

References

Adebamowo, C.A., et al. 2005. High school dietary dairy intake and teenage acne. *Journal of the American Academy of Dermatology*, vol. 52, no 2: 207–14.

Akiba, S., et al. 1999. Influence of chronic UV exposure and lifestyle on facial skin photo-aging — results from a pilot study, *Journal of Epidemiology*, vol. 9, no. 6: S136–42.

American Family Physician. 2003. Tea tree oil shampoo in treatment of dandruff. Retrieved 6 September 2006: http://www.aafp.org/afp/20030501/tips/2.html.

Andersen, F.A. 1999. Final report on the safety assessment of cocamide MEA. *International Journal of Toxicology*, vol. 18, no. 2 suppl.: 9–16.

ARL Pathology. 2006. *Practitioner Manual*. Melbourne, Australia.

Armstrong, S.M., and Redman, J.R. 1991. Melatonin: A chronobiotic with anti-aging properties? *Medical Hypotheses*, vol. 34, no. 4: 300–309.

Athar, M., and Nasir, S.M. 2005. Taxonomic perspective of plant species yielding vegetable oils used in cosmetics and skin care products, *African Journal of Biotechnology*, vol. 4, no. 1: 36–44.

Australasian College of Dermatologists. 2006. *What is Rosacea?* Retrieved 23 March 2006: http://www.dermcoll.asn.au/rosacea.pdf.

Australian Institute of Health and Welfare. 2004. Heart, stroke and vascular diseases, Australian facts 2004. Cardiovascular disease series no. 22, cat. no. CVD 27. Canberra: AIHW.

Bangyan, L., et al. 1994. Antithetic relationship of dietary arachidonic acid and eicosapentaenoic acid on eicosanoid production in vivo. *Journal of Lipid Research*, vol. 35: 1869–77.

Banni, S., et al. 1996. Characterization of conjugated diene fatty acids in milk, dairy products, and lamb tissues. *The Journal of Nutritional Biochemistry*, vol. 7, no. 3: 150–55.

Barham, J.B., et al. 2000. Addition of eicosapentaenoic acid to y-linolenic acid-supplemented diets prevents serum arachidonic acid accumulation in humans. *Journal of Nutrition*, vol. 130: 1925–31.

Baugh, C.M., Malone, J.H., and Butterworth, C.E. 1968. Human biotin deficiency. *American Journal of Clinical Nutrition*, vol. 21: 173–82.

Baumann, L. 2005. How to prevent photoaging? *Journal of Investigative Dermatology*, vol. 125, no. 4: xii–xiii.

BBC News. 2006. Exercise 'cuts skin cancer risk.' Retrieved 12 May 2006: http://news.bbc.co.uk/2/hi/health/4764535.stm.

Begoun, P. 2002. *The Beauty Bible*, 2nd ed., chapter 2. Seattle: Beginning Press.

Berbis, P., et al. 1990. Essential fatty acids and the skin. *Allergie et Immunologie*, vol. 22, no. 6: 225–31.

Birt, D.F., et al. 1999. Glucocorticoid mediation of dietary energy restriction inhibition of mouse skin carcinogenesis. *Journal of Nutrition*, vol. 129, no. 2 suppl.: 571S–74S.

Boelsma, E. 2003. Human skin condition and its association with nutrient concentrations in serum and diet. *American Journal of Clinical Nutrition*, vol. 77, no. 22: 348–55.

Boreham, D.R, Gasmann, H.C., and Mitchel, R.E. 1995. Water bath hyperthermia is a simple therapy for psoriasis and also stimulates skin tanning in response to sunlight. *International Journal of Hyperthermia*, vol. 11, no. 6: 745–54.

Brand-Miller, J., Foster-Powell, K., and Colagiuri, S. 2002. *The New Glucose Revolution*. Sydney: Hodder Headline Australia.

Breedlove, G. 1998. *The Herbal Home Spa*. North Adams, MA: Storey Books.

Briozzo, J., et al. 1989. Antimicrobial activity of clove oil dispersed in a concentration of sugar solution. *The Journal of Applied Bacteriology*, vol. 66, no. 1: 69–75.

British Association of Dermatologists. Social importance of skin. Retrieved 17 March 2006: http://www.bad.org.uk/public/skin/social/.

British Association of Dermatologists, Nottingham Eczema Team. 2000. Salt water baths and eczema. Retrieved 17 March 2006: www.bad.org.uk.

Budiyanto, A., et al. 2000. Protective effect of topically applied olive oil against photocarcinogenesis following UVB exposure of mice. *Carcinogenesis*, vol. 21, no. 11: 2085–90.

Buttriss, J., ed. 2002. *Adverse Reactions to Food*. London: British Nutrition Foundation, Blackwell Science.

Caili, F., et al. 2006. A review on pharmacological activities and utilization technologies of pumpkin. *Plant Foods for Human Nutrition*, vol. 61, no. 2: 70–77.

Cancer Council Australia. 2004. All about skin cancer. Retrieved 21 September 2006: http://www.cancer.org.au/content.cfm?randid=960742.

Carstens, J. 2006. The ugly side of beauty products. *Nature & Health*, October/November issue: 24–27.

Cassavant, M.C., et al. 2006. Investigation of antibiotic and antioxidant properties of leaf extracts from *Juglans nigra, Quercus alba*, and *Quercus rubra*. OLCC-McClain. Retrieved 21 January 2007: http://acs.confex.com/acs/mwrm06/techprogram/P38759.htm.

Chek, P. 2004. *How to Eat, Move and Be Healthy!*, chapter 6. San Diego: C.H.E.K Institute.

Christman, B.W., et al. 1992. An imbalance between the excretion of thromboxane and prostacyclin metabolites in pulmonary hypertension. *New England Journal of Medicine*, vol. 327, no. 2: 70–75.

Clark, A.M., et al. 2006. Antimicrobial activity of juglone. *Phytotherapy Research*, vol. 4, no. 1: 11–14.

Coeliac Society of Australia. Information about coeliac disease. Retrieved 20 November 2006: http://www.coeliac.org.au/index.htm.

Cohen, D. Complete psoriasis relief. Retrieved 16 August 2006: http://newyorkbodyscan.com/psoriasis.html.

Cordain. L. 2005. Implications for the role of diet in acne. *Seminars in Cutaneous Medicine and Surgery*, vol. 24, no. 2: 84–91.

Cordain, L., et al. 2002. Acne vulgaris: A disease of western civilization. *Archives of Dermatology*, vol. 138, no. 12: 1584–90.

Cordain, L., et al. 2005. Origins and evolution of the Western diet: Health implications for the 21st century. *American Journal of Clinical Nutrition*, vol. 81, no. 2: 341–54.

Cork, M., 2006. Emollients information sheet. National Eczema Society (UK). Retrieved 27 November 2006: http://www.eczema.org/emolienttherapy.pdf.

Cork, M., et al. 2005. New understanding of the predisposition to atopic eczema and sensitive skin. Allergy UK factsheet. Retrieved 27 November 2006: www.allergyuk.org.

Cotterill, J.A., and Cunliffe, W.J. 1997. Suicide in dermatological patients. *British Journal of Dermatology*, vol. 137, no. 2: 246.

Cowley, N.C., and Farr, P.M. 1992. A dose-response study of irritant reactions to sodium lauryl sulphate in patients with seborrhoeic dermatitis and atopic eczema. *Acta Dermato-Venereologica*, vol. 72, no. 6: 432–35.

Crossroads Institute. Brainwaves and EEG: The language of the brain. Retrieved 20 June 2006: www.crossroadsinstitute.org/eeg.html.

Darbre, P.D., et al. 2004. Concentrations of parabens in human breast tumours. *Journal of Applied Toxicology*, vol. 24, no. 1: 5–13.

David, T.J. 2000. Adverse reactions and intolerances to foods. *British Medical Bulletin*, vol. 56, no. 1: 34–50.

Daviglus, M.L., et al. 1997. Fish consumption and the 30-year risk of fatal myocardial infarction. *New England Journal of Medicine*, vol. 336, no. 15: 1046–53.

De, M., et al. 1999. Antimicrobial screening of some Indian spices. *Phytotherapy Research*, vol. 13, no. 7: 616–18.

De Groot, A.C., et al. 1987. Contact allergy to cocamide DEA and lauramide DEA in shampoos. *Contact Dermatitis*, vol. 16, no. 2: 117.

De Groot, A.C., and Frosch, P.J. 1997. Adverse reactions to fragrance. *Contact Dermatitis*, vol. 36, no. 2: 57.

De Paepe, K., et al. 2002. Repair of acetone- and sodium lauryl sulphate-damaged human skin barrier function using topically applied emulsions containing barrier lipids. *Journal of the European Academy of Dermatology and Venereology*, vol. 16, no. 6: 587–94.

Deiana, M., et al. 1999. Inhibition of peroxynitrite dependent DNA base modification and tyrosine nitration by the extra virgin olive oil-derived antioxidant hydroxytyosol. *Free Radical Biology & Medicine*, vol. 26, no. 5–6: 762–69.

Dengate, S. 2001. *The Failsafe Cookbook: Reducing Food Chemicals for Calm, Happy Families*, chapter 1. Sydney: Random House Australia.

Diegelmann, R.F. 2001. Collagen metabolism. *Wounds*, vol. 13, no. 5: 177–82.

Dixon, R.A.F., et al. 1990. Requirement of 5-lipoxygenase-activating protein for leukotriene synthesis. *Nature*, vol. 343: 282–84.

Dorman, H.J.D., and Deans, S.G. 2000. Antimicrobial agents from plants: Antibacterial activity of plant volatile oils. *Journal of Applied Microbiology*, vol. 88: 308–16.

Dr.Hauschka Skin Care. Viewing cellulite holistically (booklet).

Dweck, A.C. 2000. Functional botanicals — their chemistry and effects. International Cosmetic Expo, Miami, Florida.

Eczema Association of Australasia Inc. 2006. Facts about eczema. Retrieved 23 March, 2006: http://www.eczema.org.au/info/facts.html.

Enshaieh, S., et al. 2007. The efficacy of 5% topical tea tree oil gel in mild to moderate acne vulgaris: A randomized double-blind placebo-controlled study. *Indian Journal of Dermatology, Venereology and Leprology*, vol. 73, no 1: 22–25.

Erasmus, U. 1993. *Fats That Heal, Fats That Kill*. Burnaby, BC: Alive Books.

Eskew, M.L., et al. 1989. Effects of inadequate vitamin E and/or selenium nutrition on the release of arachidonic acid metabolites in rat alveolar macrophages. *Prostaglandins*, vol. 38, no. 1: 79–89.

Fartasch, M., et al. 1997. Mode of action of glycolic acid on human stratum corneum: Ultrastructural and functional evaluation of the epidermal barrier. *Archives of Dermatological Research*, vol. 289, no. 7: 404–9.

Fauler, J., and Frolich, J.C. 1989. Cardiovascular effects of leukotrienes. *Cardiovascular Drugs and Therapy*, vol. 3, no. 4: 499–505.

Ferrandiz, M.L., and Alcaraz, M.J. 1991. Anti-inflammatory activity and inhibition of arachidonic acid metabolism by flavonoids. *Inflammation Research*, vol. 32, no. 3–4: 283–88.

Fito, M., et al. 2000. Protective effect of olive oil and its phenolic compounds against low density lipoprotein oxidation. *Lipids*, vol. 35, no. 6: 6333–38.

Fogh, K., et al. 1989. Eicosanoids in skin of patients with atopic dermatitis: Prostaglandin E2 and leukotrienes B4 are present in biologically active concentrations. *Journal of Allergy and Clinical Immunology*, vol. 83, no. 2, pt. 1: 450–55.

Fortin, P.R., et al. 1995. Validation of a meta-analysis: The effects of fish oil in rheumatoid arthritis. *Journal of Clinical Epidemiology*, vol. 48, no. 11: 1379–90.

Gabriel, S. 2000. *Breathe for Life*. South Yarra, Australia: Hardie Grant Books.

Gehring, W., et al. 1999. Effect of topically applied evening primrose oil on epidermal barrier function in atopic dermatitis as a function of vehicle. *Arzneimittel-forschung*, vol. 49, no. 7: 635–42.

Ghersetich, I., et al. 1994. Hyaluronic acid in cutaneous intrinsic aging. *International Journal of Dermatology*, vol. 33, no. 2: 119–22.

Gloor, M., et al. 2004. On the course of the irritant reaction after irritation with sodium lauryl sulphate. *Skin Research & Technology*, vol. 10, no. 3: 144–48.

Gong, H., et al. 2004. Ocular surface in Zn-deficient rats. *Ophthalmic Research*, vol. 36, no. 3: 129–38.

Griffiths, C.E.M. 2001. The role of retinoids in the prevention and repair of aged and photoaged skin. *Clinical and Experimental Dermatology*, vol. 26, no. 7: 613–18.

Guerrero, A. 2005. *In Balance for Life*, chapters 1, 3 and 5. New York: Square One Publishing.

Harvey, P.W., and Everett, D.J. 2004. Significance of the detection of esters of p-hydroxybenzoic acid (parabens) in human breast tumours. *Journal of Applied Toxicology*, vol. 24, no. 1: 1–4.

Hawrelak, J. 2003. Probiotics: Choosing the right one for your needs. *Journal of the Australian Traditional-Medicine Society*, vol. 9, no. 2: 67–75.

Haywood, R., et al. 2003. Sunscreens inadequately protect against ultraviolet-A-induced free radicals in skin: Implications for skin aging and melanoma? *Journal of Investigative Dermatology*, vol. 121, no. 4: 862–68.

Higgins, E.M., and du Vivier, A.W.P. 1994. Cutaneous disease and alcohol misuse. *British Medical Bulletin*, vol. 50, no. 1: 85–98.

Hong, J., et al. 2004. Modulation of arachidonic acid metabolism by curcumin and related beta-diketone derivatives: Effects on cytosolic phospholipase A(2), cyclooxygenases and 5-lipoxygenase. *Carcinogenesis*, vol. 25, no. 9: 1671–79.

Horrobin, D.F. 1989. Essential fatty acids in clinical dermatology. *Journal of the American Academy of Dermatology*, vol. 20, no. 6: 1045–53.

Horrobin, D.F. 2000. Essential fatty acid metabolism and its modification in atopic eczema. *American Journal of Clinical Nutrition*, vol. 71, no. 1 suppl.: 367S–72S.

Horrocks, L.A., and Yeo, Y.K. 1999. Health benefits of docosahexaenoic acid (DHA). *Pharmacological Research*, vol. 40, no. 3: 211–25.

Hoyt, G., Hickey, M.S., and Cordain, L. 2005. Dissociation of the glycaemic and insulinaemic responses to whole and skimmed milk. *British Journal of Nutrition*, vol. 93: 175–77.

Jaivin, L. 2006. Let's sleep on it. *Sunday Telegraph*, 13 August 2006.

Janssen Pharmaceuticals, Inc. 2007. Ortho Evra. Retrieved 13 March 2007: www.orthoevra.com.

Jayaprakasam, B., et al. 2003. Anticancer and antiinflammatory activities of cucurbitacins from *Cucurbita andreana*. *Cancer Letters*, vol. 189, no. 1: 11–16.

Jones, M. 1998. *Your Child: Eczema*, chapter 5. Shaftesbury, Dorset, UK: Element Books.

Kang, Y., et al. 1999. Hyaluronan suppresses fibronectin fragment-mediated damage to human cartilage explant cultures by enhancing proteoglycan synthesis. *Journal of Orthopaedic Research*, vol. 17, no. 6: 858–69.

Kern, D. 2006. What is acne? Acne.org. Retrieved 23 August 2006: http://www.acne.org/whatisacne.html.

Kilkenny, M., et al. 1998. The prevalence of common skin conditions in Australian school children: 3. Acne vulgaris. *British Journal of Dermatology*, vol. 139, no. 5: 840–45.

Kirschmann, G.J., and Kirschmann, J.D. 1996. *Nutrition Almanac*, 4th ed., section VIII. Singapore: McGraw Hill Book Co.

Kitigawa, S., Li, H., and Sato, S. 1997. Skin permeation of parabens in excised guinea pig dorsal skin, its modification by penetration enhancers and their relationship with n-octanol/water partition coefficients. *Chemical & Pharmaceutical Bulletin* (Tokyo), vol. 45, no. 8: 1354–57.

Kritchevsky, D. 1995. The effect of over- and undernutrition on cancer. *European Journal of Cancer Prevention*, vol. 4, no. 6: 445–51.

Kritchevsky, D. 1999. Caloric restriction and experimental carcinogenesis. *Toxicological Sciences*, vol. 52, no. 2 suppl.: 13–16.

Leitzmann, M.F., et al. 2004. Dietary intake of n-3 and n-6 fatty acids and the risk of prostate cancer. *American Journal of Clinical Nutrition*, vol. 80, no. 1: 204–16.

Leveque, J.L., et al. 1993. How does sodium lauryl sulfate alter the skin barrier function in man? A multiparametric approach. *Skin Pharmacology*, vol. 6, no. 2: 111–15.

Levin, C., and Maibach, H. 2002. Exploration of "alternative" and "natural" drugs in dermatology. *Archives of Dermatology*, vol. 138, no. 2: 207–11.

Linus Pauling Institute, Oregon State University. 2005. Essential fatty acids. Retrieved 13 November 2006: http://lpi.oregonstate.edu/infocenter/othernuts/omega3fa.

Lubit, R.H., Bonds, C.L., and Lucia, M.A. 2006. Sleep disorders. Medscape Reference: Drugs, Diseases & Procedures website. Retrieved 2 March 2007: http://emedicine.medscape.com/article/287104-overview.

Lumb, K., and Tan, K. 2007. Melanoma — anyone can be affected. Sunday program. Retrieved 12 March 2007: www.ninemsn.com.au.

Manku, M.S., et al. 1982. Reduced levels of prostaglandin precursors in the blood of atopic patients: Defective delta-6-desaturase function as a biochemical basis of atopy. *Prostaglandins, Leukotrienes &?Medicine*, vol. 9, no. 6: 615–28.

Manku, M.S., et al. 1984. Essential fatty acids in the plasma phospholipids of patients with atopic eczema. *British Journal of Dermatology*, vol. 110, no. 6: 64–68.

Mansburg, G. 2004. Eczema and psoriasis. *Journal of Complementary Medicine*, vol. 3, no. 3: 26–32.

Masumura, S., et al. 1992. The effects of season and exercise on the levels of plasma polyunsaturated fatty acids and lipoprotein cholesterol in young rats. *Biochimica et Biophysica Acta*, vol. 1125, no. 3: 292–96.

Mattison, J.A., et al. 2003. Calorie restrictions in rhesus monkeys. *Experimental Gerontology*, vol. 38, no 1–2: 35–46.

McCarthy, M.F. 1996. Glucosamine for wound healing. *Medical Hypotheses*, vol. 47, no. 4: 273–75.

McDevitt, C.A., et al. 1989. Cigarette smoke degrades hyaluronic acid. *Lung*, vol. 167, no. 4: 237–45.

Medem: Medical Library. 2005. News from the American Medical Association: Smoking associated with the severity of psoriasis. Retrieved 28 March 2006: http://www.medem.com/medlb/article_detaillb.cfm.

Merck Manual, section 10, chapter 111. Retrieved 23 March 2006: http://www.merck.com/mrkshared/mmanual/section10/chapter111/111d.jsp.

Michaelsson, G., Juhlin, L., and Vahlquist, A. 1977. Effects of oral zinc and vitamin A in acne. *Archives of Dermatology*, vol. 113, no. 1: 31–36.

Moreno, J.A., et al. 2003. Effect of phenolic compounds of virgin olive oil on LDL oxidation resistance. *Medicina Clinica*, vol. 120, no. 4: 128–31.

Moscatelli, D., and Rubin, H. 1977. Hormonal control of hyaluronic acid production in fibroblasts and its relation to nucleic acid and protein synthesis. *Journal of Cellular Physiology*, vol. 91, no 1: 79–88.

Muhlebach, S., et al. 1996. Successful therapy of salicylate poisoning using glycine and activated charcoal. *Schweisische Medizinische Wochenschrift*, vol. 126, no. 49: 2127–29. Abstract retrieved 28 November 2006: www.ncbi.nlm.nih.gov.

Murad, H. 2005. *The Cellulite Solution*, Introduction. London: Piatkus.

Murakoshi, M., et al. 1992. Inhibition by squalene of the tumor-promoting activity of 12-0-tetradecanolyphorbol-13-acetate in mouse skin carcinogenesis. *International Journal of Cancer*, vol. 52, no. 6: 950–52.

Murray, M., and Pizzorno, J. 1998. *Encyclopedia of Natural Medicine*, 2nd ed. London: Little, Brown & Company.

Nase, G. 2005. Beating rosacea: Vascular, ocular and acne forms. Retrieved 16 August 2006: http://www.drnase.com/research_rosacea_articles.htm.

Nase, G. 2005. Facial rosacea: Vascular basis of the disorder. Retrieved 18 August 2006: http://www.drnase.com/vascular_basis.htm.

National Cancer Institute. 2005. What you need to know about skin cancer. Retrieved 21 September 2006: http://www.cancer.gov/cancertopics/wyntk/skin/page13

National Institute of Arthritis and Musculoskeletal and Skin Diseases. Questions and answers about acne. Retrieved 24 August 2006: http://www.niams.nih.gov/hi/topics/acne/acne.htm.

National Institute of Arthritis and Musculoskeletal and Skin Diseases. Questions and answers about rosacea. Retrieved 23 March 2006: http://www.niams.nih.gov/Health_Info/Rosacea/default.asp.

National Psoriasis Foundation. 2006. About psoriasis: Statistics. Retrieved 23 March 2006: www.psoriasis.org/about/stats/.

Nijveldt, R.J., et al. 2001. Flavonoids: A review of probable mechanisms of action and potential applications. *American Journal of Clinical Nutrition*, vol. 74, no. 4: 418–25.

Östman, E.M., et al. 2001. Inconsistency between glycemic and insulinemic responses to regular and fermented milk products. *American Journal of Clinical Nutrition*, vol. 74, no. 1: 96–100.

Pareja, B., and Kehl, H. 1990. Contribution to the identification of the active principles of Rosa aff Rubiginosa L. Anales de la Real Academia de Farmacia, Instituto de Espana, vol. 56, no. 2: 283–94.

Pashko, L.L., and Schwartz, A.G. 1992. Reversal of food restriction-induced inhibition of mouse skin tumour promotion by adrenalectomy. *Carcinogenesis*, vol. 13, no. 10: 1925–28.

Patel, D.K., et al. 1990. Depletion of plasma glycine and effect of glycine by mouth on salicylate metabolism during aspirin overdose. *Human & Experimental Toxicology*, vol. 9, no. 6: 389–95.

Patils, S., et al. 1995. Quantification of sodium lauryl sulfate penetration into the skin and underlying tissue after topical application — pharmacological and toxicological implications. *Journal of Pharmaceutical Sciences*, vol. 84, no. 10: 1240–44.

PDRhealth. 2006. Phosphatidylcholine. Retrieved 5 October 2006: www.pdrhealth.com/drug_info/nmdrugprofiles/ nutsupdrugs/pho_0288.shtml.

Pennisi, E. 2005. Why do humans have so few genes? *Science*, vol. 309, no. 5731: 80.

Persson, E., et al. 2003. Influence of antioxidants in virgin olive oil on the formation of heterocyclic amines in fried beefburgers. *Food & Chemical Toxicology*, vol. 41, no. 11: 1587–97.

Petrik, M.B., et al. 2000. Antagonism of arachidonic acid is linked to the antitumorigenic effect of dietary eicosapentaenoic acid in Apc (Min/+) mice, *Journal of Nutrition*, vol. 130, no. 5: 1153–58.

Pierpaoli, W., and Maestroni, G.J. 1987. Melatonin: A principal neuroimmuno-regulatory and anti-stress hormone: Its anti-aging effects. *Immunology Letters*, vol. 16, no. 3–4: 355–61.

Pitchford, P. 1993. *Healing with Whole Foods*, rev. ed., chapter 7. Berkeley, CA: North Atlantic Books.

Plunkett, A., et al. 1999. The frequency of non-malignant skin conditions in adults in central Victoria, Australia. *International Journal of Dermatology*, vol. 38, no. 12: 901.

Podda, M., and Grundmann-Kollmann, M. 2001. Low molecular weight antioxidants and their role in skin ageing. *Clinical & Experimental Dermatology*, vol. 26, no. 7: 578–82.

Proksch, E., et al. 2006. Skin barrier function, epidermal proliferation and differentiation in eczema. *Journal of Dermatological Science*, vol. 43, no. 3: 159–69.

Psoriasis Association (UK). 2006. What is psoriasis? Retrieved 23 March 2006: www.psoriasis-association.org.uk/ultra.html.

Pugazhendhi, D., et al. 2005. Oestrogenic activity of p-hydroxybenzoic acid (common metabolite of parabens esters) and methylparaben in human breast cancer cell lines. *Journal of Applied Toxicology*, vol. 25, no. 4: 301–9.

Purba, M., et.al. 2001. Skin wrinkling: Can food make a difference? *Journal of the American College of Nutrition*, vol. 20, no. 1: 71–80.

Purvis, D., et al. 2006. Acne, anxiety, depression and suicide in teenagers: A cross-sectional survey of New Zealand secondary school students. *Journal of Paediatrics and Child Health*, vol. 42, no. 12: 793–96.

Qiu, H., et al. 2006. Expression of 5-lipoxygenase and leukotrienes A4 hydrolase in human atherosclerotic lesions correlates with symptoms of plaque instability. *Proceedings of the National Academy of Sciences*, vol. 103, no. 21: 8161–66.

Reiter, R.J. 1995. Oxygen radical detoxification process during aging: The functional importance of melatonin. *Aging*, vol. 7, no. 5: 340–51.

Reiter, R.J. 1995. The pineal gland and melatonin in relation to aging: A summary of the theories and of the data. *Experimental Gerontology*, vol. 30, no. 3–4: 199–212.

Reiter, R.J., et al. 1995. A review of the evidence supporting melatonin's role as an antioxidant. *Journal of Pineal Research*, vol. 18, no. 1: 1–11.

Rexbye, H., et al. 2006. Influence of environmental factors on facial ageing. *Oxford Journals*, vol. 35, no. 2: 110–15.

Robbins, A. 2001. *Get the Edge: A 7-Day Program to Transform Your Life*. San Diego: Robbins Research International.

Rosacea Support Group. 2006. Exercise influence. Retrieved 18 August 2006: http://www.rosacea-research.org/wiki/index.php/Exercise_Influence.

Rosacea Support Group. 2006. Histamine containing or triggering foods. Retrieved 18 August 2006: http://rosacea-research.org/wiki/index.php/Histamine_Containing_or_Triggering_Foods.

Rosenbaum, M., et al. 1998. An exploratory investigation of the morphology and biochemistry of cellulite. *Plastic and Reconstructive Surgery*, vol. 101, no. 7: 1934–39.

Roth, G.S., et al. 2001. Dietary caloric restriction prevents the age-related decline in plasma melatonin levels of rhesus monkeys. *Journal of Endocrinology & Metabolism*, vol. 86, no. 7: 3292–95.

Ruzicka, T. 1989. Leukotrienes in atopic eczema. *Acta Dermato-Venereologica Supplementum*, vol. 144: 48–49.

Saavedra, J.M., Harris, G.D., and Finberg, L. 1991. Capillary refilling (skin turgor) in the assessment of dehydration. *Archives of Pediatrics & Adolescent Medicine*, vol. 145, no. 3: 296–298.

Samuelsson, B. 1983. Leukotrienes: Mediators of immediate hypersensitivity reactions and inflammation. *Science*, vol. 220, no 4597: 568–75.

SanGiovanni, J.P., and Chew, E.Y. 2005. The role of omega-3 long-chain polyunsaturated fatty acids in health and disease of the retina. *Progress in Retinal & Eye Research*, vol. 24, no. 1: 87–138.

Santosh, K., et al. 2000. Green tea and skin. *Archives of Dermatology*, vol. 136, no. 8: 989–94.

Sardi, B. 2004. Yuzurihara, the village of long life, reveals its secrets. Knowledge of Health Inc. Retrieved 10 April 2006: http://www.knowledgeofhealth.com/pdfs/yuzurihara.pdf.

Sarin, C.L., Austin, J.C., and Nickel, W.O. 1974. Effects of smoking on digital blood-flow velocity. *Journal of the American Medical Association*, vol. 229, no. 10: 1327–28.

Sausenthaler, S., et al. 2006. Margarine and butter consumption, eczema & allergic sensitization in children. *Pediatric Allergy and Immunology*, vol. 17, no. 2: 85–93.

Seville, R.H. 1997. Psoriasis and stress. *British Journal of Dermatology*, vol. 97, no. 3: 297–302.

Shelef, L.A. 1984. Antimicrobial effects of spices. *Journal of Food Safety*, vol. 6, no. 1: 29–44.

Siddappa, K. 2003. Dry skin conditions, eczema and emollients in their management. *Indian Journal of Dermatology, Venereology and Leprology*, vol. 69, no. 2: 69–75.

Siebecker, A. 2005. Traditional bone broth in modern health and disease. *Townsend Letter*, Feb/Mar issue.

Smith, R., et al. 2004. The effect of short-term altered macronutrient status on acne vulgaris and biochemical markers of insulin sensitivity. *Asia Pacific Journal of Clinical Nutrition*, vol. 13 (supplement): S67.

Snyder, P. 1997. Antimicrobial effects of spices and herbs. Hospitality Institute of Technology and Management, St Paul, Minnesota.

Srivastava, K.C. 1984. Aqueous extracts of onion, garlic and ginger inhibit platelet aggregation and alter arachidonic acid metabolism. *Biomedica Biochimica Acta*, vol. 43, no. 8–9: S335–46.

Staberg, B., et al. 1987. Abnormal vitamin D metabolism in patients with psoriasis. *Acta Dermato-Venereologica*, vol. 67, no. 1: 65–68. Abstract retrieved 22 August 2006: http://www.ncbi.nlm.nih.gov.

Stokkan, K.A., et al. 1991. Food restriction retards aging of the pineal gland. *Brain Research*, vol. 545, no. 1–2: 66–72.

Swain, A.R., Soutter, V.L., and Loblay, R.H. Royal Prince Alfred Hospital Allergy Unit. 2002. *Friendly Food: The Essential Guide to Avoiding Allergies, Additives and Problem Chemicals*. Sydney: Murdoch Books.

Thompson, R.W., et al. 1975. Alterations of porcine skin acid mucopolysaccharides in zinc deficiency. *Journal of Nutrition*, vol. 105, no 2: 154–60.

Thomsen, M. 2001. *Phytotherapy Desk Reference*, 2nd ed. Dee Why, Australia: Institute for Phytotherapy.

Tidwell, J. 2006. Allergies: Histamine in food. Retrieved 18 August 2006: http://allergies.about.com/cs/histamine/a/aa071000a.htm.

Tortora, G.J., and Grabowski, S. 2000. *Principles of Anatomy and Physiology*, 9th ed., chapters 17 and 22. New York: John Wiley & Sons.

Treffers, S. 1999. *Food Additives: A Guide to Their Use, Origin and Effects*. Brisbane: Hartrade.

Tung, R.C., et al. 2000. Alpha-hydroxy acid-based cosmetic procedures: Guidelines for patient management. *American Journal of Clinical Dermatology*, vol. 1, no. 2: 81–88.

Uauy, R., et al. 2000. Essential fatty acids in visual and brain development. *Lipids*, vol. 36, no. 9: 885–95.

U.S. Department of Energy Genome Programs. 2006. How many genes are in the human genome? Retrieved 18 March 2006: http://www.ornl.gov/sci/techresources/Human_Genome/faq/genenumber.shtml.

U.S. Department of Health & Human Services. 2007. Household Products Database. Retrieved 4 March 2007: http://hpd.nlm.nih.gov/cgi-bin/household/brands?tbl=chem&id=711.

Vander Straten, M., et al. 2001. Tobacco use and skin disease. *Southern Medical Journal*, vol. 94, no. 6: 621–34.

Walsh, S.W. 1984. Pre-eclampsia: An imbalance in placental prostacyclin and thromboxane production. *American Journal of Obstetrics and Gynecology*, vol. 152, no. 3: 335–40.

Wang, Z.Y., et al. 1991. Protection against ultraviolet B radiation-induced photocarcinogenesis in hairless mice by green tea polyphenols. *Carcinogenesis*, vol. 12, no. 8: 1527–30.

Weimar, V.M., et al. 1978. Zinc sulfate in acne vulgaris. *Archives of Dermatology*, vol. 114, no. 12: 1776–78. Abstract retrieved 24 August 2006: http://archderm.ama-assn.org/cgi/content/abstract/144/12/1776.

Wilkin, J., et al. 2002. Standard classification of rosacea: Report of the National Rosacea Society expert committee on the classification and staging of rosacea. *Journal of the American Academy of Dermatology*, vol. 46, no. 4: 584–87.

Wille, J., et al. 2003. Palmitoleic acid isomer in human skin sebum is effective against gram-positive bacteria. *Skin Pharmacology and Physiology*, vol. 16, no. 3: 176–87.

Williams, H.C., et al. 1995. Skin moisturisers in atopic eczema. British Association of Dermatologists website. Retrieved 27 November 2006: http://www.bad.org.uk/public/leaflets/other_atopic_-_skin.asp.

Winkler, C., et al. 2005. Extracts of pumpkin (*Cucurbita pepo* L.) seeds suppress stimulated peripheral blood mononuclear cells in vitro. *American Journal of Immunology*, vol. 1, no. 1: 6–11.

Wooltorton, E. 2003. Accutane (isotretinoin) and psychiatric adverse effects. *Canadian Medical Association Journal*, vol. 168, no. 1: 66.

World Health Organization. 2007. Soil-transmitted helminths. Retrieved 21 January 2007: http://www.who.int/wormcontrol/statistics/f1062-EXP-HS-Finalppqxp6.52:Layout 1 30/6/11 2:55 PM Page 373aqs/en/index1.html.

Wrong Diagnosis. 2006. Prevalence of eczema. Retrieved 12 January 2006: http://www.wrongdiagnosis.com/e/eczema/stats-country.htm.

Young, P. 2006. Salicylate summary for UKPID. IPCS INTOX Databank. Retrieved 13 September 2006: http://www.intox.org/databank/documents/pharm/salicy/ukpid14.htm.

Zlatkov, N.B., et al. 1984. Free fatty acids in the blood serum of psoriatics. *Acta Dermato-Venereologica*, vol. 64, no. 1: 22–25.

About the Nutrient Analyses

Computer-assisted nutrient analysis of the recipes was prepared by Kimberly Zammit, HBSc (the project supervisor was Len Piché, PhD, RD, Division of Food & Nutritional Sciences, Brescia University College, London, ON), using Food Processor® SQL, version 10.9, ESHA Research Inc., Salem OR (this software contains over 35,000 food items based largely on the latest USDA data and the entire Canadian Nutrient File, 2007b). The database was supplemented when necessary with data from the Canadian Nutrient File (version 2010) and documented data from other reliable sources.

The analysis was based on:

- imperial weights and measures (except for foods typically packaged and used in metric quantities);
- the larger number of servings (i.e., the smaller portion) when there is a range;
- the smaller ingredient quantity when there was a range;
- the first ingredient listed when there was a choice of ingredients.

Calculations involving meat and poultry use lean portions without skin and with visible fat trimmed. A pinch of salt was calculated as $1/8$ tsp (0.5 mL). All recipes were analyzed prior to cooking. Optional ingredients and garnishes, and ingredients that are not quantified, were not included in the calculations.

All percent daily values (% DVs) and nutrition claims that appear in the recipes are based on U.S. standards.

Library and Archives Canada Cataloguing in Publication

Fischer, Karen, 1972-
    The 8-week healthy skin diet : includes more than 100 recipes for beautiful skin / Karen Fischer.

Includes index.
First published in Australia under title: The healthy skin diet.
ISBN 978-0-7788-0440-6

    1. Skin — Care and hygiene. 2. Skin — Diseases — Diet therapy. 3. Skin — Diseases — Diet therapy — Recipes. 4. Cookbooks. I. Fischer, Karen, 1972- . Healthy skin diet. II. Title. III. Title: Eight-week healthy skin diet.

RL87.F58 2013   646.7'26   C2012-907486-1

Index

A

Accutane. *See* Roaccutane
ACE Smoothie, 355
acidosis, 31–33
acne, 147–66
  aggravation of, 149, 153
  diet and, 27, 164–65
  drug therapies, 111, 149
  supplements for, 156, 158
  topical treatments, 153–54, 155
ACV Drink, 344
additives
  in beauty products, 126–30
  in foods, 38, 263, 275–76, 459
aging, 141, 204
  foods that combat, 91–94, 392
AHA (alpha hydroxy acid), 131
Aïoli, 383
alcohol, 35–36, 160, 195, 228, 253
alkalosis, 33
allergies, 17, 203, 208–9, 263. *See also* histamine reactions
Almond Milk, 356. *See also* almonds
  Berry Beauty Smoothie, 348
  Skin-Firming Drink, 350
  Vitamin E Muesli, 370
almond oil, 131, 236
almonds. *See also* Almond Milk
  ACE Smoothie, 355
  Amine-Free Fruit Salad, 363
  Bircher Muesli, 371
  Designer Muesli, 368
  French Toast with Berries and Almonds, Delicious, 359
  Gluten-Free Muesli, 369

alpha-linolenic acid (ALA), 56, 60. *See also* omega-3 EFAs
Amine-Free Fruit Salad, 363
amines. *See* histamine reactions
amino acids, 86, 87, 91, 254
Anti-Aging Broth, 93, 392
  Beef Barley Soup, 425
  Herb and Garlic Chicken Casserole, 399
  Roasted Corn and Cauliflower Soup, 439
  Seafood Hotpot, 420
  Slow-Cooked Lamb Casserole, 427
  Sweet Chicken Stir-Fry, 400
  Therapeutic Chicken Soup, 396
  Therapeutic Veggie Soup, 438
antibiotics, 149, 195
antihistamines, 259–60. *See also* histamine reactions
antioxidants, 182, 229, 459
anxiety, 125, 192. *See also* stress
apple cider vinegar. *See* vinegar, apple cider
apple juice
  ACV Drink (variation), 344
  Apple Omega Juice, 354
  Bircher Muesli, 371
  Papaya Beauty Smoothie, 349
  Stewed Pears with Vanilla Soy Custard, 452
apples, 163. *See also* apple juice
  Amine-Free Fruit Salad, 363
  Berry Beauty Porridge (tip), 358
  Carrot Cake, 457

Poached Apple Surprise, 453
Spinach Salad, Tasty, 432
Spot-Free Skin Juice, 351
Apricot Chicken, C-Rich, 402
arachidonic acid (AA), 56, 62, 63–64, 227
ascorbic acid. *See* vitamin C
aspirin, 203, 217. *See also* salicylates
avocado, 324
  Avocado Beauty Snack, 390
  Avocado Dip with Dipping Sticks, 391
  Avocado on Toast, 360
  Avocado Salsa, 390
  Chicken and Salad Sandwich, 397
  Chicken and Salad Wrap, 398
  Falafel Wraps, 444
  Perfect Poached Eggs, 364
  Salad Sandwiches with Creamy Mayo, 442
  Salmon and Salad Sandwich, 410
  Smoked Salmon and Avocado on Toast, 361
  Smoked Salmon and Eggs, 365
  Sweet Raspberry, Avocado and Watercress Salad, 431
  Tuna and Avocado Wrap, 409

B

babies. *See also* breastfeeding; children
  cradle cap in, 183–85, 217
  eczema in, 205, 211, 268
  feeding, 272, 273–74
  and supplements, 269
bananas
  Avocado on Toast, 360
  Banana Cake, 458

bananas (*continued*)
Bircher Muesli, 371
Fruit Salad with Flax Seeds, 363
Gluten-Free Muesli, 369
Papaya Beauty Smoothie, 349
Skin-Firming Drink, 350
Sweet Banana and Carob Spread, 455
Sweet Banana Porridge, 360
Tangy Papaya Cups, 454
Vitamin E Muesli, 370
Whole Fruit Jam on Toast, 361
bandaging (wet), 213
barbecuing, 71
baths, 322
for acne, 153–54
for children, 211, 264–65
for eczema, 208, 210–12
for psoriasis, 235
as relaxation technique, 227, 242
beans. *See also* beans, green/yellow; bean sprouts
Beans on Toast, 376
Falafel, 443
Kids' Creamy Beans on Toast, 378
beans, green/yellow
Chicken and Three Veg, 406
Lean Lamb and Three Veg, 426
Omega Niçoise Salad, 408
Skin Juice for Sensitive Skin No. 2, 353
Spicy Green Papaya Salad, 436
bean sprouts
Lamb Stir-Fry, 428
Seafood Hotpot, 420
Shrimp and Sweet Chile Vegetable Stir-Fry, 418
Spicy Green Papaya Salad, 436
Thai Fish with Corn, 411
Vegetable Hand Rolls, 388
beauty, 293–310. *See also* beauty products

actions as revealing, 302–10
appreciating, 124, 298–301, 306–7
exercises, 306–8
feelings and, 303, 305, 309–10
good energy as, 296–98, 307–8
inner, 294–98, 302–10
subconscious mind and, 299–301, 302
The Beauty Bible (Begoun), 131
beauty products, 16, 126–42, 145. *See also* skin care
bad additives, 126–30
cleansers, 137–38, 151
good additives, 130–36
makeup, 138–39
moisturizers, 138, 139
toners, 138, 150
beef
Anti-Aging Broth, 392
Beef Barley Soup, 425
Healthy Hamburger, 422
Steak Sandwiches, 424
beets
Chicken and Salad Wrap, 398
Healthy Hamburger, 422
Salad Sandwiches with Creamy Mayo, 442
Spot-Free Skin Juice, 351
Begoun, Paula, 131
benzoyl peroxide (BP), 155
berries. *See also* raspberries
Amine-Free Fruit Salad, 363
Berry Beauty Porridge, 358
Berry Beauty Smoothie, 348
French Toast with Berries and Almonds, Delicious, 359
Skin-Firming Drink, 350
Strawberry Rehydration Water, 348
Vitamin E Muesli, 370
beta-carotene, 216, 243. *See also* vitamin A

beta glucan, 132
beverages, 343–56. *See also* alcohol; water; *specific beverages*
alkalizing, 314, 318–19, 320
BHA (beta hydroxy acid), 131
biotin, 60, 198, 222–24
Bircher Muesli, 371
birch oil, 171
blackcurrant seed oil, 132
black walnut extract, 47
blood cells (red), 31
blood circulation, 257, 259–60
blood sugar (glucose), 77, 80, 81, 84
bowel health, 40, 163, 180, 240–41, 258. *See also* digestion
brain, 77, 297
bread, 68. *See also* sandwiches and wraps
Avocado on Toast, 360
Avocado Salsa, 390
Beans on Toast, 376
Egg Soldiers, 366
French Toast with Berries and Almonds, Delicious, 359
Kids' Creamy Beans on Toast, 378
Kids' Scrambled Eggs, 377
Perfect Poached Eggs, 364
Sardines and Lemon on Whole-Grain Toast, 362
Smoked Salmon and Avocado on Toast, 361
Smoked Salmon and Eggs, 365
Whole Fruit Jam on Toast, 361
breakfasts, 314–15, 319, 321, 357–78
breast cancer, 128
breastfeeding. *See also* babies
diet during, 87, 185, 271
supplements during, 39, 65, 156, 218, 267, 268
Breathe for Life (Gabriel), 282–92

breathing, 281–92
abdominal, 289–91
diaphragm, 288–89
exercises, 282–91, 322, 323
as immune booster, 177, 192
as relaxation technique, 123, 243
throat, 283–87
broccoli
Chicken and Three Veg, 406
Fish and Steamed Vegetables, 375
Lean Lamb and Three Veg, 426
Marinated Whole Steamed Trout, 414
broths and soups, 93–94, 389, 392, 438–39
buckwheat, 324–25
Mango and Buckwheat Crêpes, 372
Pear and Buckwheat Crêpes, 373
Rich Mineral Salad with Papaya, Dill and Baby Spinach, 435
butter, 53

C

cabbage
Garden Salad, 437
Lamb Stir-Fry, 428
Shrimp and Sweet Chile Vegetable Stir-Fry, 418
Skin Juice for Sensitive Skin No. 1, 352
Skin Juice for Sensitive Skin No. 2, 353
Spot-Free Skin Juice, 351
Sweet Chicken Stir-Fry, 400
Therapeutic Chicken Soup, 396
Tropical Vegetarian Stir-Fry, 447
Vegetable Casserole, Tasty, 450

caffeine, 43, 97
Cajun Chicken, 404
Cajun Seasoning, 405
calcium, 65, 66, 160, 218, 272
Calcium-Rich Smoothie, 351
calendula, 132
calories, 73, 74, 75, 76, 144
Candida albicans, 48–49, 52
candies, 275–76
carbohydrates, 15, 77–86, 144
commitment (low GI), 81–82
hit and run (high GI), 78–80, 179, 194, 205
kinds, 78–79
sources, 79, 81
carrots
Anti-Aging Broth, 392
Avocado Dip with Dipping Sticks, 391
Beef Barley Soup, 425
Carrot Cake, 457
Chicken and Salad Sandwich, 397
Colorful Non-Fried Rice, 449
C-Rich Apricot Chicken, 402
Fish and Steamed Vegetables, 375
Healthy Hamburger, 422
Lamb Stir-Fry, 428
Rainbow Trout with Honey-Roasted Vegetables, 412
Salad Sandwiches with Creamy Mayo, 442
Salmon and Salad Sandwich, 410
Spinach Salad, Tasty, 432
Spot-Free Skin Juice, 351
Steak Sandwiches, 424
Therapeutic Chicken Soup, 396
Therapeutic Veggie Soup, 438
Tropical Vegetarian Stir-Fry, 447
Vegetable Hand Rolls, 388

carrot seed oil, 132
case studies, 6–9, 74, 118, 136, 238, 256. *See also specific concerns*
of beauty, 294, 296, 299
of breathing, 283, 284
of children, 269, 275
cashews
Spicy Green Papaya Salad, 436
Tropical Vegetarian Stir-Fry, 447
cauliflower
Creamy Chickpea Curry, 441
Herb and Garlic Chicken Casserole, 399
Roasted Corn and Cauliflower Soup, 439
Slow-Cooked Lamb Casserole, 427
Therapeutic Chicken Soup, 396
Therapeutic Veggie Soup, 438
Vegetable Casserole, Tasty, 450
celery
Anti-Aging Broth, 392
Avocado Dip with Dipping Sticks, 391
Beef Barley Soup, 425
Detox Dal, 440
Skin Juice for Sensitive Skin No. 1, 352
Skin Juice for Sensitive Skin No. 2, 353
Sweet Chicken Stir-Fry, 400
Therapeutic Chicken Soup, 396
Therapeutic Veggie Soup, 438
celiac disease, 84–86
cells, 175
blood, 31
fat, 168, 169–70
skin, 5, 22
cellulite, 167–82
anatomy, 168–70
diet strategies, 181–82

cellulite (continued)
exercise and, 173, 176–78, 180
management program, 171–82
cereals, 358, 360, 368–71. See also grains
chamomile, 132, 228
charisma, 297
chemical exposure, 37–39, 207–8, 218–19, 238, 263
chicken, 88–89
Anti-Aging Broth, 392
Cajun Chicken, 404
Chicken and Salad Sandwich, 397
Chicken and Salad Wrap, 398
Chicken and Three Veg, 406
C-Rich Apricot Chicken, 402
Herb and Garlic Chicken Casserole, 399
Sweet Chicken Stir-Fry, 400
Therapeutic Chicken Soup, 396
Vegetable Hand Rolls, 388
chickpeas
Chickpea Beauty Salad, 430
Creamy Chickpea Curry, 441
Hummus, 382
children, 263–79. See also babies
diet for, 270–77
eczema in, 9, 13, 268
elimination diet, 272–75, 278–79
inflammation prevention, 275–76
supplements for, 266–72
topical treatments, 264–65
chlorophyll, 50–51, 325
for children, 266, 269
Green Water, 344
as supplement, 163, 221–22, 260

chlorpromazine, 62
chromium, 82–84, 162, 194
cilantro
Creamy Chickpea Curry, 441
C-Rich Apricot Chicken, 402
Falafel, 443
Seafood Hotpot, 420
Shrimp and Sweet Chile Vegetable Stir-Fry, 418
Spicy Green Papaya Salad, 436
Vegetable Hand Rolls, 388
cinnamon, 194
citrus seed extract, 188
cleaning products, 37
cleansers, 137–38, 151
clove oil, 48
coal tar products, 237
cocamide DEA, 129
coconut milk
Berry Beauty Smoothie, 348
Creamy Chickpea Curry, 441
Seafood Hotpot, 420
coconut oil, 133, 236
coffee, 14, 43–44, 174
collagen, 21, 91, 175
Colorful Non-Fried Rice, 449
connective tissue, 168–69, 175–76
constipation, 39–41
Cordain, Loren, 26–27
corn
Colorful Non-Fried Rice, 449
Roasted Corn and Cauliflower Soup, 439
Salmon Steaks with Peas and Mash, 416
Thai Fish with Corn, 411
corticosteroids, 213
cortisol, 43
cortisone creams, 212
cradle cap, 183–85, 217
Creamy Chickpea Curry, 441
Creamy Mayonnaise, 380
Aïoli, 383
Tartar Sauce, 381
Tuna Dip, 381

C-Rich Apricot Chicken, 402
cysteine, 94

D
dairy products, 65. See also Almond Milk; soy milk
and acne, 161–62, 165
avoiding, 178–79, 194
sensitivity to, 161, 272
d-alpha tocopherol. See vitamin E
dandelion root, 325
Dandelion Tea, 345
Soy Dande', 345
dandruff, 186–99
diet for, 197–99
exercise and, 196–97
treatment recipes, 189–90
DEA (diethanolamine), 129, 183
dehydration, 42–44
Delicious French Toast with Berries and Almonds, 359
d-5-desaturase, 60
demineralization, 30, 31
dermatitis, 86, 116
atopic (eczema), 200–231
seborrheic (dandruff), 186–99
dermis, 21
Designer Muesli, 368
desserts, 316–17, 451–58
detox. See liver detoxification
Detox Dal, 440
DGLA (dihomo-gamma-linolenic acid), 56
diabetes, 16, 84. See also hypoglycemia
diet. See also foods; Healthy Skin Diet
and acne, 27, 164–65
calorie-restricted, 73, 75, 76
and connective tissue, 169
as eczema cause, 200, 203, 204, 206–7
elimination, 225–26, 231, 272–75, 278–79
and skin health, 24–27
vegetarian, 91

digestion, 17, 53, 240–41, 268. *See also* bowel health
dinners, 316, 320, 321
dips, 381–83, 390–91
DMDM hydantoin, 127
docosahexaenoic acid (DHA), 56
dressings, 386
drinks. *See* alcohol; beverages

E

eczema, 200–231
  aggravation of, 206–7, 208, 209, 215
  allergies and, 203, 208–9
  bath treatments, 208, 210–12
  in children, 9, 13, 268
  diet as cause, 200, 203, 204, 206–7
  diet for managing, 225–26, 228–29
  drug therapies, 212–14
  glycine for, 216–17, 218–19, 222, 228
  short-term relief, 201, 207–8
  supplements for, 216–24
  topical treatments, 201, 209–15, 265
  triggers, 202–8
edema, 170, 177
eggplant
  Creamy Chickpea Curry, 441
  Herb and Garlic Chicken Casserole, 399
  Slow-Cooked Lamb Casserole, 427
eggs, 89
  Boiled Eggs, Vegetables and Rice, 374
  Colorful Non-Fried Rice, 449
  Creamy Mayonnaise, 380
  Egg Soldiers, 366
  French Toast with Berries and Almonds, Delicious, 359

Kids' Scrambled Eggs, 377
Mango and Buckwheat Crêpes, 372
Omega Niçoise Salad, 408
Omelet, Tasty, 367
Pear and Buckwheat Crêpes, 373
Perfect Poached Eggs, 364
Smoked Salmon and Eggs, 365
Stewed Pears with Vanilla Soy Custard, 452
egg white injury, 24, 222, 223
eicosapentaenoic acid (EPA), 56, 60, 65, 66
elastin, 21, 175
emotions, 122–23, 125, 323
  and beauty, 303, 305, 309–10
endorphins, 119, 277
epidermis, 20–21
Erasmus, Udo, 68
essential fatty acids (EFAs), 56, 60. *See also* omega-3 EFAs; omega-6 EFAs
estrogen, 169
evening primrose oil (EPO), 62–63, 133, 265
exercise, 15, 101–8, 145, 197, 322
  and acne, 164
  benefits, 102–3, 257
  and cellulite, 173, 176–78, 180
  C.H.E.K. method, 108
  and dandruff, 196–97
  program, 106–7
  and stress, 227, 243
  and toxins, 173
  types, 103–4
exfoliation, 141–42, 322
eyeshadow, 138

F

Falafel, 443
Falafel Wraps, 444
fat cells, 168, 169–70
fats, 15, 55–72, 143–44. *See also* fatty acids; prostaglandins

saturated, 56, 63–64, 204
trans, 56, 204
unsaturated, 56
Fats That Heal, Fats That Kill (Erasmus), 68
fatty acids, 55, 170. *See also* essential fatty acids
feelings. *See* emotions
fiber, 27, 163
fish, 68, 90, 326. *See also* fish oils; salmon; seafood; tuna
  Fish and Steamed Vegetables, 375
  Marinated Whole Steamed Trout, 414
  Omega Niçoise Salad, 408
  Rainbow Trout with Honey-Roasted Vegetables, 412
  Sardines and Lemon on Whole-Grain Toast, 362
  Seafood Hotpot, 420
fish oils, 198, 241
  cautions, 67, 271
  for children, 266, 269–71
flavonoids, 259
flaxseed oil, 67, 68, 270–71, 326–27. *See also* flax seeds
  Berry Beauty Smoothie, 348
  Calcium-Rich Smoothie, 351
  Creamy Mayonnaise, 380
  Flaxseed Lemon Drink, 346
  Omega Salad Dressing, 386
  Tasty Salad Dressing, 386
flax seeds, 70, 164, 270–71, 326–27. *See also* flaxseed oil
  ACE Smoothie, 355
  Amine-Free Fruit Salad, 363
  Apple Omega Drink, 354
  Berry Beauty Porridge, 358
  Bircher Muesli, 371
  Designer Muesli, 368
  French Toast with Berries and Almonds, Delicious, 359

flax seeds (*continued*)
 Fruit Salad with Flax Seeds, 363
 Gluten-Free Muesli, 369
 Ground Flax Seeds, 358
 Mango and Buckwheat Crêpes, 372
 Mango Ice, 454
 Papaya Beauty Smoothie, 349
 Pear and Buckwheat Crêpes, 373
 Pear Flaxseed Drink for Sensitive Skin, 347
 Skin-Firming Drink, 350
 Sweet Banana Porridge, 360
 Tangy Papaya Cups, 454
fluid retention, 170, 177
fluids, 165. *See also* beverages; hydration
foods. *See also* diet
 acid-forming, 33–35
 additives in, 38, 263, 275–76, 459
 alkali-forming, 52, 53
 amine-free, 252, 262
 anti-aging, 91–94, 392
 anti-parasitic, 46–47
 histamines in, 251–53
 intolerances to, 84–86, 161, 203, 272
 sulfur-rich, 254
formaldehyde, 127
fragrance, 128
French Toast with Berries and Almonds, Delicious, 359
fruit, 35. *See also* berries; *specific fruits*
 Amine-Free Fruit Salad, 363
 C-Rich Apricot Chicken, 402
 Fruit Salad with Flax Seeds, 363
 Rhubarb Crumble, 456
 Tropical Vegetarian Stir-Fry, 447
fungal infections, 48–49, 189–90, 194–95, 213. *See also* yeast infections

G

Gabriel, Sophie, 282–92
Garden Salad, 437
garlic, 47, 48
 Aïoli, 383
 Anti-Aging Broth, 392
 Creamy Chickpea Curry, 441
 Hummus, 382
 Omega Salad Dressing, 386
 Rich Mediterranean Pasta, 448
 Sweet Chutney, 384
 Thai Fish with Corn, 411
 Vegetable Casserole, Tasty, 450
genetics, 24, 169
ginger
 Anti-Aging Broth, 392
 Apple Omega Juice, 354
 Flaxseed Lemon Drink, 346
 Marinated Whole Steamed Trout, 414
 Pear Flaxseed Drink for Sensitive Skin, 347
 Seafood Hotpot, 420
 Skin Juice for Sensitive Skin No. 1, 352
 Sweet Chutney, 384
 Therapeutic Chicken Soup, 396
 Tropical Vegetarian Stir-Fry, 447
GLA (gamma-linolenic acid), 56, 60, 61, 132
glucosamine, 92, 175–76
 Skin-Firming Drink, 350
glucose, 77, 80, 81, 84
glutathione, 239
gluten, 84–86
Gluten-Free Muesli, 369
glycemic index (GI), 79–80, 82
glycemic load, 26
glycine
 for children, 266, 267
 deficiency, 217, 219
 for eczema, 216–17, 218–19, 222, 228
 Green Water (tip), 344

glycolic acid, 131
grains, 81–82, 86. *See also specific grains*
 Beef Barley Soup, 425
 Tabbouleh, 446
grape seed extract, 48
grape seed oil, 189
gratitude, 123–24, 307–8
greens, 326. *See also* spinach
 Chicken and Salad Sandwich, 397
 Chicken and Salad Wrap, 398
 Falafel Wraps, 444
 Fish and Steamed Vegetables, 375
 Garden Salad, 437
 Marinated Whole Steamed Trout, 414
 Omelet, Tasty, 367
 Roasted Sweet Potato Salad, 434
 Salad Sandwiches with Creamy Mayo, 442
 Salmon and Salad Sandwich, 410
 Sardines and Lemon on Whole-Grain Toast, 362
 Steak Sandwiches, 424
 Sweet Raspberry, Avocado and Watercress Salad, 431
 Tuna and Avocado Wrap, 409
 Green Water, 344

H

Hagan, James, 286
hand scrubs, 215
Healthy Hamburger, 422
Healthy Skin Diet, 13–14, 16–17, 312–39, 340–41. *See also* supplements; 3-Day Alkalizing Cleanse
 eating habits, 314–17
 and eating out, 14, 35, 94, 314, 315, 316
 fish days, 334–35, 336–37, 338–39
 gluten-free days, 334–35, 336, 338–39

guidelines, 12–16, 143–45

meal options, 329–31

meat days, 335, 337–38

menu and activity plan, 329, 332–39

planning for, 312–17

poultry days, 333–34, 336, 338

top 12 ingredients, 323–28

vegetarian days, 335, 337, 339

herbs, 47. *See also* cilantro; parsley

Herb and Garlic Chicken Casserole, 399

Rich Mineral Salad with Papaya, Dill and Baby Spinach, 435

Spicy Green Papaya Salad, 436

Vegetable Hand Rolls, 388

histamine reactions, 249–54. *See also* allergies; antihistamines

honey

Flaxseed Lemon Drink (tip), 346

Pear Flaxseed Drink for Sensitive Skin (tip), 347

Sweet Chile Sauce, 383

hormones, 130, 154–56, 169

hug therapy, 277

Hummus, 382

hyaluronan, 92, 175

hydration, 42–44, 180, 229, 240. *See also* beverages; water

hypoglycemia, 16, 80, 315. *See also* blood sugar

I

immune system, 53, 192–96, 199. *See also* lymphatic system

infections, 203, 264–65

fungal, 48–49, 189–90, 194–95, 213

yeast, 48–49, 52, 192, 196

insomnia, 96–97. *See also* sleep

insulin, 80. *See also* blood sugar

isopropyl alcohol (isopropanol), 129

isotretinoin (Roaccutane), 111, 149

itch relief, 201, 255, 264–65

J

Jam on Toast, Whole Fruit, 361

jealousy, 303–5. *See also* self-sabotage

jojoba oil, 133

Jung, Carl, 304–5

K

kelp, 328

Kids' Creamy Beans on Toast, 378

Kids' Scrambled Eggs, 377

kindness, 303

kombu, 174, 328

Detox Dal, 440

Miso Soup, 389

Therapeutic Chicken Soup, 396

L

lactic acid, 131

lamb

Lamb Stir-Fry, 428

Lean Lamb and Three Veg, 426

Slow-Cooked Lamb Casserole, 427

laughter, 122–23, 323

lecithin, 133, 170, 175, 181, 327

Apple Omega Juice, 354

Berry Beauty Smoothie, 348

Calcium-Rich Smoothie, 351

Designer Muesli, 368

Flaxseed Lemon Drink, 346

Gluten-Free Muesli, 369

Papaya Beauty Smoothie, 349

Pear Flaxseed Drink for Sensitive Skin, 347

Skin-Firming Drink, 350

lemon, 53, 328

Avocado Dip with Dipping Sticks, 391

Flaxseed Lemon Drink, 346

Green Water (tip), 344

Hummus, 382

lentils

Detox Dal, 440

Therapeutic Veggie Soup, 438

lettuce. *See* greens

leukotrienes, 63–64

lime, 53, 3278

Avocado Salsa, 390

Marinated Whole Steamed Trout, 414

Papaya Beauty Smoothie, 349

Rich Mineral Salad with Papaya, Dill and Baby Spinach, 435

Salmon Steaks with Peas and Mash, 416

Spicy Green Papaya Salad, 436

Sweet Chile Sauce, 383

Tangy Papaya Cups, 454

Thai Fish with Corn, 411

linoleic acid. *See* omega-6 EFAs

linolenic acid, 56, 60

liver detoxification, 16, 17, 154–57, 238–39, 261

cautions, 156, 217

glycine and, 216–17, 218–19, 222, 228

sulfation and, 253, 254

supplements for, 173, 218–19, 239, 254, 317

lunches, 315, 319, 321

lymphatic system, 101–2, 172, 176–78. *See also* immune system

M

macronutrients, 26, 57. *See also* carbohydrates; protein

magnesium, 92
    food sources, 164–65, 182
    as supplement, 60, 175–76, 218
makeup, 138–39. *See also* beauty products
malic acid, 131
mangos
    ACE Smoothie, 355
    Amine-Free Fruit Salad, 363
    Bircher Muesli, 371
    Mango and Buckwheat Crêpes, 372
    Mango Ice, 454
    Sweet Chicken Stir-Fry, 400
    Sweet Chutney, 384
maple syrup
    Omega Salad Dressing, 386
    Stewed Pears with Vanilla Soy Custard, 452
    Sweet Banana and Carob Spread, 455
    Sweet Banana Porridge, 360
margarine, 68
Marinated Whole Steamed Trout, 414
mascara, 139
massage, 171–74, 176–78, 184, 277
MEA, 129
meat, 71, 89. *See also specific meats*
medications, 39, 97, 195–96
melanoma. *See* skin cancer
melatonin, 75–76, 95–96
mercury contamination, 90
methylparaben, 128
micronutrients, 26–27, 57, 60. *See also specific nutrients*
mineral oil, 127–28
Miso Soup, 389
moisturizers. *See also* fats
    for acne, 150–52
    as beauty products, 138, 139
    for children, 184, 265
    for eczema, 209–15, 265

MSG (monosodium glutamate), 38
music, 121–22

N

The New Glucose Revolution, 79
nuts. *See specific types of nuts*

O

oats (rolled)
    Berry Beauty Porridge, 358
    Bircher Muesli, 371
    Designer Muesli, 368
    Fruit Salad with Flax Seeds, 363
    Rhubarb Crumble, 456
    Sweet Banana Porridge, 360
    Vitamin E Muesli, 370
oils, 171–72, 204. *See also specific types of oil*
ointments
    for eczema, 201, 209, 210, 214, 215
    for psoriasis, 236, 237
    for rosacea, 255
olive oil, 71, 134
    for cellulite, 174
    for dandruff, 189, 190
    in hand scrub, 215
    for psoriasis, 234–37, 242
olives
    Omega Niçoise Salad, 408
    Rich Mediterranean Pasta, 448
    Tuna and Avocado Wrap, 409
omega-3 EFAs, 26, 55, 56, 66–71, 181. *See also* alpha-linolenic acid; fish oils; prostaglandins
    and acne, 158
    for children, 185, 266, 269–71
    for dandruff, 198
    for eczema, 228–29
    food sources, 68–70, 164, 175, 261, 270–71
    for psoriasis, 241, 244
    for rosacea, 260

omega-6 EFAs, 56, 60, 61–63, 64
omega-9 fats, 71
Omega Niçoise Salad, 408
Omega Salad Dressing, 386
onions
    Anti-Aging Broth, 392
    Detox Dal, 440
    Lamb Stir-Fry, 428
    Rainbow Trout with Honey-Roasted Vegetables, 412
    Roasted Corn and Cauliflower Soup, 439
    Seafood Hotpot, 420
    Steak Sandwiches, 424
    Sweet Chicken Stir-Fry, 400
    Sweet Chutney, 384
    Therapeutic Veggie Soup, 438
    Tropical Vegetarian Stir-Fry, 447
oxygen, 31. *See also* breathing
Oysters with Dipping Sauce, 393

P

papayas
    ACE Smoothie, 355
    Berry Beauty Porridge (tip), 358
    Calcium-Rich Smoothie, 351
    Fruit Salad with Flax Seeds, 363
    Papaya Beauty Smoothie, 349
    Rich Mineral Salad with Papaya, Dill and Baby Spinach, 435
    Spicy Green Papaya Salad, 436
    Sweet Chicken Stir-Fry, 400
    Tangy Papaya Cups, 454
parabens, 128
parasites, 44–48, 319, 321

parsley
  Avocado Salsa, 390
  Chickpea Beauty Salad,
    430
  Skin Juice for Sensitive
    Skin No. 1, 352
  Skin Juice for Sensitive
    Skin No. 2, 353
  Tabbouleh, 446
Pasta, Rich Mediterranean,
    448
pears, 163
  Fruit Salad with Flax Seeds,
    363
  Pear and Buckwheat
    Crêpes, 373
  Pear Flaxseed Drink for
    Sensitive Skin, 347
  Skin Juice for Sensitive
    Skin No. 1, 352
  Skin Juice for Sensitive
    Skin No. 2, 353
  Spot-Free Skin Juice, 351
  Stewed Pears with Vanilla
    Soy Custard, 452
peas (green)
  Chicken and Three Veg,
    406
  Colorful Non-Fried Rice,
    449
  Salmon Steaks with Peas
    and Mash, 416
  Tropical Vegetarian Stir-Fry,
    447
peppers, bell
  Avocado Dip with Dipping
    Sticks, 391
  Colorful Non-Fried Rice,
    449
  C-Rich Apricot Chicken,
    402
  Garden Salad, 437
  Lamb Stir-Fry, 428
  Rich Mediterranean Pasta,
    448
  Seafood Hotpot, 420
  Shrimp and Sweet Chile
    Vegetable Stir-Fry, 418
  Thai Fish with Corn, 411
  Tropical Vegetarian Stir-Fry,
    447

peppers, chile
  Salmon Steaks with Peas
    and Mash, 416
  Shrimp and Sweet Chile
    Vegetable Stir-Fry, 418
  Spicy Green Papaya Salad,
    436
  Sweet Chile Sauce, 383
  Sweet Chutney (variation),
    384
  Thai Fish with Corn, 411
perspiration, 103–4
pH balance, 27, 29–54, 143,
    221–22, 314
phenothiazine, 62
pityrosporum (yeast), 192
Poached Apple Surprise, 453
Poached Eggs, Perfect, 364
pollution, 169, 208. See also
    chemical exposure
polyamines, 240
potassium, 27
pregnancy, 13, 63
  and diet, 70, 87, 90, 95,
    216, 315
  and supplement use, 39,
    65, 156, 172, 218
probiotics, 45, 51–53, 316
  for children, 266, 267–68
  for dandruff, 195, 198
  for eczema, 220–21
prostaglandins, 57–71,
    157–58
  series 1 (good), 58–59,
    61–63, 157
  series 2 (bad), 58–59,
    63–66
  series 3 (beautiful), 58–59,
    60, 66–71
protein, 15, 86–94, 144
  food sources, 70, 88–91, 165
psoriasis, 9–10, 232–45. See
    also dandruff
  diet for, 243–44
  topical treatments, 189–90,
    235, 236
  triggers, 232–33, 242
  WOL therapy, 234–37, 242
pumpkin seeds, 319, 321
  Designer Muesli, 368
  Gluten-Free Muesli, 369

  Rich Mineral Salad with
    Papaya, Dill and Baby
    Spinach, 435

Q
quercetin, 259, 261
questionnaires
  acidosis, 32
  biotin deficiency, 224
  bowel health, 40, 241
  Candida, 49
  celiac disease, 85
  chromium deficiency, 82
  histamine/amine sensitivity,
    250
  immune system, 193
  omega-3, 67
  omega-6, 61
  parasites, 46
  protein deficiency, 87
  skin health, 11–12
  stress, 117
  zinc deficiency, 159

R
Rainbow Trout with
  Honey-Roasted
  Vegetables, 412
raisins
  Bircher Muesli, 371
  Spinach Salad, Tasty, 432
  Sweet Chutney, 384
rashes, 211. See also eczema;
  psoriasis
raspberries
  Berry Beauty Porridge,
    358
  Designer Muesli, 368
  Sweet Raspberry, Avocado
    and Watercress Salad,
    431
relationships, 302–3, 305–6
relaxation, 15, 115–25, 145,
  192. See also stress
  techniques, 116–18, 227,
    242
restaurant dining, 14, 35, 94,
  314, 315, 316
retinol. See vitamin A
Rhubarb Crumble, 456

rice. *See also* rice bran
    Boiled Eggs, Vegetables and
        Rice, 374
    Colorful Non-Fried Rice,
        449
    Creamy Chickpea Curry, 441
    C-Rich Apricot Chicken,
        402
    Herb and Garlic Chicken
        Casserole, 399
    Marinated Whole Steamed
        Trout, 414
    Shrimp and Sweet Chile
        Vegetable Stir-Fry, 418
    Slow-Cooked Lamb
        Casserole, 427
    Sweet Chicken Stir-Fry,
        400
    Tropical Vegetarian Stir-Fry,
        447
rice bran
    ACE Smoothie (tip), 355
    Bircher Muesli, 371
    Designer Muesli, 368
    Fruit Salad with Flax Seeds,
        363
    Gluten-Free Muesli, 369
    Rich Mediterranean Pasta,
        448
    Rich Mineral Salad with
        Papaya, Dill and Baby
        Spinach, 435
Roaccutane, 111, 149
Robbins, Anthony, 123
rosacea, 13, 246–62
    diet for, 261–62
    exercise and, 256–57
    and flushing, 255, 256
    supplements for, 259–60
    topical treatments, 254–55
rosehip oil, 134
rosemary oil, 171–72
rose oil, 212

S

salads, 430–37
Salad Sandwiches with
    Creamy Mayo, 442
salicylates, 203–4, 209,
    216–18, 267, 269

salicylic acid, 131, 155
salmon
    Salmon and Salad
        Sandwich, 410
    Salmon Steaks with Peas
        and Mash, 416
    Smoked Salmon and
        Avocado on Toast, 361
    Smoked Salmon and Eggs,
        365
    Thai Fish with Corn, 411
salt, 27, 160
    for acne, 153–54, 155
    for eczema, 208
    for hand scrub, 215
sandwiches and wraps, 397–
    98, 409–10, 442–45
Sardines and Lemon on
    Whole-Grain Toast, 362
sauces, 380–81, 383–85
sea buckthorn berry oil, 134
seafood. *See also* fish
    Oysters with Dipping
        Sauce, 393
    Seafood Hotpot, 420
    Shrimp and Sweet Chile
        Vegetable Stir-Fry, 418
seaweed, 328. *See also* kombu
sebum, 148
seeds, 70. *See also* flax seeds;
        pumpkin seeds
    Hummus, 382
    Lamb Stir-Fry, 428
    Vitamin E Muesli, 370
selenium, 239
self-compliments, 120–21
self-confidence, 174, 181
self-esteem, 119–25
self-sabotage, 76, 300–301,
    304–5. *See also* jealousy
shadow self, 304–5
shampoos, 183–84, 187,
    191, 192
shea butter, 135
Shrimp and Sweet Chile
    Vegetable Stir-Fry, 418
silver (colloidal), 213
sisterhood, 305–6
skin. *See also* skin cancer;
    skin care
    anatomy, 19–22

cell regeneration, 5, 22
    diet and, 24–27
    health of, 11–12, 24
    oil production, 148,
        157–62
    problem causes, 23–27
    self-examination, 112
    types, 22, 137
skin cancer, 102, 109–10,
    111, 112–13
skin care, 16, 126–42, 145.
        See also beauty products
    for acne, 150–54
    for cradle cap, 183–84
    exfoliation, 141–42, 322
Skin-Firming Drink, 350
Skin Juice for Sensitive Skin
    No. 1, 352
Skin Juice for Sensitive Skin
    No. 2, 353
sleep, 15, 95–100, 144,
        192, 243, 323. *See also*
        relaxation
Smoked Salmon and Avocado
    on Toast, 361
Smoked Salmon and Eggs,
        365
smoking, 36
snacks, 316, 319–20, 387–94
snow peas. *See* peas
soap products, 211
sodium, 27, 160. *See also* salt
sodium lauryl sulfate (SLS),
    126–27, 183, 187, 211
soups and broths, 93–94,
    389, 392, 438–39
Soy Dande', 345
soy lecithin. *See* lecithin
soy milk
    Berry Beauty Porridge, 358
    Calcium-Rich Smoothie, 351
    Designer Muesli, 368
    French Toast with Berries
        and Almonds, Delicious,
        359
    Gluten-Free Muesli, 369
    Kids' Creamy Beans on
        Toast, 378
    Soy Dande', 345
    Stewed Pears with Vanilla
        Soy Custard, 452

Sweet Banana Porridge, 360

spelt flour
  Rhubarb Crumble, 456
  Spelt Wraps, 445
Spicy Green Papaya Salad, 436
spinach. *See also* greens
  Rich Mineral Salad with Papaya, Dill and Baby Spinach, 435
  Smoked Salmon and Avocado on Toast, 361
  Tasty Spinach Salad, 432
Spot-Free Skin Juice, 351
Steak Sandwiches, 424
steroids, 212–13
stocks. *See* broths and soups
Strawberry Rehydration Water, 348
stress, 115–16, 117, 277. *See also* anxiety; relaxation
  and immune system, 192–93
  relieving, 227, 242–43
  and skin, 141, 153, 169, 192, 205, 250
subconscious mind, 299–301, 302
sugar, 179, 194–95. *See also* glycemic index
sulfates, 127
sulfation, 253, 254
sunlight (as psoriasis treatment), 190, 235
sunscreens, 113–14, 136, 153
supplements, 14, 60, 322. *See also specific supplements*
  for acne, 156–57, 158
  for children, 266–70
  for dandruff, 197–99
  for eczema, 216–24
  for rosacea, 259–60
sweating, 103–4, 155, 164. *See also* exercise
sweet almond oil, 131, 236
Sweet Banana and Carob Spread, 455
Sweet Banana Porridge, 360

Sweet Chicken Stir-Fry, 400
Sweet Chile Sauce, 383
Sweet Chutney, 384
  Sweet Chutney Dressing, 433
  Tasty Salad Dressing, 386
sweet potatoes
  Chicken and Three Veg, 406
  Herb and Garlic Chicken Casserole, 399
  Lean Lamb and Three Veg, 426
  Rainbow Trout with Honey-Roasted Vegetables, 412
  Roasted Sweet Potato Salad, 434
  Salmon Steaks with Peas and Mash, 416
  Slow-Cooked Lamb Casserole, 427
  Tasty Vegetable Casserole, 450
Sweet Raspberry, Avocado and Watercress Salad, 431
sweets, 275–76, 316–17, 451–58

T

Tabbouleh, 446
  Falafel Wraps, 444
Tangy Papaya Cups, 454
tanning, 111, 173
Tartar Sauce, 381
Tasty Omelet, 367
Tasty Salad Dressing, 386
Tasty Spinach Salad, 432
Tasty Vegetable Casserole, 450
taurine, 272
tea, 14, 43–44, 133
TEA (triethanolamine), 183
tea tree oil, 155, 188
teenage acne, 27, 148, 155, 158
Thai Fish with Corn, 411
Therapeutic Chicken Soup, 396

Therapeutic Veggie Soup, 438
3-Day Alkalizing Cleanse, 41, 317–23
  cold weather version, 320–21
  complementary activities, 322–23
  menu and activity plan, 332–33
  preparing for, 318
  supplements during, 322
  warm weather version, 318–20
thromboxanes, 63–64
thrush. *See Candida albicans*
thyme oil, 48
tofu
  Colorful Non-Fried Rice (variation), 449
  Miso Soup, 389
  Tropical Vegetarian Stir-Fry, 447
  Vegetable Hand Rolls, 388
tomatoes, 53
  Avocado Salsa, 390
  Beans on Toast, 376
  Falafel Wraps (variation), 444
  Garden Salad, 437
  Omega Niçoise Salad, 408
  Omelet, Tasty, 367
  Rich Mediterranean Pasta, 448
  Spicy Green Papaya Salad, 436
  Steak Sandwiches, 424
  Tabbouleh, 446
  Thai Fish with Corn, 411
  Tomato Sauce, 385
toners, 138, 150
topical treatments, 132, 133. *See also specific ingredients*
  for children, 264–65
  for eczema, 201, 209–15, 265
  for psoriasis, 236, 237
  for rosacea, 254–55
tortillas
  Chicken and Salad Wrap, 398
  Falafel Wraps, 444

tortillas (*continued*)
Tuna and Avocado Wrap, 409
toxins, 172–73. *See also* liver detoxification
tretinoin. *See* vitamin A
trifluorperperazine, 62
Tropical Vegetarian Stir-Fry, 447
tryptophan, 98
tuna
Avocado Beauty Snack, 390
Omega Niçoise Salad, 408
Tuna and Avocado Wrap, 409
Tuna Dip, 381
turmeric, 328

U

urination (frequent), 44
UV (ultraviolet) radiation, 15, 109–14, 145

V

vegetables, 50. *See also* greens; *specific vegetables*
Anti-Aging Broth, 392
Boiled Eggs, Vegetables and Rice, 374
Falafel Wraps, 444
Lamb Stir-Fry, 428
Omega Niçoise Salad, 408
Rainbow Trout with Honey-Roasted Vegetables, 412
Roasted Corn and Cauliflower Soup, 439
Vegetable Hand Rolls, 388

vinegar, 38, 53, 93, 191. *See also* vinegar, apple cider
vinegar, apple cider, 53, 132, 323–24
for dandruff, 189, 190
for eczema, 212, 222
ACV Drink, 344
Omega Salad Dressing, 386
Oysters with Dipping Sauce, 393
Salad Dressing, Tasty, 386
Skin Juice for Sensitive Skin No. 1, 352
Skin Juice for Sensitive Skin No. 2, 353
Sweet Chile Sauce, 383
Sweet Chutney, 384
vitamin A, 45, 135, 156, 162, 243
vitamin B, 60, 198, 218. *See also* biotin
vitamin C (ascorbic acid), 60, 135, 259–60
vitamin D, 111, 235
vitamin E, 135
Vitamin E Muesli, 370
vulvovaginitis, 265

W

walnuts, 70. *See also* black walnut extract
wasabi, 47
water, 42–44, 318, 320
weight loss, 14. *See also* diet, calorie-restricted
wheat germ
ACE Smoothie, 355
Bircher Muesli, 371
Vitamin E Muesli, 370

Williams, Hywel C., 214
willpower, 76, 301
wine, 36
World Health Organization (WHO), 45
worms, 45. *See also* parasites
worry, 192, 194. *See also* stress
wraps. *See* sandwiches and wraps

X

xanthan gum, 135

Y

yeast infections, 48–49, 52, 192, 196
Yuzurihara (Japan), 92

Z

zinc, 92, 158–61
food sources, 161, 164–65, 182, 198, 244
as supplement, 60, 160, 175–76
zinc oxide, 136
zucchini
Boiled Eggs, Vegetables and Rice, 374
Chickpea Beauty Salad, 430
Rainbow Trout with Honey-Roasted Vegetables, 412
Rich Mediterranean Pasta, 448
Shrimp and Sweet Chile Vegetable Stir-Fry, 418